Management of Pituitary Tumors

Guest Editors

MANISH K. AGHI, MD, PhD
LEWIS S. BLEVINS Jr, MD

NEUROSURGERY CLINICS OF NORTH AMERICA

www.neurosurgery.theclinics.com

Consulting Editors
ANDREW T. PARSA, MD, PhD
PAUL C. McCORMICK, MD, MPH

October 2012 • Volume 23 • Number 4

SAUNDERS an imprint of ELSEVIER, Inc.

W.B. SAUNDERS COMPANY
A Division of Elsevier Inc.

1600 John F. Kennedy Blvd. • Suite 1800 • Philadelphia, PA 19103-2899

http://www.theclinics.com

NEUROSURGERY CLINICS OF NORTH AMERICA Volume 23, Number 4
October 2012 ISSN 1042-3680, ISBN-13: 978-1-4557-4946-1

Editor: Jessica McCool
Developmental Editor: Teia Stone

Neurosurgery Clinics of North America (ISSN 1042-3680) is published quarterly by Elsevier Inc., 360 Park Avenue South, New York, NY 10010-1710. Months of issue are January, April, July, and October. Business and Editorial Offices: 1600 John F. Kennedy Blvd., Suite 1800, Philadelphia, PA 19103-2899. Customer Service Office: 11830 Westline Industrial Drive, St. Louis, MO 63146. Periodicals postage paid at New York, NY, and additional mailing offices. Subscription prices are $360.00 per year (US individuals), $552.00 per year (US institutions), $393.00 per year (Canadian individuals), $674.00 per year (Canadian institutions), $502.00 per year (international individuals), $674.00 per year (international institutions), $144.00 per year (US students), and $208.00 per year (international students). International air speed delivery is included in all *Clinics* subscription prices. All prices are subject to change without notice. **POSTMASTER:** Send address changes to *Neurosurgery Clinics of North America*, Elsevier Periodicals Customer Service, 11830 Westline Industrial Drive, St. Louis, MO 63146. **Customer Service: 1-800-654-2452 (US and Canada). From outside the US and Canada, call: 1-314-453-7041. Fax: 1-314-453-5170. E-mail: JournalsCustomerService-usa@elsevier.com (for print support) and journalsonlinesupport-usa@elsevier.com (for online support).**

Reprints. For copies of 100 or more, of articles in this publication, please contact the Commercial Reprints Department, Elsevier Inc., 360 Park Avenue South, New York, NY 10010-1710. Tel. (212) 633-3812; Fax: (212) 462-1935; E-mail: reprints@elsevier.com.

Neurosurgery Clinics of North America is covered in *MEDLINE/PubMed (Index Medicus), EMBASE/Excerpta Medica, and Current Contents/Clinical Medicine (CC/CM).*

Printed and bound by CPI Group (UK) Ltd, Croydon, CR0 4YY

Transferred to digital print 2012

Cover image from the American Association for Cancer Research: Vredenburgh JJ, Desjardins A, Herndon JE, et al. Bevacizumab plus irinotecan in recurrent glioblastoma multiforme. J Clin Oncol 2007;25(30):4722–9; with permission for print use only.

Contributors

CONSULTING EDITORS

ANDREW T. PARSA, MD, PhD
Associate Professor, Principal Investigator,
Brain Tumor Research Center, Reza and
Georgianna Khatib Endowed Chair in Skull
Base Tumor Surgery, Department of
Neurological Surgery, University of California,
San Francisco, San Francisco, California

PAUL C. McCORMICK, MD, MPH, FACS
Herbert & Linda Gallen Professor of
Neurological Surgery, Department of
Neurological Surgery, Columbia University
Medical Center, New York, New York

GUEST EDITORS

MANISH K. AGHI, MD, PhD
Associate Professor, UCSF Neurosurgery,
Co-Director, Center for Minimally Invasive Skull
Base Surgery, Department of Neurological
Surgery, California Center for Pituitary
Disorders at UCSF, San Francisco, California

LEWIS S. BLEVINS Jr, MD
Clinical Professor of Neurological Surgery
and Medicine, UCSF, Medical Director,
Department of Neurological Surgery, Clinical
Professor of Neurological Surgery and
Medicine, California Center for Pituitary
Disorders at UCSF, San Francisco, California

AUTHORS

MANISH K. AGHI, MD, PhD
Associate Professor, UCSF Neurosurgery,
Co-Director, Center for Minimally Invasive Skull
Base Surgery, Department of Neurological
Surgery, California Center for Pituitary
Disorders at UCSF, San Francisco, California

VALÉRIE BIOUSSE, MD
Cyrus H. Stoner Professor of Ophthalmology,
Professor of Ophthalmology and Neurology,
Emory University School of Medicine,
Atlanta, Georgia

LEWIS S. BLEVINS Jr, MD
Clinical Professor of Neurological Surgery
and Medicine, UCSF, Medical Director,
Department of Neurological Surgery,
Clinical Professor of Neurological Surgery
and Medicine, California Center for Pituitary
Disorders at UCSF, San Francisco,
California

SARAH K. BOURNE, BA
Department of Neurosurgery, Massachusetts
General Hospital, Boston, Massachusetts

JESSICA K. DEVIN, MD
Faculty Physician, Division of Diabetes,
Endocrinology and Metabolism, Vanderbilt
University Medical Center, Nashville,
Tennessee

WILLIAM P. DILLON, MD
Chief, Neuroradiology, Professor of Radiology,
Neurology and Neurosurgery, Department of
Radiology and Biomedical Imaging, University
of California, San Francisco, San Francisco,
California

MARIA FLESERIU, MD, FACE
Associate Professor of Medicine and
Neurological Surgery; Director Northwest
Pituitary Center, Oregon Health and Science
University, Portland, Oregon

CLARE LOUISE FRASER, MBBS, MMed, FRANZCO
Neuro-Ophthalmology Fellow, Emory University School of Medicine, Atlanta, Georgia

CHRISTOPHER P. HESS, MD, PhD
Associate Professor, Division of Neuroradiology, Department of Radiology and Biomedical Imaging, University of California, San Francisco, San Francisco, California

ADRIANA G. IOACHIMESCU, MD, PhD, FACE
Assistant Professor, Departments of Medicine and Neurosurgery, Emory University, Atlanta, Georgia

SANDEEP KUNWAR, MD
Department of Neurological Surgery, California Center for Pituitary Disorders, University of California, San Francisco, San Francisco, California

MARK J. LOBO, MD
Senior Resident Physician, Department of Radiation Oncology, University of Virginia, Charlottesville, Virginia

JOSHUA W. LUCAS, MD
Department of Neurosurgery, University of Southern California, Los Angeles, California

NESTORAS MATHIOUDAKIS, MD
Assistant Professor of Medicine, Division of Endocrinology and Metabolism, Department of Medicine, Johns Hopkins University School of Medicine, Baltimore, Maryland

BRANDON A. MILLER, MD, PhD
Resident, Department of Neurosurgery, Emory University, Atlanta, Georgia

MARK E. MOLITCH, MD
Martha Leland Sherwin Professor of Endocrinology, Division of Endocrinology, Metabolism and Molecular Medicine, Northwestern University Feinberg School of Medicine, Chicago, Illinois

NANCY J. NEWMAN, MD
Leo Delle Jolley Professor of Ophthalmology, Professor of Ophthalmology and Neurology, Instructor in Neurological Surgery, Department of Neuro-Ophthalmology, Emory Eye Center, Emory University School of Medicine, Emory University, Atlanta, Georgia

MICHAEL C. OH, MD, PhD
Department of Neurological Surgery, California Center for Pituitary Disorders, University of California, San Francisco, San Francisco, California

NELSON M. OYESIKU, MD, PhD, FACS
Al Lerner Chair and Vice-Chairman, Department of Neurosurgery; Professor, Departments of Neurosurgery and Medicine, Emory University, Atlanta, Georgia

W. CALEB RUTLEDGE, MD, MS
Medical Student, Department of Neurosurgery, Emory University, Atlanta, Georgia

ROBERTO SALVATORI, MD
Medical Director, Pituitary Center, Associate Professor of Medicine, Johns Hopkins University School of Medicine, Baltimore, Maryland

JASON P. SHEEHAN, MD, PhD
Professor, Departments of Neurological Surgery and Radiation Oncology, University of Virginia, Charlottesville, Virginia

SAMEER A. SHETH, MD, PhD
Department of Neurosurgery, Massachusetts General Hospital, Boston, Massachusetts

BROOKE SWEARINGEN, MD
Department of Neurosurgery, Massachusetts General Hospital, Boston, Massachusetts

TARIK TIHAN, MD, PhD
Department of Pathology, University of California, San Francisco, San Francisco, California

NICHOLAS A. TRITOS, MD, DSc
Department of Medicine, Neuroendocrine Clinical Center, Massachusetts General Hospital, Boston, Massachusetts

ZHIYUAN XU, MD
Instructor, Department of Neurological Surgery, University of Virginia, Charlottesville, Virginia

GABRIEL ZADA, MD
Department of Neurosurgery, University of Southern California, Los Angeles, California

Contents

Magnetic resonance imaging is the fundamental imaging tool for the evaluation of tumors and other lesions of the pituitary gland and infundibulum. Abnormalities may arise within the pituitary itself, from vestigial embryologic remnants, or from surrounding tissues. Correct diagnosis rests on accurate assessment of lesion location, imaging appearance, and clinical presentation. This article reviews the radiologic evaluation of lesions within the sella and suprasellar cistern, focusing on common masses and pseudomasses of the pituitary and sellar region that neurosurgeons are most likely to encounter in clinical practice.

Clinically nonfunctioning pituitary adenomas range from those causing significant hypothalamic/pituitary dysfunction and visual field compromise to those being completely asymptomatic, detected either at autopsy or as incidental findings on imaging scans performed for other reasons (often referred to as pituitary incidentalomas). Growth of nonfunctioning pituitary adenomas without treatment occurs in about 10% of microadenomas and 24% of macroadenomas. In the absence of hypersecretion, hypopituitarism, or visual-field defects, periodic screening by magnetic resonance imaging may detect enlargement. Potential indications for surgery are growth of a pituitary incidentaloma, the development of visual-field defects, or the development of hypopituitarism.

The endoscopic transsphenoidal approach to the sella turcica has been developed and refined for the treatment of pituitary lesions. Studies comparing endoscopic transsphenoidal surgery with the traditional microscopic transsphenoidal technique have found equivalent or improved rates of tumor resection and hormonal remission, and equal or lower rates of complications. This procedure affords improved panoramic visualization, illumination, surgical freedom, and mobility. This approach facilitates two-handed microdissection and the ability to look around corners using angled lenses, promoting maximal tumor resection and preservation of the pituitary gland. Experience, technologic advancements, and improved instrumentation are likely to contribute to improved surgical outcomes.

This article discusses contemporary use of external beam radiotherapy and stereotactic radiosurgery for pituitary adenoma patients. Specific techniques are discussed. In addition, indications and outcomes, including complications, are detailed.

Pituitary adenomas are generally considered benign tumors; however, a subset of these tumors displays aggressive behavior and are not easily cured. The protocol for nonsurgical treatment of aggressive pituitary lesions is less standardized than that of other central nervous system tumors. Aggressive surgical treatment, radiation, dopamine agonists, antiangiogenic drugs, and other chemotherapeutics all have roles in the treatment of aggressive pituitary tumors. More studies are needed to improve outcomes for patients with aggressive pituitary tumors.

Pituitary carcinomas are defined as malignant primary neoplasms of the adenohypophysis with either systemic or craniospinal metastases. Although pituitary adenomas are common, pituitary carcinomas only make up 0.1% to 0.2% of all pituitary tumors. Prognosis is very poor with approximately 66% mortality in the first year of diagnosis. Although effective medical and surgical treatments are available for pituitary adenomas, pituitary carcinomas require a multimodality treatment including surgery, hormonal therapy, cytotoxic chemotherapy, and radiation with limited success. Here we review the clinical behavior and pathologic characteristics of pituitary carcinomas and the recent advances in potential therapies for this malignant disease.

Pituitary adenomas frequently manifest with neuro-ophthalmic symptoms and signs. The location of the pituitary gland makes involvement of both the visual pathways and the ocular motor cranial nerves likely when there is adenomatous expansion. A sudden expression of visual loss or diplopia commonly accompanies pituitary apoplexy. Several preoperative neuro-ophthalmic indicators help predict posttreatment outcomes and help determine the best intervention. Treatments themselves may also cause neuro-ophthalmic complications. The current literature and avenues of future research are reviewed.

This article presents management options for the patient with acromegaly after non-curative surgery. The current evidence for repeat surgery, adjuvant medical therapy with somatostatin analogues, dopamine agonists, the growth hormone receptor antagonist pegvisomant, combination medical therapy, and radiotherapy in the context of persistent postoperative disease are summarized. The relative advantages and disadvantages of each of these treatment modalities are explored, and a general treatment algorithm that integrates these modalities is proposed.

Cushing disease (CD) is caused by overproduction of adrenocorticotropin by a pituitary adenoma (or, rarely, carcinoma). The diagnosis of CD requires distinguishing it from other hypercortisolemic states with a thorough endocrine workup. CD remains a primarily surgical disease, with remission rates of 70% to 95% following microscopic or endoscopic transsphenoidal surgery.

Recent evidence supports the notion that the incidence of Cushing disease is higher than previously thought. Transphenoidal surgery, in the hands of experienced neurosurgeons, is currently considered the first-line treatment of choice. However, an examination of remission and recurrence rates in long-term follow-up studies reveals that potentially up to 40% to 50% of patients could require additional treatment. If left untreated, the resultant morbidity and mortality are high. Successful clinical management of patients with Cushing disease remains a challenge. The development of new therapeutic agents has been eagerly anticipated. This article discusses the results of currently available and promising new therapeutic agents used to treat this challenging disease.

Prolactinomas are the most common hormone-secreting pituitary adenomas, comprising 40% of all pituitary tumors. Prolactinomas present a unique challenge for clinicians, as these tumors are amenable to either medical or surgical treatments based on patients' comorbidities, tolerance to medical treatment, and the response of tumors to medical treatment. Rare prolactinomas that are unresponsive to either medical or surgical treatment modalities may be responsive to radiation therapy. This article reviews the recent advancements in the management of prolactinomas.

Pituitary tumors are a unique class of intracranial neoplasms with the potential to disrupt hormone function and water metabolism. Preoperative and postoperative endocrine assessment is mandatory to recognize and promptly treat new deficiencies and identify those that have resolved. Close collaboration among neurosurgical, endocrine, and anesthetic teams is equally vital during the perioperative period. Appropriate patient education at the time of discharge regarding the symptoms of diabetes insipidus, hyponatremia, and adrenal insufficiency is increasingly important.

NEUROSURGERY CLINICS OF NORTH AMERICA

Preface

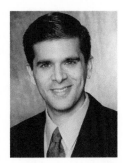 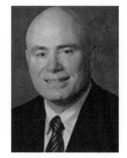

Manish K. Aghi, MD, PhD   Lewis S. Blevins Jr, MD
Guest Editors

Pituitary tumors can be found in nearly one in five people based on autopsy studies and MRI studies of healthy volunteers. The majority of these tumors are asymptomatic, slow-growing pituitary adenomas or Rathke's cleft cysts. When symptomatic, the challenge involves treatment in a manner that alleviates symptoms without compromising a patient's endocrine function or exposing the patient to other morbidities such as meningitis, arterial injury, or CSF leak. When asymptomatic and incidentally found, the challenge involves weighing the natural history of the lesion and its consequences versus the risks of surgery.

Over the past few decades, treatment of pituitary tumors has evolved to include new medications, the use of endoscopic endonasal surgical techniques, and increasing ability to use radiosurgery to deliver high doses of radiation selectively to the tumor.

This issue of *Neurosurgery Clinics* aims to provide an organized and expansive overview of the latest advances in the diagnosis, natural history, and management of pituitary tumors. Specifically, we present an overview of imaging of the pituitary gland, an area with imaging properties distinct from the rest of the central nervous system. We then relate the management of incidentally found pituitary tumors, followed by details of endoscopic surgery for pituitary tumors. The role of external beam radiation therapy and radiosurgery in the management of pituitary tumors is then reviewed, followed by management strategies for large nonfunctional adenomas. The clinical management of rare pituitary tumors that become malignant pituitary carcinomas is discussed, followed by strategies for managing hormonally active tumors like prolactinomas, growth hormone-secreting adenomas causing acromegaly, and ACTH-secreting adenomas causing Cushing's disease. The issue concludes with a discussion of diabetes insipidus, the most common morbidity seen with the treatment of pituitary tumors.

These contributions are presented by some of the world's foremost experts in endocrinology, neurosurgery, and radiation oncology. We hope the combined perspective of these experts will make this issue a valuable resource for physicians caring for patients with pituitary tumors.

Manish K. Aghi, MD, PhD
UCSF Neurosurgery
Center for Minimally Invasive Skull Base Surgery
California Center for Pituitary Disorders at UCSF
505 Parnassus Avenue, Room M779
San Francisco, CA 94143-0112, USA

Lewis S. Blevins Jr, MD
California Center for Pituitary Disorders at UCSF
400 Parnassus Avenue, Room A-808
San Francisco, CA 94143-0350, USA

E-mail addresses:
AghiM@neurosurg.ucsf.edu (M.K. Aghi)
BlevinsL@neurosurg.ucsf.edu (L.S. Blevins)

Neurosurg Clin N Am 23 (2012) ix
http://dx.doi.org/10.1016/j.nec.2012.06.007
1042-3680/12/$ – see front matter © 2012 Elsevier Inc. All rights reserved.

neurosurgery.theclinics.com

Preface

Manish K. Aghi, MD, PhD   Lewis S. Blevins Jr, MD
Guest Editors

Imaging the Pituitary and Parasellar Region

Christopher P. Hess, MD, PhD*, William P. Dillon, MD

KEYWORDS

• Pituitary gland • Infundibulum • Sella • Suprasellar cistern • Magnetic resonance imaging

KEY POINTS

• Key distinguishing features for lesions arising in and around the sella on magnetic resonance imaging (MRI) include the site of origin, intrinsic signal and enhancement pattern, and the presence or absence of distinguishing features including cysts, calcification, and fluid-fluid levels.
• Although adenoma is by far the most common abnormality of the pituitary gland, there are several mimics of adenoma that should be considered when reviewing MRI of the sella.
• Pituitary infundibular masses invoke a specific differential diagnosis, depending on the imaging abnormalities present, the presence or absence of the posterior pituitary bright spot, clinical history and demographics, and the presence or absence of other lesions.

Imaging remains the cornerstone of diagnosis for lesions arising in and around the sella. Exquisite soft-tissue contrast and the ability to interrogate the pituitary gland and parasellar anatomy with high spatial resolution and without artifacts from surrounding bony structures have made magnetic resonance imaging (MRI) the primary modality for evaluation of sellar, parasellar, and suprasellar lesions, with computed tomography (CT) reserved for patients with contraindications to MRI and for those undergoing emergent evaluation. This article focuses on the use of MRI to distinguish among common masses and pseudomasses that arise within the sella and parasellar regions. Primary disorders of other surrounding structures that may present with similar clinical symptoms are not discussed.

DIAGNOSTIC APPROACH TO THE SELLA AND INFUNDIBULAR REGION
Imaging Technique

MRI evaluation of the pituitary and parasellar region is best undertaken on modern 1.5-T or 3-T scanners using a protocol that includes both noncontrast and gadolinium-enhanced sequences. Sagittal and coronal planes are most useful, using 3-mm or thinner slices without any interslice gap to adequately evaluate small structures that may be involved in the diseases that occur in this region.

The intrinsic composition of lesions, as characterized based on their T1-weighted and T2-weighted relaxation properties without contrast, usually differs significantly from the pituitary gland, cerebrospinal fluid (CSF), and brain because of the presence of intralesional fluid, protein, hemorrhage, or tumor. Imaging performed after the administration of gadolinium chelate may increase contrast between abnormalities and normal tissues, show otherwise occult disease, and allow one to more confidently differentiate between solid and cystic lesions. Fat suppression is recommended for both T2-weighted and gadolinium-enhanced images, as normal high T2 and T1 signal within the bones of the central skull base may obscure a pathologically high T2 signal or enhancement.

In addition to T1-, T2-, and gadolinium-enhanced T1-weighted images, dynamic contrast-enhanced imaging, gradient-echo T2*-weighted imaging,

Disclosures: None.
Neuroradiology Division, Department of Radiology & Biomedical Imaging, University of California, 505 Parnassus Avenue, San Francisco, CA 94143-0628, USA
* Corresponding author.
E-mail address: christopher.hess@ucsf.edu

Neurosurg Clin N Am 23 (2012) 529–542
http://dx.doi.org/10.1016/j.nec.2012.06.002
1042-3680/12/$ – see front matter © 2012 Elsevier Inc. All rights reserved.

and diffusion-weighted imaging play an important role in the diagnosis of certain disorders and should be added when these disorders are suspected. These abnormalities are discussed individually in subsequent sections.

Normal MRI Appearance of the Pituitary and Infundibulum

The identification of abnormalities in the sella and parasellar region requires familiarity with normal anatomy and biological variability. The normal size of the gland varies with age, measuring up to 12 mm in height in lactating women, 10 mm in menstruating women, 8 mm in males and postmenopausal women, and 6 mm in infants (**Table 1**).

The anterior aspect of the gland, or adenohypophysis, comprises roughly 70% of its volume, and should appear uniform in signal on both unenhanced and enhanced images. Posteriorly within the gland, the neurohypophysis exhibits intrinsic T1 hyperintensity on unenhanced images referred to as the posterior pituitary bright spot (PPBS). The pituitary stalk comprises pars tuberalis cells from the adenohypophysis that surround neurohypophyseal axons descending from the hypothalamus. The normal pituitary infundibulum is wider at its origin from the hypothalamus and tapers inferiorly, reaching its minimum thickness at the level of the pituitary gland. The upper limit for stalk thickness has been reported as 3.5 mm near the median eminence, 2.8 mm at its midpoint, and 2.0 mm at its most inferior aspect. In children, the maximum thickness of the infundibulum is somewhat less, around 2.5 mm.[1]

Interpretative Strategy

A systematic approach to image interpretation is required to develop an accurate differential diagnosis for lesions within or intimately associated with the pituitary gland and/or infundibulum. Key considerations include the following:

- Verification of the normal imaging appearance of the gland and infundibulum, noting its size, enhancement pattern, and presence or absence of the PPBS
- Localization of abnormalities as entirely intrasellar, both sellar and intrasellar, or entirely suprasellar, and as within or separate from the pituitary gland
- Characterization of lesions as entirely solid, entirely cystic, or mixed solid and cystic
- Evaluation of lesion margins (circumscribed or invasive), morphology, and relationship to the normal pituitary
- Distinguishing imaging features that are unique or highly suggestive of certain lesions, such as cysts, low T2 signal, calcification, and fluid-fluid levels
- Presence or absence of mass effect on the optic apparatus, invasion of the cavernous sinuses, and abnormalities located elsewhere in the brain

LESIONS PRIMARY TO THE PITUITARY GLAND
Pituitary Adenoma

Adenoma is the most common abnormality of the pituitary gland and represents 15% of all intracranial neoplasms. It is a slowly growing, benign tumor that almost exclusively arises within the sella and occasionally from the pituitary stalk. Adenomas are rarely found in ectopic sites such as the sphenoid sinus, nasopharynx, cavernous sinuses, and sphenoid bone. Whereas small tumors become clinically manifest owing to excess hormone secretion, larger tumors are more frequently nonsecreting, and tend to present

Table 1
University of California San Francisco magnetic resonance imaging protocol for imaging of the sella

Pulse Sequence	Slice/Gap	Parameters
1. Coronal and sagittal T1	2.7 mm no skip	TR/TE = 600 ms/min, NEX = 3
2. Fat-suppressed coronal T2	2.0 mm no skip	TR/TE = 3000/100 ms, ETL = 16, NEX = 3
3. Dynamic gadolinium-enhanced T1[a]	2.0 mm no skip	TR/TE = 600 ms, ETL = 8, NEX = 2
4. Postgadolinium coronal and sagittal T1	2.7 mm no skip	TR/TE = 800 ms/min, NEX = 3
5. Coronal T2* gradient echo[b]	3.0 mm no skip	TR/TE = 800 ms/25 ms, NEX = 2
6. Axial and coronal diffusion (b = 1000)[c]	2.0 mm no skip	TR/TE = 8000 ms/min, NEX = 1

Abbreviations: ETL, echo train length; NEX, number of excitations; TE, echo time; TR, repetition time.
  [a] Dynamic gadolinium-enhanced imaging performed in cases of suspected adenoma and postoperatively after macroadenoma resection.
  [b] T2*-weighted (susceptibility sensitive) imaging used for suspected or known hemorrhage or calcification (ie, pituitary apoplexy and craniopharyngioma).
  [c] Diffusion-weighted imaging used in cases with suspected or known infection.

with symptoms related to compression of adjacent structures or elevated intracranial pressure.

Prolactin-secreting and growth hormone–secreting adenohypophyseal cells are located more laterally within the normal pituitary gland and corticotropin-secreting, thyroid-stimulating hormone–secreting, and gonadotropin-secreting cells are located more medially. This inherent spatial organization of adenotrophs within the gland imparts a similar spatial distribution to the origin of hormone-secreting adenomas. Pathologically, adenomas are circumscribed and contained within a pseudocapsule of compressed surrounding pituitary tissue, or are locally invasive, equipped on a molecular basis with microscopic machinery that facilitates contiguous spread through the dura into adjacent bone or cavernous sinus.

Microadenomas, tumors that measure less than 1 cm in diameter, exhibit T1 signal on MRI that is the same as or lower than the gland signal unless intratumoral hemorrhage is present (**Fig. 1**). T2 signal is more variable. Most tumors exhibit high T2 signal, and tend to be softer and more readily resected at surgery. Low-T2–signal tumors are less common, but as a group tend to be firmer and more adherent to surrounding tissue on surgical manipulation. Approximately 80% of prolactinomas have high T2 signal, and between 40% and 60% of growth hormone–secreting adenomas have low T2 signal.[2,3] Most tumors are round or discoid in morphology. Subtle contour deformity of the pituitary gland may be present, as may displacement of the infundibulum. The direction of infundibular displacement is usually opposite the side of the tumor, but this finding is only variably seen and is considered unreliable.

Following administration of intravenous gadolinium chelate, microadenomas are relatively hypoenhancing or isoenhancing relative to the normal pituitary gland during the wash-in phase of contrast. Dynamic imaging, whereby high-resolution pituitary images are obtained immediately following bolus injection of contrast, is useful for illustrating the differential uptake of contrast between a microadenoma and normal pituitary gland, and is used to enhance sensitivity to small tumors by up to 10%.[4] Some tumors retain contrast on delayed imaging more avidly than does the gland, such that MRI obtained during the washout phase of contrast may also increase sensitivity, revealing tumors as hyperenhancing relative to the gland.

Tumors larger than 1 cm are referred to as macroadenomas or, if larger than 4 cm, giant adenomas. Slow tumor growth results in progressive enlargement of the sella. The direction of growth is variable. Approximately 80% extend superiorly into the suprasellar cistern, but the remaining 20% grow in any of the remaining 5 directions to invade the cavernous sinuses, sphenoid sinus, or dorsum sella. MRI often reveals more heterogeneous intrinsic signal than microadenoma on both T1-weighted and T2-weighted images, especially when internal tumor cysts, necrosis, and/or hemorrhage develop within the tumor (**Fig. 2**). Enhancement is moderate to avid; rare hypoenhancement has been described as a feature of thyrotropin-secreting tumors.[5] The normal pituitary gland, often compressed around large

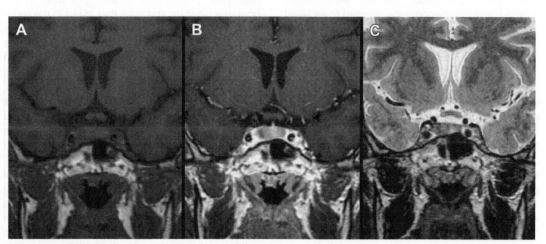

Fig. 1. Microadenoma. Subtle intrinsic low T2 signal in the right lobe of the pituitary (*A*), seen to better advantage on gadolinium-enhanced T1-weighted image as hypoenhancing relative to the surrounding gland (*B*). This growth hormone–secreting microadenoma appears relatively T2 hypointense compared with normal adenohypophyseal tissue (*C*).

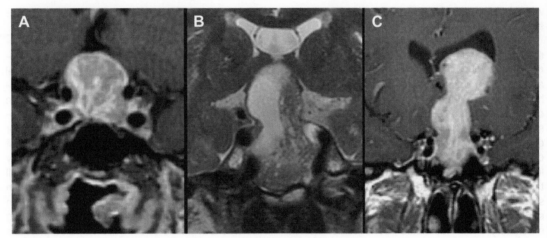

Fig. 2. Macroadenoma. "Dumbbell" or "snowman" appearance of a typical macroadenoma, which shows a narrower waist as it passes through the sellar diaphragm (*A*). Larger macroadenomas are frequently more heterogeneous and contain areas of cystic degeneration (*B*). Tumor growth in adenomas occurs in any direction and may be dramatic, as illustrated in this case in which the superior tumor extends into the third and left lateral ventricle (*C*).

adenomas, is important to identify preoperatively, as preservation of this tissue is a surgical goal in preventing pituitary insufficiency. The PPBS may be difficult to see or even absent, although it is rare for patients with macroadenoma to have central diabetes insipidus (DI).

Pituitary apoplexy is due to acute intratumoral hemorrhage or bland tumor infarction. Although uncommon, it is a surgical emergency with specific features on MRI. The term apoplexy refers to the clinical syndrome that results when hemorrhage causes compression of parasellar structures, especially the optic nerve or chiasm, and/or meningismus.[6] Acute presentation distinguishes this entity from subclinical tumoral hemorrhage, a more common phenomenon referred to as silent apoplexy by some investigators. It is also considered a separate entity from postischemic pituitary hemorrhage in patients with prolonged hypotension, referred to as Sheehan syndrome and classically occurring in women with severe postpartum bleeding. Both are more common in patients with known adenomas.

As rapid loss of vision or acute cranial neuropathy may occur, any mass effect on the optic chiasm should be sought on imaging and discussed as an indication for emergent neurosurgical decompression. Subarachnoid and retroclival hemorrhage may also be present. MRI in the acute setting may be subtle, particularly on the routine T1-weighted images. If blood is present, this appears as intratumoral heterogeneous signal and occasionally fluid-fluid levels, which may be T1 hyperintense owing to the presence of methemoglobin. T2-weighted images typically show hypointensity within hemorrhagic areas, which evolves with time into hyperintensity. T2*-weighted gradient-echo images are more sensitive to the presence of blood products and may demonstrate areas of "blooming," signal loss around areas of hemorrhage. CT is useful to confirm the presence of blood products in acute or equivocal cases.

Nonadenomatous Tumors of the Pituitary Gland

Pituicytomas are histologically benign, World Health Organization Grade 1 tumors derived from pituicytes, populations of astroglial cells in the posterior pituitary and stalk that assist in the regulation of oxytocin and vasopressin secretion. The controversial pathology of these rare tumors is evident from the range of names they have been assigned, including infundibuloma, choristoma, and pilocytic astrocytoma of the neurohypophysis. Clinical presentation varies with location, with sellar tumors most commonly found incidentally or as a result of hypopituitarism, and suprasellar tumors usually present with visual symptoms related to mass effect.

Although most pituicytomas are located in the suprasellar cistern or have both sellar and suprasellar components, it is the only nonadenomatous primary pituitary tumor that has been reported with a purely intrasellar presentation.[7] The tumor is solid and frequently infiltrative, and inseparable from the pituitary gland. Intrinsic signal on MRI is isointense to cortex on unenhanced T1-weighted images and hyperintense to cortex on T2-

weighted images. Pituicytoma is more vascular than adenoma, and enhancement is more frequently uniformly homogeneous than heterogeneous. Primarily because of their posterior location and vascularity, gross total resection of pituicytomas may be difficult or impossible.

Spindle-cell oncocytoma and granular cell tumor of the neurohypophysis are pathologically distinct nonadenomatous tumors of the pituitary gland that are less common even than pituicytoma. The former arises from the adenohypophysis, is commonly both sellar and suprasellar, and is radiologically indistinguishable from the far more common adenoma or lymphocytic hypophysitis. Granular cell tumors, in contradistinction, arise from the neurohypophysis and are entirely suprasellar in most cases, with a smaller number reported with simultaneous sellar and suprasellar location. Hyperdensity on CT may also be a useful distinguishing feature.[7]

Pituitary Carcinoma

Unlike locally invasive adenomas, pituitary carcinomas are rare, with a reported incidence of only 0.2%.[8] These tumors arise from the adenohypophysis and are frequently hormonally active, most commonly secreting corticotropin, prolactin, or growth hormone. Pituitary carcinomas are indistinguishable from adenomas using histologic criteria, and are currently diagnosed only when systemic or craniospinal metastatic disease is identified.

Most pituitary carcinomas present initially as invasive macroadenomas greater than 1 cm in size, demonstrate an aggressive course with rapid growth and multiple recurrences, and are typically diagnosed as carcinomas some 4 to 7 years later when metastases are identified.[9] Central nervous system (CNS) metastases, which are less common than systemic metastases, usually involve the cortex, the cerebellum, the cerebellopontine angle, or the CSF. Outside of the CNS, the liver, lymph nodes, bones, and lung are the most frequent sites of disease. Although most pituitary carcinomas are locally invasive, there are no distinguishing features by imaging save for the presence of metastatic disease.

Pituitary Hyperplasia

Pituitary hyperplasia is a nonneoplastic, polyclonal proliferation of one or more functionally distinct adenohypophyseal cells that results in enlargement of the gland. Hyperplasia can be physiologically normal, for example during pregnancy or lactation, or may be pathologic, either primary or secondary to endocrine gland failure. Most cases are found in hypothyroid patients, in whom the lack of thyroxine from the nonfunctioning thyroid gland results in overproduction of hypothalamic thyrotropin-releasing hormone. Excess of this hormone, in turn, stimulates the pituitary to produce thyroid-stimulating hormone but also results in excess prolactin secretion. Clinically the symptoms of hypothyroidism may be minimal, and masked by symptoms of hyperprolactinemia. MRI in pituitary hyperplasia shows symmetric enlargement of an otherwise normal-appearing, homogeneously enhancing gland (**Fig. 3**). The gland may be mildly or markedly enlarged, and can occasionally enlarge to a point at which adjacent structures including the optic chiasm are compressed.[10] However, in contrast to macroadenoma, there is no remodeling of the sella, and the gland homogeneously enhances.

Lymphocytic Hypophysitis

Lymphocytic hypophysitis is an autoimmune disorder of the pituitary gland that occurs 5 to 8 times more frequently in women than in men, often occurring in the time period 6 months before to 6 months after pregnancy. Clinically, patients present with hypopituitarism, pituitary insufficiency, DI, and/or symptoms related to mass effect on surrounding structures. Many patients have a personal or family history of autoimmune disease, such as Hashimoto or Graves thyroiditis, systemic lupus erythematosus, or primary biliary cirrhosis. The disease is associated with HLA DR4 and DR5.

MRI findings mirror microscopic pathology, which shows edema and infiltration of the pituitary gland by lymphocytes and plasma cells with areas of glandular fibrosis. Although neurohypophysisitis has been described, the disease is more often confined to the adenohypophysis. The normal PPBS may be absent. The pituitary gland and/or infundibulum may be enlarged within a normal volume sella (see **Fig. 3**). Uncommonly, inflammation may be cystic or necrotic, resulting in areas with higher T2 signal and hypoenhancement within the pituitary. Enhancement may be homogeneous or heterogeneous, and an adjacent enhancing dural tail (thought to represent enhancement of adjacent inflamed diaphragma sellae) is a useful secondary finding. Inflammation infrequently extends to secondarily involve the clivus and/or cavernous sinuses, where narrowing of the lumen of the internal carotid arteries can occur.

Because of its relative infrequency, lymphocytic hypophysitis is often mistaken on MRI for adenoma or other disorders. Symmetric suprasellar extension and midline pituitary stalk position

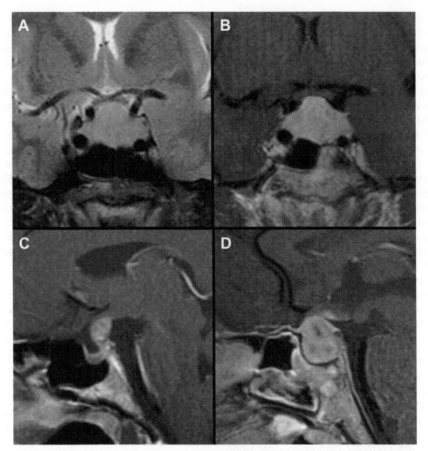

Fig. 3. Pituitary hyperplasia (*A, B*) and lymphocytic hypophysitis (*C, D*). Both T2-weighted (*A*) and gadolinium-enhanced T1-weighted (*B*) images show enlargement the pituitary gland with uniform T2 signal intensity and enhancement, without sellar enlargement, in a 28-year-old woman presenting with hyperprolactinemia and hypothyroidism. (*C, D*) Two cases of lymphocytic hypophysitis, one with infundibular thickening (*C*) and the other showing heterogeneous enhancement within an enlarged pituitary gland (*D*). In *D*, note subtle thickening of the sellar diaphragm with adjacent "tails" of inflammatory dural enhancement anterior and posterior to the gland along the planum sphenoidale and dorsum sellae.

help to differentiate this disorder from adenoma. Nakata and colleagues[11] have also recently described low signal on T2-weighted images around the pituitary gland and in the cavernous sinus as uncommon but highly specific to lymphocytic hypophysitis. Although the disease usually responds to immunotherapy, the natural history is usually one of multiple remissions and relapses.

NONPITUITARY SELLAR LESIONS
Intrasellar Meningioma

Intrasellar meningiomas arising from the inferior layer of the diaphragma sellae or along the anterior wall of the sella from the periosteal meningeal layer of the tuberculum sella, limbus sphenoidale, or the chiasmatic sulcus can masquerade as macroadenomas.[12] Similar to large adenomas, these tumors present more frequently with changes in vision or signs of elevated intracranial pressure than with pituitary dysfunction. However, mechanical compression of the pituitary infundibulum may be associated with a "stalk effect" whereby the loss of normal dopaminergic inhibition from the hypothalamus results in mild pituitary hypersecretion of prolactin.

Intrasellar meningiomas may reside entirely within the sella or extend superiorly into the suprasellar cistern. Tumors that arise from the inferior surface of the diaphragma sellae displace the normal pituitary inferiorly, and the more common tumors arising from the anterior wall of the sella displace the gland posteriorly. Meningiomas calcify more frequently than adenomas, and may show a "tail" of contiguous thickened dura that extends peripherally from the edges of the mass, along the dural reflections of the cavernous sinuses or planum sphenoidale (**Fig. 4**). Bony hyperostosis and pneumosinus dilatans (focal enlargement of adjacent air-filled paranasal sinus), if present, are useful distinguishing features. Enhancement on MRI is variable, but meningiomas typically enhance slightly less than the pituitary gland. A cleavage plane between the tumor and the pituitary assists in its differentiation from macroadenoma. Meningiomas that extend into the cavernous sinus narrow the lumen of the cavernous internal carotid artery more frequently than invasive adenomas.

Lymphoma

Sellar presentation of lymphoma is exceedingly rare. Primary CNS lymphoma, which most frequently has a B-cell non-Hodgkin histology, most commonly arises in the periventricular white matter and corpus callosum. Low T2 signal and reduced diffusion are typical features on MRI. Leptomeningeal and intraventricular spread of lymphoma may involve the chiasmatic, infundibular, and suprasellar cisterns. Multifocal disease can help to distinguish this disorder from the far more common adenoma. Although CNS lymphoma usually enhances homogeneously elsewhere in the brain, more heterogeneous enhancement has been described in primary sellar lymphoma.[13]

Metastasis

Although metastases to the pituitary gland or stalk are frequent in autopsy studies of patients with widely disseminated cancer, antemortem diagnosis of pituitary metastases is uncommon. Breast and bronchogenic carcinoma are the most common primary cancers, with pituitary metastases more common in patients with concomitant osseous metastases or with multifocal metastatic disease in 5 or more locations.[14] Asymptomatic lesions are now commonly identified with 3-T MRI techniques; symptomatic lesions are

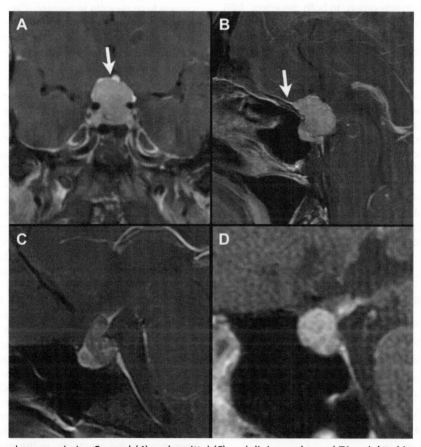

Fig. 4. Macroadenoma mimics. Coronal (*A*) and sagittal (*B*) gadolinium-enhanced T1-weighted images showing sellar and suprasellar mass with portions of the residual pituitary displaced superiorly by the mass (*A, arrow*) and anterior dural tail along the planum sphenoidale (*B, arrow*). Breast (*C*) and bronchogenic (*D*) carcinoma metastatic disease may also mimic adenoma.

associated with DI, anterior pituitary insufficiency, or retro-orbital pain. Because of its direct blood supply, the posterior lobe of the gland is involved more frequently than the anterior lobe. Imaging shows locally invasive and rapidly growing lesions within or separable from the pituitary (see **Fig. 4**). Erosion of the dorsum sella or the inferior sellar wall may help to distinguish metastases from other adenomas or craniopharyngiomas, which are more typically invasive than destructive.

INFUNDIBULAR ABNORMALITY

Lymphocytic hypophysitis, metastatic disease, and rarely primary pituitary tumors may show isolated involvement of the pituitary infundibulum. The differential diagnosis of lesions is broad, however, and several other disorders also frequently affect this structure (**Box 1**).

Germinoma

Germinoma and Langerhans cell histiocytosis (LCH) are the most common causes of central DI in the pediatric age group. In both disorders, MRI reveals absence of the normal PPBS in more than 90% of children presenting with this symptom, and infundibular thickening in roughly one-third.[15] When the infundibulum is normal and DI persists, serial reimaging at 3- to 6-month intervals is indicated, as a time lag of up to 14 months has been reported between the initial onset of symptoms and development of lesions on MRI.[16]

Pineal and hypothalamic tumor locations are more common than infundibular disease in germinoma. Isolated sellar disease is rare, although infundibular tumors may extend inferiorly into the posterior sella.[17] The PPBS is characteristically absent on MRI in patients presenting with central DI. High cellularity results in hyperdensity relative to the normal brain on CT (**Fig. 5**) as well as low

signal on T2-weighted MRI, although both intrinsic T1 and T2 signals are variable. Tumor cysts may be present in some cases. Because synchronous tumors in the pineal gland are not uncommon, this region should be critically scrutinized. Leptomeningeal dissemination may also occur, resulting in tumoral studding of the ventricular surface or CSF spaces. Measurement of serum and CSF β–human chorionic gonadotropin and α-fetoprotein may assist in diagnosis of germinoma and sometimes obviate biopsy.

Langerhans Cell Histiocytosis and Other Histiocytoses

LCH is a rare disorder of unknown etiology, characterized by localized or systemic clonal proliferation of antigen-presenting cells derived from the monocyte-macrophage system. The hypothalamic-pituitary axis is the most common site of intracranial disease. Although most frequently observed in the pediatric age group, the disorder can present at any age from neonate to geriatric. Central DI occurs as the initial presentation in up to 25% of patients, followed by a deficit in at least one other anterior pituitary hormone in many patients at some point during the disease course.

The most common MRI finding in LCH is absence of the normal PPBS. Nearly an equal proportion of patients show diffuse or focal thickening of the pituitary infundibulum (see **Fig. 5**). Rarely, infundibular thinning is observed. Lesions may extend to involve the hypothalamus superiorly and/or the sella and pituitary inferiorly. Except in cases of large masses, the stalk remains midline. T1 signal is usually low relative to cortex, although subtle T1 hyperintensity has been described and can be useful for differential diagnosis. Lesions are T2 hyperintense and enhance homogeneously. Rarely, LCH occurs as a separate lesion in the meninges, choroid plexus, or brain parenchyma.

Both absence of the PPBS and infundibular thickening are not specific to LCH, and can be found in germinoma and other infiltrative diseases. When one or both of these findings is present, however, other imaging abnormalities may suggest LCH. In a series of 163 patients with LCH,[18] craniofacial osseous lesions were seen in 56%, nonspecific paranasal sinus and/or mastoid opacification in 55%, enlarged Virchow-Robin spaces in 70%, and leukoencephalopathy in 36%. The skull base, especially the temporal bone around the mastoids, is the most frequent site of osseous craniofacial disease,[19] with lytic "punched-out" lesions showing characteristic beveled edges at their periphery. These locations

---

Box 1
Infundibular mass differential

Germinoma

Lymphocytic hypophysitis

Langerhans cell histiocytosis

Adenoma or nonadenomatous pituitary tumors

Granulomatous disease (sarcoid, Wegener granulomatosis, tuberculosis)

Lymphoma

Metastatic disease

Other infiltrative disease: Erdheim-Chester, Rosai-Dorfman

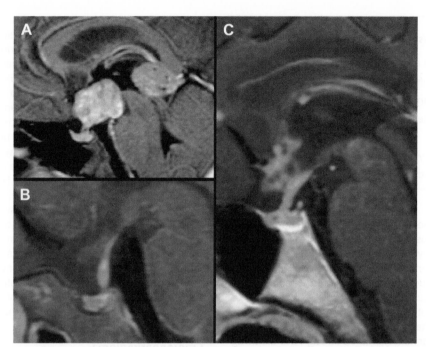

Fig. 5. Infundibular disease. (*A*) Infundibular and pineal masses in a patient with germinoma. (*B*) Subtle thickening of the infundibulum in a child with diabetes insipidus and Langerhans cell histiocytosis. (*C*) Thickening of the pituitary stalk accompanied by irregular enhancement along the anterior recesses of the third ventricle (and inferiorly in the tectal plate) in a patient with neurosarcoid.

may be better than CNS lesions for obtaining histologic confirmation.

Rarely, non–Langerhans cell histiocytoses may also involve the pituitary. Erdheim-Chester disease is a lipogranulomatous disorder in which abnormal lipid-laden macrophages accumulate in various body systems, most commonly the musculoskeletal system. Isolated pituitary infundibular disease has been reported, although hypothalamic disease and dural disease are more common in the CNS.[20,21] Similarly, Rosai-Dorfman disease is an unusual proliferative disease of histiocytes characterized by pale eosinophilic cytoplasm that usually presents with cervical lymphadenopathy or nasal obstruction and, rarely, extranodal disease, including the sella.[22,23]

Granulomatous Hypophysitis

Granulomatous hypophysitis is a less common but histologically distinct variant of adenohypophysitis that may be idiopathic or associated with granulomatous inflammatory disease (tuberculosis, sarcoid, or syphilis, for example), or systemic diseases such as Takayasu arteritis, Crohn disease, Wegener granulomatosis, and thyroiditis. Granulomatous inflammation can also result after rupture of Rathke cleft cyst. Unlike lymphocytic hypophysitis,

granulomatous hypophysitis occurs with roughly equal incidence in men and women. The imaging appearance overlaps that of lymphocytic hypophysitis, although high T2 signal may be more common in Wegener granulomatosis.[24,25] Concomitant disease elsewhere in the CNS is common in cases of tuberculosis and sarcoidosis, with characteristic nodular leptomeningeal enhancement present in the basilar cisterns, perivascular spaces, or along cranial nerves in many cases (see **Fig. 5**).

CYSTIC LESIONS

Different lesions with cystic composition that arise in the sella are given in (**Box 2**).

Arachnoid Cyst

The pituitary gland and stalk are enveloped within a thin membranous capsule that is derived from the pia, but the sella does not normally contain arachnoid cells.[26] True arachnoid cysts in this location that are isolated from the subarachnoid space are thus distinctly uncommon, hypothesized to arise either as obstructed herniations through the sellar diaphragm or de novo from subarachnoid rests within the sella. Pathologically, the cyst wall comprises a single layer of mesothelial cells surrounded by a collagenous layer. The

> **Box 2**
> **Cystic mass differential**
>
> Arachnoid cyst
>
> Rathke cleft cyst
>
> Craniopharyngioma
>
> Cystic or hemorrhagic adenoma
>
> Abscess
>
> Dermoid cyst
>
> Epidermoid cyst

clinical presentation mimics that of a nonsecreting adenoma, usually in older patients. On imaging, arachnoid cysts approximate CSF signal intensity on all sequences. A discrete cyst wall is not identified, although the normal gland is compressed posteriorly and inferiorly.

Similar but distinct from true arachnoid cysts of the sella, the so-called empty sella results when the subarachnoid herniates through the diaphragmatic hiatus and enlarges over time. More common in middle-aged and elderly women, it has been speculated that empty sella "syndrome" results from enlargement of the diaphragmatic hiatus by physiologic enlargement of the pituitary gland during pregnancy and later herniation of the arachnoid through the secondarily incompetent hiatus.

Rathke Cleft Cyst

Nonneoplastic cysts arising from embryonic Rathke cleft, which normally regresses following development of the adenohypophysis, are most often discovered incidentally during cranial imaging for other causes. Clinical symptoms arise from mass effect; headache and visual symptoms are more common than hypopituitarism. Histologically, a single layer of columnar or cuboidal epithelial cells envelops the fluid within the cyst. The natural history is one of slow growth over time. A roughly 20% recurrence rate is documented following surgical resection and is increased by fat graft, which is consequently avoided by most surgeons. Squamous metaplasia within the epithelial layer of the cyst on pathologic examination also makes recurrence more likely.

MRI of Rathke cleft cyst demonstrates a sharply circumscribed, unilocular cyst, which (unlike cystic adenoma) is usually located in the midline. The cysts are more commonly intrasellar but sometimes sellar and suprasellar. Purely suprasellar cysts are unusual. Within the sella, cysts arise between the anterior and posterior lobes of the adenohypophysis, within the pars intermedia region of the gland. In cases of suprasellar extension, cysts are located along the anterior aspect of the infundibulum. Intrinsic signal varies based on cyst contents, with roughly two-thirds containing "machine oil" fluid with high T1 and variable T2 signal, and the other third containing simple serous fluid that more closely approximates the composition and signal intensity of normal CSF (**Fig. 6**). Of the roughly 70% cysts with high T2 signal, an intracystic, T2 hypointense and nonenhancing mural nodule is diagnostic. Hemorrhage within Rathke cysts is extremely rare, but when it occurs patients may present with symptoms of apoplexy, and fluid-fluid levels may be identified within cysts with hemorrhage. Thin or absent cyst-wall enhancement is characteristic of these lesions. Infection of Rathke cleft cyst is also a rare complication. Features suggestive of infection include rapid enlargement of the cyst, enhancement, and surrounding edema.

Craniopharyngioma

Unlike most other cystic sellar and suprasellar lesions, craniopharyngioma is a true neoplasm of epithelial cells.[27] Presenting clinical symptoms are related to elevated intracranial pressure, visual changes, hypopituitarism, and, interestingly, neuropsychiatric deficits related to compression or invasion of frontal or temporal lobe structures. Pathologically these tumors are divided into 2 subtypes, adamantinomatous and squamous-papillary; it is speculated that the former originate from squamous cell rests along the involuted embryologic craniopharyngeal duct and the latter arise in squamous metaplasia of cells deriving from the pars tuberalis of the adenohypophysis. The adamantinomatous variant occurs in adults but is far more common in children, and with rare exception the squamous-papillary type is seen only in adults. Tumors with adamantinomatous histology (or mixed or transitional histology) are histologically benign but biologically aggressive, and their tendency to invade surrounding structures often prevents gross total surgical resection. Gross total resection of squamous-papillary craniopharyngioma is curative.

Adamantinomatous craniopharyngiomas arise from anywhere along the primitive craniopharyngeal duct, but in contrast to Rathke cleft cyst, 90% to 95% have a suprasellar component; pure intrasellar tumors are rare, seen in 5% or fewer of cases. Unlike Rathke cleft cysts, which are smaller and most commonly intrasellar, craniopharyngiomas are larger (>2 cm) and typically centered in the suprasellar cistern with inferior extension into

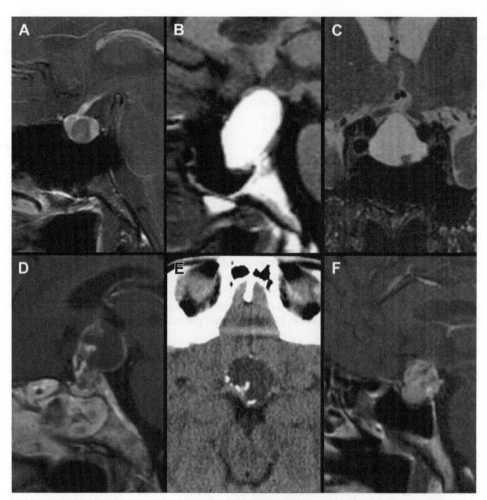

Fig. 6. Rathke cleft cysts (*A–C*) and craniopharyngioma (*D–F*). (*A*) Classic Rathke cleft cyst seen as a rounded, non-enhancing sellar mass within the pars intermedia. (*B*) "Machine oil" cyst with uniform high T1 signal on unenhanced T1-weighted image. (*C*) Fluid-type Rathke cyst with high T2 signal and eccentric mural nodule. (*D*) Adamantinomatous craniopharyngioma gadolinium-enhanced MRI and (*E*) unenhanced CT in the same pediatric patient, showing solid and cystic mass with eccentric mural calcification. (*F*) Note the more solid appearance of squamous-papillary craniopharyngioma in an adult.

the sella (see **Fig. 6**). A single unilocular cyst is less common than multiple conglomerate cysts, the former characterized by a smooth contour and the latter by a lobulated contour. High T1 signal is evident within one or more cysts in 80% of cases. Unlike Rathke cleft cysts, enhancement of cyst walls can be prominent, and a solid enhancing component, although typically small, is usually present.

Calcification, present in 90% of cases and seen at the periphery of individual cystic components, can be challenging to identify on MRI. Low T1 and T2 signal that blooms on gradient-echo images is typical, although calcification may also be seen with high T1 or T2 signal or may be occult if present in low concentrations. CT obtained in equivocal cases can assist in distinguishing these tumors from Rathke cleft cysts and macroadenomas, in which calcification is far less common. Hydrocephalus may be present when there is significant invasion of surrounding structures or extension into the third ventricle. Although uncommon, malignant transformation may occur after irradiation, and dissemination through the CSF or along the surgical tract are known complications.

Tumors with squamous-papillary and mixed histology have a less prominent cystic component and a spherical morphology, and may be entirely solid. Calcification is atypical, and tumor infiltration of surrounding structures is less frequent than with the adamantinomatous subtype. Papillary tumors may occasionally arise in ectopic locations such as the floor of the third ventricle, the posterior fossa, and the nasopharynx.

Cystic and Hemorrhagic Adenoma

Microadenoma may occasionally present with intrapituitary hemorrhage or tumor cyst formation, without a discrete solid enhancing component on MRI. Although the former may contain fluid levels or heterogeneous signal intensity to suggest the presence of intralesional hemorrhage, a unilocular cyst without enhancement may also be observed. Unlike Rathke cleft cysts, adenomas are almost always off midline (**Fig. 7**). However, follow-up MRI in 1 to 3 months to characterize the temporal evolution of lesions may be the only method to distinguish hemorrhagic and cystic adenomas from other pituitary cysts. Specifically, hemorrhage typically evolves in signal over time, becomes smaller, and may result in spontaneous obliteration of the adenoma. Adenomas with tumor

cysts, by contrast, remain similar in signal and either increase in size or develop a solid enhancing component that can be more readily visualized on follow-up.

Pituitary Abscess

The diagnosis of abscess within the pituitary gland is seldom made prospectively; pus is more commonly identified during transsphenoidal resection of preoperatively presumed cystic neoplasms. An underlying lesion such as adenoma, Rathke cyst, or craniopharyngioma can serve as the initial nidus for infection, but abscess is more commonly the result of either contiguous or hematogenous spread from a separate nidus of infection. Prior surgery and radiation are the major risk factors. Only one-third of patients have fever and/or leukocytosis; one-fourth present with frank meningitis. Hypopituitarism is frequent, leading to clinical suspicion for other pituitary abnormalities.

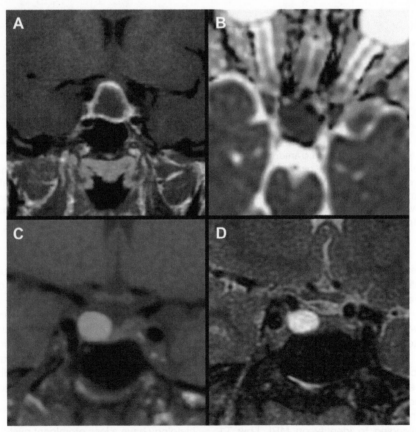

Fig. 7. Cystic sellar masses. Gadolinium-enhanced T1 (*A*) and axial apparent diffusivity map (*B*) in a patient with intrapituitary abscess. Irregular enhancement of the abscess wall and reduced diffusion distinguish this lesion from other cystic lesions in the pituitary gland. (*C*) High T1 signal within a hemorrhagic adenoma on unenhanced T1-weighted image, which resolved on follow-up. (*D*) Cystic adenoma showing high T2 signal laterally within the pituitary. Only 10% of Rathke cleft cysts are located off the midline.

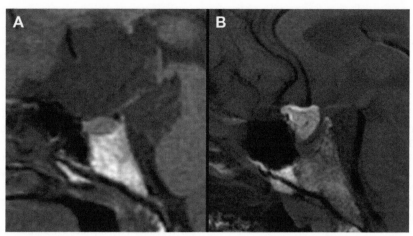

Fig. 8. Epithelial cysts. Unenhanced T1-weighted image shows multilobulated epidermoid cyst (*A*) with subtle T1 hyperintensity relative to normal prepontine CSF surrounding the sella and displacing surrounding structures. The same sequence in a patient with a sellar dermoid cyst (*B*) illustrates intrinsic T1 hyperintensity caused by fat within the tumor.

MRI appearance of pituitary infection overlaps with the appearance of other pituitary cystic disease. Subtle T1 hyperintensity and slightly heterogeneous T2 hyperintensity may herald the presence of infectious debris and trace blood products often seen with infections (see **Fig. 7**). Reduced diffusion on diffusion-weighted imaging, when performed, is very suggestive of infection, and may be useful in monitoring treatment. Furthermore, the peripherally enhancing rim of pyogenic abscess is less commonly smooth and thin than with cystic neoplasm, and abscesses may instead show subtle indistinctness and nonuniform thickness of the enhancing wall.

Epidermoid and Dermoid Cysts

Epidermoid tumors usually present in adults because of local mass effect. Unlike dermoid cysts, these tumors are often either off midline or asymmetric to one side of the midline. These cysts frequently insinuate around local anatomic structures, including the skull base and cranial nerves. MRI shows relatively circumscribed lesions with signal intensity that differs slightly from CSF, often slightly higher than CSF on T1-weighted and T2-weighted images (**Fig. 8**). Similar to the case of infection, high signal on diffusion-weighted images can be an important finding for differentiating epidermoid from other cystic lesions.

Dermoid cysts are up to 10 times less common than epidermoid cysts. Almost always found in the midline, these tumors represent congenital inclusion cysts that result when ectodermal and mesodermal epithelial elements remain trapped intracranially during embryonic closure of the neural tube. Dermoid cysts often contain fat,

calcification, and fluid in various proportions, and may present with cyst rupture and chemical meningitis. High T1 signal caused by lipids within the tumor (see **Fig. 8**), or within the CSF spaces in cases of rupture, are characteristic.

REFERENCES

1. Atkins D, Sanford R. Infundibuloneurohypophysitis in children. Padiatr Neurosurg 1999;30:267–71.
2. Lundin P, Nyman R, Burman P, et al. MRI of pituitary macroadenomas with reference to hormonal activity. Neuroradiology 1992;34:43–51.
3. Hagiwara A, Inoue Y, Wakasa K, et al. Comparison of growth hormone-producing and non-growth hormone-producing pituitary adenomas: imaging characteristics and pathologic correlation. Radiology 2003;228:533–8.
4. Bartynski WS, Lin L. Dynamic and conventional spin-echo MR of pituitary microlesions. AJNR Am J Neuroradiol 1997;18:965–72.
5. Sarlis NJ, Gourgiotis L, Koch CA, et al. MR imaging features of thyrotropic-secreting pituitary adenomas at initial presentation. AJR AM J Roentgenol 2003; 181:577–82.
6. Nawar RN, Abdel Mannan D, Selman WR, et al. Pituitary tumor apoplexy: a review. J Intensive Care Med 2008;23:75–89.
7. Covington MF, Chin SS, Osborn AG. Pituicytoma, spindle cell oncocytoma, and granular cell tumor: clarification and meta-analysis of the world literature since 1893. AJNR Am J Neuroradiol 2011;32:2067–72.
8. Kaltsas GA, Nomikos P, Kontogeorgos G, et al. Clinical review: diagnosis and management of pituitary carcinomas. J Clin Endocrinol Metab 2005;90: 3089–99.

9. Pernicone PJ, Scheithauer BW, Sebo TJ, et al. Pituitary carcinoma: a clinicopathologic study of 15 cases. Cancer 1997;79:804–12.

10. Wolansky LJ, Leavitt GD, Elias BJ, et al. MRI of pituitary hyperplasia in primary hypothyroidism. Neuroradiology 1996;38:50–2.

11. Nakata Y, Sato N, Masumoto T, et al. Parasellar T2 dark sign on MR imaging in patients with lymphocytic hypophysitis. AJNR Am J Neuroradiol 2010; 31:1944–50.

12. Chi JH, McDermott M. Tuberculum sellae meningiomas. Neurosurg Focus 2003;14:1–6.

13. Kaufmann TJ, Lopes MB, Laws ER, et al. Primary sellar lymphoma: radiologic and pathologic findings in two patients. AJNR Am J Neuroradiol 2002;23: 364–7.

14. Morita A, Meyer F, Laws E. Symptomatic pituitary metastases. J Neurosurg 1998;89:69–73.

15. Alter CA, Bilaniuk LT. Utility of magnetic resonance imaging in the evaluation of the child with central diabetes insipidus. J Pediatr Endocrinol Metab 2002;15(Suppl 2):681–7.

16. Mootha SL, Barkovich AJ, Grumbach MM, et al. Idiopathic hypothalamic diabetes insipidus, pituitary stalk thickening, and the occult intracranial germinoma in children and adolescents. J Clin Endocrinol Metab 1997;82:1362–7.

17. Kanagakia M, Mikia Y, Takahashib JA, et al. MRI and CT findings of neurohypophyseal germinoma. Eur J Radiol 2004;49:204–11.

18. Prayer D, Grois N, Prosch H, et al. MR imaging presentation of intracranial disease associated with Langerhans cell histiocytosis. AJNR Am J Neuroradiol 2004;25:880–91.

19. D'Ambrosio N, Soohoo S, Warshall C, et al. Craniofacial and intracranial manifestations of Langerhans cell histiocytosis: report of findings in 100 patients. Am J Roentgenol 2008;191:589–97.

20. Wright RA, Hermann RC, Parisi JE. Neurological manifestations of Erdheim-Chester disease. J Neurol Neurosurg Psychiatr 1999;66(1):72–5.

21. Adem C, Hélie O, Lévêque C, et al. Case 78: Erdheim-Chester disease with central nervous system involvement. Radiology 2005;234:111–5.

22. Kelly WF, Bradey N, Scoones D. Rosai-Dorfman disease presenting as a pituitary tumour. Clin Endocrinol 1999;50:133–7.

23. Woodcock RJ, Mandell JW, Lipper MH. Sinus histiocytosis (Rosai-Dorfman disease) of the suprasellar region: MR imaging findings—a case report. Radiology 1999;213:808–10.

24. Katzman GL, Langford CA, Sneller MC, et al. Pituitary involvement by Wegener's granulomatosis: a report of two cases. AJNR Am J Neuroradiol 1999;20:519–23.

25. Goyal M, Kucharczyk W, Keystone E. Granulomatous hypophysitis due to Wegener's granulomatosis. AJNR Am J Neuroradiol 2000;21:1466–9.

26. Dubuisson AS, Stevenaert A, Martin D, et al. Intrasellar arachnoid cysts. Neurosurgery 2007;61:505–13.

27. Zada G, Lin N, Ojerholm E, et al. Craniopharyngioma and other cystic epithelial lesions of the sellar region: a review of clinical, imaging and histopathological relationships. Neurosurg Focus 2010;28:E4.

Management of Incidentally Found Nonfunctional Pituitary Tumors

Mark E. Molitch, MD

KEYWORDS

- Adenoma • Pituitary • Incidentaloma • Tumor • Transsphenoidal surgery

KEY POINTS

- Patients with pituitary incidentalomas should be evaluated for tumor hypersecretion.
- Those with macroadenomas should be evaluated for hypopituitarism, visual-field defects, and other mass effects.
- Visual-field defects, tumor growth, and hypopituitarism are indications for surgery.
- Deficiencies in corticotropin/cortisol and thyrotropin/thyroxine should be corrected before any surgery.
- Tumor growth in patients who do not undergo surgery can be expected in 10.6% of microadenomas and 24.1% of macroadenomas.
- For patients without specific indications for surgery, surveillance magnetic resonance imaging may need to be performed for up to 20 years.

INTRODUCTION

Clinically nonfunctioning adenomas (CNFA) of the pituitary, by definition, produce no clinical syndrome related to overproduction of tumor hormones. Studies have shown, however, that 70% to 80% of CNFAs produce gonadotropins or their subunits, and thus are actually gonadotroph adenomas.[1] A few per cent also stain for corticotropin, growth hormone (GH), prolactin (PRL), or thyrotropin; because these hormones are not secreted in sufficient quantities to cause clinical syndromes, such tumors are referred to as "silent" corticotroph, somatotroph, lactotroph, or thyrotroph adenomas.[2]

Although large CNFAs often present because they cause significant hypothalamic/pituitary dysfunction or visual symptoms, others may be completely asymptomatic, being detected either at autopsy or as incidental findings on magnetic resonance imaging (MRI) or computed tomography (CT) scans performed for other reasons. These asymptomatic adenomas are referred to as pituitary incidentalomas. Several other lesions also may be found in the sellar area and may mimic a pituitary adenoma, including craniopharyngiomas, Rathke cleft cysts, meningiomas, gliomas, dysgerminomas, cysts, hamartomas, metastases, and focal areas of infarction.[3–6] Lymphocytic infiltration of the pituitary can also masquerade as a pituitary adenoma.[7]

Statistically, some normal individuals must have pituitaries that exceed the normal size boundary of 9 mm (+3 standard deviations in healthy subjects[8–10]). Chanson and colleagues[11] reported several patients with "normal pituitary hypertrophy"; on MRI, these pituitaries had homogeneous isointense signals, enhanced homogeneously with

Disclosure: The author has served as a Consultant for Abbott Laboratories and receives research support from Eli Lilly & Co. and Novo-Nordisk, companies which make various hormone replacement therapies used for hypopituitarism.
Division of Endocrinology, Metabolism and Molecular Medicine, Northwestern University Feinberg School of Medicine, 645 North Michigan Avenue, Suite 530, Chicago, IL 60611, USA
E-mail address: molitch@northwestern.edu

contrast, and in 2 cases had normal pituitary tissue found at surgery.

This article reviews the epidemiology and management of patients with pituitary mass lesions incidentally found on head MRI or CT done for some reason other than suspected pituitary disease; that is, pituitary incidentalomas.

PREVALENCE OF PITUITARY INCIDENTALOMAS
Autopsy Findings

Pituitary adenomas have been found at autopsy in 1.5% to 31% of subjects not suspected of having pituitary disease while alive (**Table 1**).[3,12–43] The average frequency of finding an adenoma for these studies, which examined a total of 19,387 pituitaries, is 10.7%. The tumors are distributed equally throughout the age groups (range 16–86 years) and between the sexes. In the studies in which PRL immunohistochemistry was performed, 22% to 66% stained positively for PRL.[18,20,21,26,29–31,33–36,38,39] Detailed immunohistochemical analysis of 334 pituitary adenomas found in 316 pituitaries of 3048 autopsy cases in one series showed that 39.5% stained for PRL, 13.8% for corticotropin, 7.2% for gonadotropins or α subunits, 1.8% for GH, 0.6% for thyrotropin, and 3.0% for multiple hormones.[39]

In these postmortem studies all but 7 of the tumors were less than 10 mm in diameter. The relative lack of macroadenomas in these autopsy studies suggests that growth from a microadenoma to a macroadenoma must be an exceedingly uncommon event, and/or that virtually all macroadenomas come to clinical attention and, therefore, are not included in autopsy findings. There is a separate report of an additional 3 macroadenomas being found at autopsy.[44]

CT and MRI Scans in Normal Individuals

Three series have evaluated CT scans of the sella in normal subjects who were having such scans for reasons unrelated to possible pituitary disease, finding discrete areas of low density greater than 3 mm in diameter in 4% to 20%.[3,45,46] Two similar studies have been performed using MRI. Chong and colleagues[47] found focal pituitary gland hypodensities of 2 to 5 mm in 20 of 52 normal subjects with nonenhanced images using a 1.5-T scanner and 3-mm thick sections. With similar scans but with gadolinium-DTPA (diethylenetriamine pentaacetic acid) enhancement, Hall and colleagues[48] found focal areas of decreased intensity 3 mm or greater in diameter in 34%, 10%, and 2% of 100 volunteers, depending on whether there was

agreement on the diagnosis between 1, 2, or 3 independent reviewing neuroradiologists.

Sellar lesions greater than 10 mm in diameter have not been found in these small studies of consecutive normal individuals, similar to the very limited number found at autopsy. However, Nammour and colleagues[49] found that of 3550 consecutive CT scans done in men with a mean age of 57 years for the symptoms of change in mental status, headache, or possible metastases, 7 (0.2%) were found to have pituitary macroadenomas ranging from 1.0 to 2.5 cm in size; all were thought to be CNFAs after hormonal evaluation. Similarly, when nonenhanced MRI scans were performed without specific views of the sellar area in asymptomatic normal subjects, macroadenomas were found in 0.16% of 3672 subjects in a study by Yue and colleagues[50] and in 0.3% of 2000 subjects in a study by Vernooij and colleagues.[51] Furthermore, macroadenomas have been reported as incidental findings.[52]

Clinical Experience with Pituitary Incidentalomas

Clinically, patients with incidental macroadenomas are commonly seen in everyday practice. In 10 series totaling 513 patients reported with pituitary CNFAs who were not treated either surgically or medically, thereby giving an indication of their natural history, 353 (68.8%) had macroadenomas and 260 (31.2%) had microadenomas (**Table 2**).[53–62] However, these were not all true incidentalomas. Many had tumors 2 cm or more in diameter and many were symptomatic with hypopituitarism or visual-field defects, but for a variety of reasons surgery was not performed. For example, in the series reported by Karavitaki and colleagues,[61] only one-half of the 24 macroadenomas were incidental findings and 11 had varying degrees of hypopituitarism. In this series, 5 of the patients had major visual-field defects but did not have surgery either because of major comorbidities (3 patients) or because the patient did not wish surgery (2 patients).[61] Similarly, in the series of 28 patients with macroadenomas reported by Dekkers and colleagues,[62] only 6 (21%) were truly incidentalomas, with 44% having hypopituitarism and 46% having visual-field defects. Nevertheless, the proportion of patients with macroadenomas found clinically as incidentalomas is much greater than would be expected based on the autopsy or radiology findings. These data suggest that the mass effects of such tumors may have caused some of the symptomatology causing the patients to have the scans in the first place, even in those in whom there were no true visual-field defects or hypopituitarism.

Table 1
Frequency of pituitary adenomas found at autopsy

Authors,[Ref.] Year	No. of Pituitaries Examined	No. of Adenomas Found	Frequency (%)	No. of Macroadenomas Found	Stain Positive for Prolactin (%)
Susman,[12] 1933	260	23	8.8	—	—
Close,[13] 1934	250	23	9.2	—	—
Costello,[14] 1936	1000	225	22.5	0	—
Sommers,[15] 1959	400	26	6.5	0	—
McCormick and Halmi,[16] 1971	1600	140	8.8	0	—
Haugen,[17] 1973	170	33	19.4	—	—
Kovacs et al,[18] 1980	152	20	13.2	2	53
Landolt,[19] 1980	100	13	13.0	0	—
Mosca et al,[20] 1980	100	24	24.0	0	23
Burrows et al,[21] 1981	120	32	26.7	0	41
Parent et al,[22] 1981	500	42	8.4	1	—
Muhr et al,[23] 1981	205	3	1.5	0	—
Max et al,[24] 1981	500	9	1.8	—	—
Schwezinger and Warzok,[25] 1982	5100	485	9.5	0	—
Chambers et al,[3] 1982	100	14	14.0	0	—
Coulon et al,[26] 1983	100	10	10.0	0	60
Siqueira and Guembarovski,[27] 1984	450	39	8.7	0	—
Char and Persaud,[28] 1986	350	35	10.0	0	—
Gorczyca and Hardy,[29] 1988	100	27	27.0	0	30
El-Hamid et al,[30] 1988	486	97	20.0	0	48
Scheithauer et al,[31] 1989	251	41	16.3	0	66
Kontogeorgos et al,[32] 1991	470	49	10.4	0	—
Marin et al,[33] 1992	210	35	16.7	0	32
Sano et al,[34] 1993	166	15	9.0	0	47
Teramoto et al,[35] 1994	1000	51	5.1	0	30
Camaris et al,[36] 1995	423	14	3.2	0	44
Tomita and Gates,[37] 1999	100	24	24.0	—	—
Kurosaki et al,[38] 2001	692	79	11.4	1	24
Buurman and Saeger,[39] 2006	3048	334	11.0	3	40
Rittierodt and Hori,[40] 2007	228	7	3.0	0	—
Furgal-Borzych et al,[41] 2007	151	47	31.1	0	21
Kim et al,[42] 2007	120	7	6.7	0	29
Adhakhani et al,[43] 2011	485	61	—	—	—
Total	19,387	2084	10.7%	7	—

The final column shows the percentage of tumors that had positive immunostaining for prolactin, indicating that they were lactotroph adenomas.

Table 2
Changes in size of pituitary incidentalomas

Authors,[Ref.] Year	Microadenomas				Macroadenomas				Years Followed
	Total	Increased	Decreased	No Change	Total	Enlarged	Decreased	No Change	
Donovan and Corenblum,[53] 1995	15	0	0	15	16	4[a]	0	12	6–7
Reincke et al,[54] 1990	7	1	1	5	7	2	0	5	8
Nishizawa et al,[55] 1998	—	—	—	—	28	2[a]	0	26	5.6
Feldkamp et al,[56] 1999	31	1	1	29	19	5	1	13	2.7
Igarashi et al,[57] 1999	1	0	0	1	22	6	10	6	5.1
Sanno et al,[58] 2003	74	10	7	57	165	20[a]	22	123	2.3
Fainstein Day et al,[59] 2004	11	1	0	10	7	1	0	6	3.2
Arita et al,[60] 2006	5	2	0	3	37	19[a]	0	18	5.2
Karavitaki et al,[61] 2007	16	2	1	13	24	12	4	8	3.6
Dekkers et al,[62] 2007	—	—	—	—	28	14	8	6	7.1
Total	160	17 (10.6%)	10 (6.3%)	133 (83.1%)	353	85 (24.1%)	45 (12.7%)	223 (63.2%)	—

[a] A total of 7 cases in these series had tumor enlargement caused by apoplexy.

EVALUATION OF PATIENTS WITH PITUITARY INCIDENTALOMAS

Endocrinologic Evaluation for Pituitary Hyperfunction

As the most common lesion in the sella is a pituitary adenoma, it is reasonable to evaluate patients for hormone oversecretion, regardless of the size of the lesion.[63,64] Many of the changes occurring with hormone oversecretion syndromes may be quite subtle and only slowly progressive; therefore, screening for hormonal oversecretion is warranted even in patients with no clinical evidence of hormone oversecretion. "Silent" somatotroph and corticotroph adenomas have been reported many times, but it is not clear whether such patients with minimal clinical evidence of hormone oversecretion are free from the increased risk for the more subtle cardiovascular, bone, oncologic, and possibly other adverse effects usually associated with such tumors. Indeed, there is emerging evidence that subclinical Cushing syndrome caused by adrenal incidentalomas is associated with significantly increased prevalence of diabetes, hypertension, obesity, osteoporosis, and cardiovascular risk.[65] Whether there is a similar increased risk for these comorbidities with silent corticotroph adenomas is unknown. Furthermore, some investigators have reported that silent corticotroph adenomas have a worse prognosis than those with overt disease with respect to aggressiveness following initial surgery,[66,67] but this has not been found in other series.[62,68,69] Progression to overt Cushing disease over time was reported in 4 of 22 (18%) of cases in one series.[70] It is not clear how many of these patients have nonsuppressible serum cortisol levels or elevated urinary free cortisol levels, but Lopez and colleagues[71] found suppressed corticotropin secretion and hypocortisolism in 2 of 12 patients following resection of silent corticotropin-secreting adenomas.

Screening for hormone oversecretion in such patients has been questioned as to its cost-effectiveness.[72–74] However, evidence from the series of Fainstein Day and colleagues[59] suggests such screening is worthwhile, as 7 of their 46 patients turned out to have prolactinomas, and of the 13 who ended up going to surgery and having immunohistochemistry performed, 2 adenomas (15%) were GH positive and 4 (31%) were plurihormonal adenomas.

A serum PRL should be obtained, but it is very important to distinguish between PRL production by a tumor versus hyperprolactinemia from stalk dysfunction caused by a macroadenoma.[75] PRL levels are usually higher than 200 ng/mL for hormone-secreting macroadenomas, and lower

numbers suggest stalk dysfunction.[76–78] For very large tumors, the sample should be diluted 1:100 to avoid the "hook effect,"[79,80] in which very high PRL levels may saturate the antibodies in 2-site assays; however, this is not necessary in all assays. An insulin-like growth factor 1 (IGF-1) test is probably sufficient to screen for acromegaly but if this cannot be performed, it may be necessary to demonstrate nonsuppression of GH levels by hyperglycemia during an oral glucose tolerance test.[81]

The best screening tests for Cushing syndrome have traditionally been the overnight dexamethasone suppression test and the 24-hour urinary free cortisol, and more recently, the assessment of a midnight salivary cortisol.[82,83] An abnormal midnight salivary cortisol has been found to have greater than 93% specificity and sensitivity for diagnosing Cushing syndrome.[84] Because the patients may have little in the way of symptoms, it is likely that the 24-hour urine free cortisol will be normal and an overnight 1-mg dexamethasone suppression test or a midnight salivary cortisol might be better tests to diagnose early Cushing disease. Because of the high variability of corticotropin levels, even in patients with overt Cushing disease, corticotropin levels are probably not worth measuring. However, some participants on The Endocrine Society Taskforce that wrote the Pituitary Incidentaloma Clinical Practice Guideline of the Society thought that measurement of corticotropin levels might be useful.[64] Any abnormality found on such screening would then need to be pursued with more definitive testing. Despite the fact that most CNFAs are gonadotroph adenomas, gonadotropin oversecretion rarely causes clinical symptoms, and such a finding would not influence therapy; therefore, there is no reason to screen for this.

Endocrinologic Evaluation for Hypopituitarism

Microadenomas have generally not been thought to cause disruption of normal pituitary function. Of the 22 patients with suspected microadenomas evaluated in the series of Reincke and colleagues[54] and Donovan and Corenblum,[53] all had normal pituitary function. However, Yuen and colleagues[85] found deficiencies of one or more pituitary hormones in 50% of 38 patients with clinically nonfunctioning microadenomas. Larger lesions are much more likely to cause varying degrees of hypopituitarism, and up to 41% of patients with macroadenomas have been found to have hypopituitarism.[50,52,56,57] Thus, all patients with macroadenomas should be screened for hypopituitarism, but whether all patients with microadenomas should be similarly screened is controversial.

Screening for deficiencies of thyrotropin, corticotropin, GH, and gonadotropins consists of assessing symptoms of possible hypopituitarism in the patient and measurement of levels of free thyroxine (thyrotropin is not sensitive for diagnosing central hypothyroidism), 8 AM cortisol, IGF-1, and testosterone or estradiol. If the 8 AM cortisol level is less than 18 μg/dL, additional measures may be necessary to diagnose a deficiency of corticotropin/cortisol.[86,87] In postmenopausal women, the finding of low gonadotropins would indicate hypopituitarism.[64] Deficiencies of thyroxine and cortisol should always be replaced when diagnosed regardless of whether surgery is to be done. Gonadal hormone and GH replacements are initiated as clinically indicated, but not necessarily before surgery and generally after more detailed testing, including GH stimulation tests.[86,87] It should be remembered that those found to be corticotropin/cortisol deficient need stress doses of steroids during surgery. Because surgery can both improve and worsen pituitary function, retesting and reassessment several weeks after any surgery is mandatory. In patients who are not hypopituitary or who have partial hypopituitarism and who do not undergo surgery, an increase in tumor size on surveillance MRI is an indication for repeat assessment for hypopituitarism. Whether repeat testing is indicated in such patients in the absence of evidence for tumor growth is controversial.[64]

NATURAL HISTORY AND FOLLOW-UP OF INCIDENTAL CNFAs

In the 10 series mentioned that reported on the follow-up of patients with pituitary CNFAs that were not treated, most were incidentalomas; however, in many cases the adenomas were symptomatic but not treated for a variety of reasons (see **Table 2**). Of the 160 patients with microadenomas reported in these series, 17 (10.6%) experienced tumor growth, 10 (6.3%) showed evidence of a decrease in tumor size, and 133 (83.1)% remained unchanged in size in follow-up MRI scans over periods of up to 8 years.[53,54,56–61] Of the 353 patients with macroadenomas, 85 (24.1%) showed evidence of tumor enlargement, 45 (12.7%) showed evidence of a decrease in tumor size, and 223 (63.2%) remained unchanged in size on follow-up MRI over periods of 8 years.[53–62] In their review of the data from these series, Fernández-Balsells and colleagues[88] expressed the incidence of tumor enlargement per

100 patient-years as 12.53 for macroadenomas and 3.32 for microadenomas. The duration of follow-up of these patients was variable and in their analysis, Dekkers and colleagues[62] suggested that with longer follow-up up to 50% of patients with macroadenomas will have an increase in tumor size. It should be mentioned that of the 59 macroadenomas with an increase in tumor size, in 7 this was due to a hemorrhage into the tumor (see **Table 2**).

The incidence of pituitary apoplexy per 100 patient-years was 1.1 for macroadenomas and 0.4 for microadenomas.[88]

MANAGEMENT OF INCIDENTAL CNFAs

Tumors found to be hypersecreting may be handled in the usual way, generally with dopamine agonists for prolactinomas and surgery for GH and corticotropin-producing tumors. Treatment guidelines for the management of such tumors are readily available.[89–91] For tumors not oversecreting these hormones, the indications for surgery are based initially on mass effects of the tumors and subsequently on tumor-size enlargement.

Microadenomas

For patients with microadenomas, significant tumor enlargement will occur in only 10.6% of patients. Therefore, surgical resection is generally not indicated, and repeated annual scanning for 3 years is indicated to detect tumor enlargement; subsequently, repeat scanning can be done less frequently (**Fig. 1**). Surgery would then be done only for significant tumor enlargement. However, the rate of growth is generally quite slow so that the decision and timing of any surgery would depend on the rate and amount of growth as well as any clinical consequences, such as the development of visual-field defects.

Macroadenomas

Tumors greater than 1 cm in diameter have already indicated a propensity for growth. A careful evaluation of the mass effects of these tumors is indicated, including evaluation of pituitary function and visual field examination if the tumor abuts the chiasm. If there are visual-field defects, surgery is certainly indicated.[64] Because hypopituitarism is potentially correctable with tumor resection, this is also a relative indication for surgery.[92] In the author's opinion, tumors larger than 2 cm should also be considered for surgery simply because of their already demonstrated propensity for growth. Similarly, if a tumor is found to be abutting the optic chiasm, even though testing shows

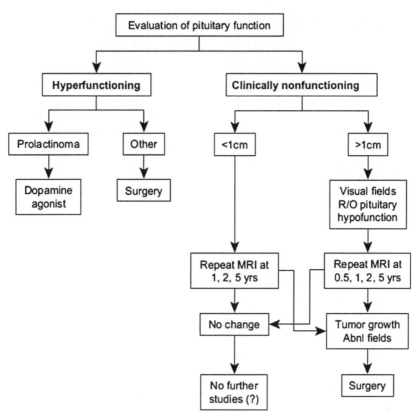

Fig. 1. Flow diagram indicating the approach to the patient found to have a pituitary incidentaloma. The first step is to evaluate patients for pituitary hyperfunction and then treat those found to be hyperfunctioning. Of patients with tumors that are clinically nonfunctioning, those with macroadenomas are evaluated further for evidence of chiasmal compression and hypopituitarism. Scans are then repeated at progressively longer intervals to assess for enlargement of the tumors. Abnl, abnormal; R/O, rule out. (*Reproduced from* Molitch ME. Nonfunctioning pituitary tumors and pituitary incidentalomas. Endocrinol Metab Clin North Am 2008;37:151–71; with permission.)

normal visual fields, consideration should be given to surgery. If surgery is not done, visual fields should be tested at 6- to 12-monthly intervals thereafter.

If a completely asymptomatic lesion is thought to be a pituitary macroadenoma based on radiologic and clinical findings, then a decision could be made to simply repeat scans on a yearly basis, surgery being deferred until there is evidence of tumor growth. Some clinicians would obtain the initial follow-up scan at 6 months to detect potential rapid growers.[64] As indicated earlier, significant tumor growth can be expected in approximately one-quarter of patients with macroadenomas. Hemorrhage into such tumors is uncommon, but anticoagulation may predispose to this complication; surgery would prevent such a complication. When there is no evidence of visual-field defects or hypopituitarism and the patient is asymptomatic, an attempt at medical therapy with a dopamine agonist or octreotide is

reasonable, realizing that only about 10% to 20% of such patients will respond with a decrease in tumor size.[93,94] Surgery may be indicated if surveillance scans show evidence of tumor enlargement. As with microadenomas, the decision to proceed with surgery is affected by the rate and extent of growth and any clinical consequences, such as compression of the optic chiasm or the development of pituitary hormone deficiencies, as well as the patient's comorbidities and risks for surgery (see **Fig. 1**).

Attempts have been made to look at the growth rates of those tumors that do grow. Dekkers and colleagues[62] estimated a growth rate of 0.6 mm per year or 236 mm^3 per year. Of their 14 patients who experienced tumor growth, 2 showed evidence of growth by 2 years, 3 more by 3 years, and then 1 each at 4, 5, 6, 7, 12, 15, 17, 20, and 22 years. By contrast, Karavitaki and colleagues[61] found that all but 4 of their 12 patients who experienced macroadenoma regrowth did so by

5 years, although patients also had evidence of tumor growth at 6 and 8 years. Honegger and colleagues[95] found tumor volume doubling times ranging from 0.8 to 27.2 years, emphasizing the tremendous variability of increases in tumor size; there was no correlation between initial tumor size and the rate of tumor-volume doubling. These data suggest that at least for patients with macroadenomas, surveillance MRI scans should be performed for at least 22 years, although the frequency of scanning can certainly be reduced after the first few years if there is no evidence of tumor growth.

SUMMARY

Pituitary incidentalomas are frequently seen in endocrine practice. Although most incidentalomas are either gonadotroph adenomas or truly nonfunctioning, some may be silent lactotroph, somatotroph, or corticotroph adenomas. For CNFAs, hypopituitarism, visual-field defects, and evidence of tumor growth are indications for surgery. Growth of nonfunctioning incidentalomas can be expected in 10.6% of microadenomas and 24% of macroadenomas. Periodic surveillance by MRI may be needed for more than 20 years to detect tumor growth.

REFERENCES

1. Young WF, Scheithauer BW, Kovacs KT, et al. Gonadotroph adenoma of the pituitary gland: a clinicopathologic analysis of 100 cases. Mayo Clin Proc 1996;71:649–56.
2. Yamada S, Kovacs K, Horvath E, et al. Morphological study of clinically nonsecreting pituitary adenomas in patients under 40 years of age. J Neurosurg 1991;75:902–5.
3. Chambers EF, Turski PA, LaMasters D, et al. Regions of low density in the contrast-enhanced pituitary gland: normal and pathologic processes. Radiology 1982;144:109–13.
4. Elster AD. Modern imaging of the pituitary. Radiology 1993;187:1–14.
5. Freda PU, Wardlaw SL, Post KD. Unusual causes of sellar/parasellar masses in a large transsphenoidal surgical series. J Clin Endocrinol Metab 1996;81:3455–9.
6. Naidich MJ, Russell EJ. Current approaches to imaging of the sellar region and pituitary. Endocrinol Metab Clin North Am 1999;28:45–79.
7. Molitch ME, Gilliam MP. Lymphocytic hypophysitis. Horm Res 2007;68(Suppl 5):145–50.
8. Doraiswamy PM, Potts JM, Axelson DA, et al. MR assessment of pituitary gland morphology in healthy volunteers: age- and gender-related differences. AJNR Am J Neuroradiol 1992;13:1295–9.
9. Elster AD, Chen MY, Williams DW, et al. Pituitary gland: MR imaging of physiologic hypertrophy in adolescence. Radiology 1999;174:681–5.
10. Tsunoda A, Okuda O, Sato K. MR height of the pituitary gland as a function of age and sex: especially physiological hypertrophy in adolescence and in climacterium. AJNR Am J Neuroradiol 1997;18:551–4.
11. Chanson P, Daujat F, Young J, et al. Normal pituitary hypertrophy as a frequent cause of pituitary incidentalomas: a follow-up study. J Clin Endocrinol Metab 2001;86:3009–15.
12. Susman W. Pituitary adenoma. Br Med J 1933;2:1215.
13. Close HG. The incidence of adenoma of the pituitary body in some types of new growth. Lancet 1934;1:732–4.
14. Costello RT. Subclinical adenoma of the pituitary gland. Am J Pathol 1936;12:205–15.
15. Sommers SC. Pituitary cell relations to body states. Lab Invest 1959;8:588–621.
16. McCormick WF, Halmi NS. Absence of chromophobe adenomas from a large series of pituitary tumors. Arch Pathol 1971;92:231–8.
17. Haugen OA. Pituitary adenomas and the histology of the prostate in elderly men. Acta Pathol Microbiol Scand A 1973;81:425–34.
18. Kovacs K, Ryan N, Horvath E. Pituitary adenomas in old age. J Gerontol 1980;35:16–22.
19. Landolt AM. Biology of pituitary microadenomas. In: Faglia G, Giovanelli MA, MacLeod RM, editors. Pituitary microadenomas. New York: Academic Press; 1980. p. 107–22.
20. Mosca L, Solcia E, Capella C, et al. Pituitary adenomas: surgical versus post-mortem findings today. In: Faglia G, Giovanelli MA, MacLeod RM, editors. Pituitary microadenomas. New York: Academic Press; 1980. p. 137–42.
21. Burrows GN, Wortzman G, Rewcastle NB, et al. Microadenomas of the pituitary and abnormal sellar tomograms in an unselected autopsy series. N Engl J Med 1981;304:156–8.
22. Parent AD, Bebin J, Smith RR. Incidental pituitary adenomas. J Neurosurg 1981;54:228–31.
23. Muhr C, Bergstrom K, Grimelius L, et al. A parallel study of the roentgen anatomy of the sella turcica and the histopathology of the pituitary gland in 205 autopsy specimens. Neuroradiology 1981;21:55–65.
24. Max MB, Deck MD, Rottenberg DA. Pituitary metastasis: incidence in cancer patients and clinical differentiation from pituitary adenoma. Neurology 1981;31:998–1002.
25. Schwezinger G, Warzok R. Hyperplasien und adenome der hypophyse im unselektierten sektionsgut. Zentralbl Allg Pathol 1982;126:495–8 [in German].

26. Coulon G, Fellmann D, Arbez-Gindre F, et al. Les adenome hypophysaires latents. Etude autopsique. Sem Hop 1983;59:2747–50 [in French].
27. Siqueira MG, Guembarovski AL. Subclinical pituitary microadenomas. Surg Neurol 1984;22:134–40.
28. Char G, Persaud V. Asymptomatic microadenomas of the pituitary gland in an unselected autopsy series. West Indian Med J 1986;35:275–9.
29. Gorczyca W, Hardy J. Microadenomas of the human pituitary and their vascularization. Neurosurgery 1988;22:1–6.
30. El-Hamid MW, Joplin GF, Lewis PD. Incidentally found small pituitary adenomas may have no effect on fertility. Acta Endocrinol 1988;117:361–4.
31. Scheithauer BW, Kovacs KT, Randall RV, et al. Effects of estrogen on the human pituitary: a clinicopathologic study. Mayo Clin Proc 1989;64:1077–84.
32. Kontogeorgos G, Kovacs K, Horvath E, et al. Multiple adenomas of the human pituitary. A retrospective autopsy study with clinical implications. J Neurosurg 1991;74:243–7.
33. Marin F, Kovacs KT, Scheithauer BW, et al. The pituitary gland in patients with breast carcinoma: a histologic and immunocytochemical study of 125 cases. Mayo Clin Proc 1992;67:949–56.
34. Sano T, Kovacs KT, Scheithauer BW, et al. Aging and the human pituitary gland. Mayo Clin Proc 1993;68:971–7.
35. Teramoto A, Hirakawa K, Sanno N, et al. Incidental pituitary lesions in 1,000 unselected autopsy specimens. Radiology 1994;193:161–4.
36. Camaris C, Balleine R, Little D. Microadenomas of the human pituitary. Pathology 1995;27:8–11.
37. Tomita T, Gates E. Pituitary adenomas and granular cell tumors. Incidence, cell type, and location of tumor in 100 pituitary glands at autopsy. Am J Clin Pathol 1999;111:817–25.
38. Kurosaki M, Saeger W, Lüdecke DK. Pituitary tumors in the elderly. Pathol Res Pract 2001;197:493–7.
39. Buurman H, Saeger W. Subclinical adenomas in postmortem pituitaries: classification and correlations to clinical data. Eur J Endocrinol 2006;154:753–8.
40. Rittierodt M, Hori A. Pre-morbid morphological conditions of the human pituitary. Neuropathology 2007;27:43–8.
41. Furgal-Borzych A, Lis GJ, Litwin JA, et al. Increased incidence of pituitary microadenomas in suicide victims. Neuropsychology 2007;55:163–6.
42. Kim JH, Seo JS, Lee BW, et al. The characteristics of incidental pituitary microadenomas in 120 Korean forensic autopsy cases. J Korean Med Sci 2007;22(Suppl):S61–5.
43. Adhakhani K, Kadivar M, Kazemi-Esfeh S, et al. Prevalence of pituitary incidentaloma in the Iranian cadavers. Indian J Pathol Microbiol 2011;54:692–4.
44. Auer RN, Alakija P, Sutherland GR. Asymptomatic large pituitary adenomas discovered at autopsy. Surg Neurol 1996;46:28–31.
45. Wolpert SM, Molitch ME, Goldman JA, et al. Size, shape and appearance of the normal female pituitary gland. AJNR Am J Neuroradiol 1984;5:263–7.
46. Peyster RG, Adler LP, Viscarello RR, et al. CT of the normal pituitary gland. Neuroradiology 1986;28:161–5.
47. Chong BW, Kucharczyk AW, Singer W, et al. Pituitary gland MR: a comparative study of healthy volunteers and patients with microadenomas. AJNR Am J Neuroradiol 1994;15:675–9.
48. Hall WA, Luciano MG, Doppman JL, et al. Pituitary magnetic resonance imaging in normal human volunteers: occult adenomas in the general population. Ann Intern Med 1994;120:817–20.
49. Nammour GM, Ybarra J, Naheedy MH, et al. Incidental pituitary macroadenoma: a population-based study. Am J Med Sci 1997;314:287–91.
50. Yue NC, Longsteth WT Jr, Elster AD, et al. Clinically serious abnormalities found incidentally at MR imaging of the brain: data from the Cardiovascular Health Study. Radiology 1997;202:41–6.
51. Vernooij MW, Ikram A, Tanghe HL, et al. Incidental findings on brain MRI in the general population. N Engl J Med 2007;357:1821–8.
52. Chacko AG, Chandy MJ. Incidental pituitary macroadenomas. Br J Neurosurg 1992;6:233–6.
53. Donovan LE, Corenblum B. The natural history of the pituitary incidentaloma. Arch Intern Med 1995;153:181–3.
54. Reincke M, Allolio B, Saeger W, et al. The 'incidentaloma' of the pituitary gland. Is neurosurgery required? JAMA 1990;263:2772–6.
55. Nishizawa S, Ohta S, Yokoyama T, et al. Therapeutic strategy for incidentally found pituitary tumors ("pituitary incidentalomas"). Neurosurgery 1998;43:1344–8.
56. Feldkamp J, Santen R, Harms E, et al. Incidentally discovered pituitary lesions: high frequency of macroadenomas and hormone-secreting adenomas - results of a prospective study. Clin Endocrinol 1999;51:109–13.
57. Igarashi T, Saeki N, Yamaura A. Long-term magnetic resonance imaging follow-up of asymptomatic sellar tumors. Their natural history and surgical indications. Neurol Med Chir (Tokyo) 1999;39:592–9.
58. Sanno N, Oyama K, Tahara S, et al. A survey of pituitary incidentaloma in Japan. Eur J Endocrinol 2003;149:123–7.
59. Fainstein Day P, Guitelman M, Artese R, et al. Retrospective multicentric study of pituitary incidentalomas. Pituitary 2004;7:145–8.
60. Arita K, Tominaga A, Sugiyama K, et al. Natural course of incidentally found nonfunctioning pituitary adenoma, with special reference to pituitary

apoplexy during follow-up examination. J Neurosurg 2006;104:884–91.

61. Karavitaki N, Collison K, Halliday J, et al. What is the natural history of nonoperated, nonfunctioning pituitary adenomas? Clin Endocrinol 2007;67: 938–43.

62. Dekkers OM, Hammer S, de Keizer RJ, et al. The natural course of non-functioning pituitary macroadenomas. Eur J Endocrinol 2007;156:217–24.

63. Dekkers OM, Pereira AM, Romijn JA. Treatment and follow-up of clinically nonfunctioning pituitary macroadenomas. J Clin Endocrinol Metab 2008;93: 3717–26.

64. Freda PU, Beckers M, Katznelson L, et al. Pituitary incidentaloma: an Endocrine Society Clinical Practice Guideline. J Clin Endocrinol Metab 2011;96: 894–904.

65. Angeli A, Terzolo M. Adrenal incidentaloma— a modern disease with old complications. J Clin Endocrinol Metab 2002;87:4869–71.

66. Scheithauer BW, Jaap AJ, Horvath E, et al. Clinically silent corticotroph tumors of the pituitary gland. Neurosurgery 2000;47:723–9.

67. Bradley KJ, Wass JA, Turner HE. Non-functioning pituitary adenomas with positive immunoreactivity for ACTH behave more aggressively than ACTH immunonegative tumours but do not recur more frequently. Clin Endocrinol 2003;58:59–64.

68. Soto-Ares G, Cortet-Rudelli C, Assaker R, et al. MRI protocol technique in the optimal therapeutic strategy of nonfunctioning pituitary adenomas. Eur J Endocrinol 2002;146:179–86.

69. Park P, Chandler WF, Barkan AL, et al. The role of radiation therapy after surgical resection of nonfunctional pituitary macroadenomas. Neurosurgery 2004;55:100–6.

70. Baldeweg SE, Pollock JR, Powell M, et al. A spectrum of behaviour in silent corticotroph pituitary adenomas. Br J Neurosurg 2005;19:38–42.

71. Lopez JA, Kleinschmidt-DeMasters BK, Sze CI, et al. Silent corticotroph adenomas: further clinical and pathological observations. Hum Pathol 2004; 35:1137–47.

72. King JT Jr, Justice AC, Aron DC. Management of incidental pituitary microadenomas: a cost-effectiveness analysis. J Clin Endocrinol Metab 1997;82:3625–32.

73. Krikorian A, Aron D. Evaluation and management of pituitary incidentalomas—revisiting an acquaintance. Nat Clin Pract Endocrinol Metab 2006;2:138–45.

74. Chanson P, Young J. Pituitary incidentalomas. Endocrinologist 2003;13:124–35.

75. Casanueva FF, Molitch ME, Schlechte JA, et al. Guidelines of the Pituitary Society for the diagnosis and management of prolactinomas. Clin Endocrinol 2006;65:265–73.

76. Molitch ME, Reichlin S. Hypothalamic hyperprolactinemia: neuroendocrine regulation of prolactin secretion in patients with lesions of the hypothalamus and pituitary stalk. In: MacLeod RM, Thorner MO, Scapagnini U, editors. Prolactin. Basic and clinical correlates. Padova (Italy): Liviana Press; 1985. p. 709–19.

77. Arafah MB, Neki KE, Gold RS, et al. Dynamics of prolactin secretion in patients with hypopituitarism and pituitary macroadenomas. J Clin Endocrinol Metab 1995;80:3507–12.

78. Karavitaki N, Thanabalasingham G, Shore HC, et al. Do the limits of serum prolactin in disconnection hyperprolactinaemia need re-definition? A study of 226 patients with histologically verified non-functioning pituitary macroadenoma. Clin Endocrinol 2006;65: 524–9.

79. St-Jean E, Blain F, Comtois R. High prolactin levels may be missed by immunoradiometric assay in patients with macroprolactinomas. Clin Endocrinol 1996;44:305–9.

80. Barkan AL, Chandler WF. Giant pituitary prolactinoma with falsely low serum prolactin: the pitfall of the "high-dose hook effect": case report. Neurosurgery 1998;42:913–5.

81. The Growth Hormone Research Society, The Pituitary Society Consensus Conference. Biochemical assessment and long-term monitoring in patients with acromegaly. J Clin Endocrinol Metab 2004;89:3099–102.

82. Arnaldi G, Angeli A, Atkinson AB, et al. Diagnosis and complications of Cushing's syndrome: a consensus statement. J Clin Endocrinol Metab 2003; 88:5593–602.

83. Findling JW, Raff H. Cushing's syndrome: important issues in diagnosis and management. J Clin Endocrinol Metab 2006;91:3746–53.

84. Carroll T, Raff H, Findling JW. Late-night salivary cortisol measurement in the diagnosis of Cushing's syndrome. Nat Clin Pract Endocrinol Metab 2008;4: 344–50.

85. Yuen KC, Cook DM, Sahasranam P, et al. Prevalence of GH and other anterior pituitary hormone deficiencies in adults with nonsecreting pituitary microadenomas and normal serum IGF-1 levels. Clin Endocrinol 2008;69:292–8.

86. Toogood AA, Stewart PM. Hypopituitarism: clinical features, diagnosis, and management. Endocrinol Metab Clin North Am 2008;37:235–71.

87. Petersenn S, Quabbe HJ, Schöfl C, et al. The rational use of pituitary stimulation tests. Dtsch Arztebl Int 2010;107:437–43.

88. Fernández-Balsells MM, Murad MH, Barwise A, et al. Natural history of nonfunctioning pituitary adenomas and incidentalomas: a systematic review and metaanalysis. J Clin Endocrinol Metab 2011;96:905–12.

89. Melmed S, Casanueva FF, Hoffman AR, et al. Diagnosis and treatment of hyperprolactinemia: an Endocrine Society Clinical Practice Guideline. J Clin Endocrinol Metab 2011;96:273–88.

90. Melmed S, Colao A, Barkan A, et al. A guideline for acromegaly management: an update. J Clin Endocrinol Metab 2009;94:1509–17.

91. Biller BM, Grossman AB, Stewart PM, et al. Treatment of adrenocorticotropin-dependent Cushing's syndrome: a consensus statement. J Clin Endocrinol Metab 2008;93:2454–62.

92. Arafah AM. Reversible hypopituitarism in patients with large nonfunctioning pituitary adenomas. J Clin Endocrinol Metab 1986;62:1173–9.

93. Shomali ME, Katznelson L. Medical therapy of gonadotropin-producing and nonfunctioning pituitary adenomas. Pituitary 2002;5:89–98.

94. Colao A, Di Somma C, Pivonello R, et al. Medical therapy for clinically non-functioning pituitary adenomas. Endocr Relat Cancer 2008;15:905–15.

95. Honegger J, Zimmermann S, Psaras T, et al. Growth modeling of non-functioning pituitary adenomas in patients referred for surgery. Eur J Endocrinol 2008; 158:287–94.

Endoscopic Surgery for Pituitary Tumors

Joshua W. Lucas, MD*, Gabriel Zada, MD

KEYWORDS

- Endoscopy • Pituitary lesions • Transsphenoidal surgery

KEY POINTS

- Endoscopic transsphenoidal surgery has proven to have similar or better results compared with traditional microsurgical techniques, with equal or reduced complication rates.
- The endoscopic technique affords the surgeon improved visualization, illumination, and surgical mobility.
- The endoscopic approach to the sella turcica can be divided into a nasal stage, a sphenoid stage, a sellar stage, and a reconstruction stage.

INTRODUCTION

In the long history of the transsphenoidal approach to the sella turcica, the use of neuroendoscopy as the sole means of visualization and surgical resection of pituitary lesions is a relatively recent technique. Despite its relatively short existence, however, this technique has been extensively refined and has become commonplace in many operating rooms around the world.

The neuroendoscopic approach to pituitary lesions has been shown in numerous studies to have tumor resection and hormonal remission rates equal to or better than the classic microsurgical transsphenoidal technique. Furthermore, the rate of complications associated with neuroendoscopic procedures has been shown to be equal to if not less than those reported from series of microsurgical procedures. The use of the endoscope for transsphenoidal surgery has provided improvements in panoramic visualization, the ability to use angled lenses to look around anatomic "corners," improved illumination, and has facilitated the development of extended approaches to the skull base. The future of neuroendoscopic resection of pituitary lesions lies in the continued miniaturization and innovation of endoscopic instrumentation, advances in optical technology, and improved visualization systems.[1]

The endonasal endoscopic transsphenoidal technique consists of four major stages: nasal, sphenoid, sellar stage, and reconstruction. In the nasal stage, the endoscope is advanced through the nasal cavity to identify the sphenoid ostium, followed by a posterior septectomy and anterior sphenoidotomy. The sphenoid stage is characterized by widening of the anterior sphenoidal exposure, removal of the sphenoid septa, and identification of key landmarks surrounding the sellar floor. The sellar stage involves removal of the bony sellar floor, dural opening, and surgical treatment of the pathologic lesion. Finally, in the reconstruction stage, prevention or repair of cerebrospinal fluid (CSF) leaks is addressed.

Funding sources: None.
Conflicts of interest: None.
Department of Neurosurgery, University of Southern California, 1200 North State Street, Suite 3300, Los Angeles, CA 90033, USA
* Corresponding author.
E-mail address: joshuawlucas@gmail.com

Neurosurg Clin N Am 23 (2012) 555–569
http://dx.doi.org/10.1016/j.nec.2012.06.008
1042-3680/12/$ – see front matter Published by Elsevier Inc.

HISTORY OF ENDOSCOPIC TRANSSPHENOIDAL SURGERY

The first documented transsphenoidal approach for resection of a pituitary lesion dates back to 1906 by Schloffer.[2,3] His efforts were soon followed by those of Kocher and von Eiselsberg in the early part of the twentieth century. Cushing introduced the sublabial transseptal technique in 1914, which reduced the degree of nasal trauma associated with earlier external rhinotomy incisions. The operative microscope, popularized by Hardy in the 1960s, revitalized the transsphenoidal procedure by providing the magnification and illumination that made precise tumor resection possible.[2]

Surgical endoscopy first emerged in the fields of otolaryngology, gastroenterology, and urology.[1,3] Early endoscopes were originally used only for visualization purposes. Endoscopic procedures, however, quickly became possible with the advent of specially designed endoscopic surgical instruments and electrocautery.[4] Walter Dandy was among the greatest pioneers of early neuroendoscopy, performing endoscopic intraventricular operations as early as 1920 and contributing greatly to the development of improved endoscopic instrumentation.[1]

The use of the endoscope in conjunction with the microsurgical approach to the sella was first proposed by Guiot and colleagues[3,5] in 1963, though he abandoned the procedure due to inadequate visualization. Apuzzo and colleagues[6] brought the procedure more recognition in 1977, reporting the use of angled (70°–120°) endoscopes to visualize the sellar contents following microsurgical dissection. In the 1990s, multidisciplinary teams of neurosurgeons and otolaryngologists developed "pure" endoscopic techniques without the use of an operating microscope for removal of sellar lesions. Jankowski and colleagues[7] published a report on their experience performing pure endoscopic transsphenoidal resections of pituitary adenomas in 1992. In 1996, Jho and Carrau[8,9] described their technique of a pure endoscopic approach in detail and, in 1997, published their report of endoscopic removal of pituitary adenomas in 44 patients. Cappabianca and colleagues[10] also helped to develop the pure endoscopic approach and introduced the concept of functional endoscopic pituitary surgery in 1998. The endoscopic approach to the sella continued to be refined during the early twenty-first century, and with technologic advancements such as neuronavigation and microvascular Doppler ultrasonography, neuroendoscopy has expanded to now include extended approaches to the skull base.[3,11] Current endoscopic endonasal approaches to the skull base can now provide access to a wide arc of pathologic conditions along the midline skull base, from the frontal sinuses to the level of the foramen magnum or even high cervical spine in selected cases (**Fig. 1**).

COMPARISON OF NEUROENDOSCOPY AND MICROSURGERY FOR PITUITARY LESIONS

Despite early skepticism regarding the application of endoscopic techniques to resection of sellar lesions, numerous studies have shown equivalent or improved rates of tumor excision and tumor remission with endoscopic approaches to pituitary lesions compared with microsurgical approaches.[12–14] It has been an ongoing challenge, however, to attempt to draw comparisons between comparable surgical approaches such as the microscopic and endoscopic transsphenoidal approaches, for several reasons. First, a lack of Class I evidence or prospective randomized studies exist in attempting to draw these conclusions. Second, many current endoscopic studies are compared with historical control series dating back several decades. As surgical technology (ie, endoscopic visualization) progresses, so do advances in neuroimaging, medical therapy, and radiosurgical options for treatment of many of the same lesions. Finally, a limited degree of selection bias exists that makes it difficult to know why certain patients underwent various procedures. Surgical series of the most experienced pituitary surgeons were primarily performed using the microscope until the last decade and these studies still define the gold standard for treatment of many of these lesions.[15]

Nevertheless, improved endocrinologic results in functioning adenoma resections have been reported using a pure endoscopic approach compared with the microsurgical technique.[16–19]

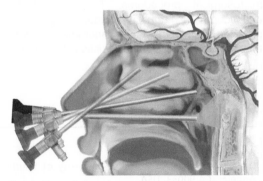

Fig. 1. Extended endoscopic approaches have been developed that allow access from the anterior skull base anteriorly to the clivus posteriorly. (*Courtesy of Luigi Cavallo, MD, PhD.*)

A meta-analysis done by Tabaee and colleagues[20] compiled data on 821 patients with pituitary adenomas treated with endoscopic pituitary surgery and found a gross tumor resection rate of 78%. The study also reported hormonal remission following endoscopic tumor resection in 81% of corticotropin-secreting tumors, 84% of growth hormone (GH)–secreting tumors, and 82% of prolactin-secreting tumors, which are equivalent to or better than rates reported in similar meta-analyses of microsurgical approaches. Another recent meta-analysis by Doward[21] included 12 additional studies and the original studies used in Tabaee's meta-analysis to assess endocrinologic outcomes after resection of functioning tumors. The overall rate of complete tumor resection associated with endoscopic resection of pituitary adenomas was 72%. Remission rates were higher for microadenomas (84% remission) than macroadenomas (69% remission) or invasive tumors (40% remission). This study also compared endocrinologic remission rates. The data showed slightly higher rates of hormonal remission associated with endoscopic procedures for functional microadenomas, as compared with microsurgical resection (84% vs 77%). For macroadenomas, the difference was more profound, with 70% remission in endoscopic procedures versus 45% remission in microsurgical procedures. It has been suggested that rates of remission in microadenoma resections, when compared with macroadenoma resections, performed via a pure endoscopic technique, would not be different from that performed with microsurgery because the expanded view gained with the endoscope does not offer a significant advantage over the standard microscopic view.[16]

In addition to similar or improved efficacy rates, endoscopic techniques may offer some distinct technical advantages over microsurgical techniques. Well-recognized drawbacks of the microsurgical approach include a narrower surgical field that is limited by the width of the nasal speculum, reduced illumination near the surgical target, the inability to visualize specific anatomic landmarks such as the carotid protuberances that define the limits of the sella, and an operative view that is limited by line of sight, making it challenging to fully inspect the resection cavity.[2,22] Pure endoscopic techniques allow improved panoramic visualization and illumination, obviating a nasal speculum. Also, the use of angled endoscopes essentially creates a surgical field limited only by the extent of dissection and available instrumentation. From this widened surgical field, modified endoscopic transsphenoidal procedures have been developed to access lesions arising or extending outside of the sella, including cavernous sinus, suprasellar, planum sphenoidale and/or olfactory groove, and retroclival lesions in which prior exposure via a microsurgical transsphenoidal approach was accompanied by formidable challenges.[23] Another advantage of the endoscopic technique includes minimal nasal mucosal trauma, thereby essentially obviating nasal packing unless a significant CSF leak or mucosal bleeding is observed intraoperatively, and reducing patient discomfort postoperatively.[2,24] Furthermore, once a surgeon overcomes the initially steep learning curve associated with endoscopic techniques for transsphenoidal surgery, a potential decrease in blood loss, operating time, and overall length of hospital stay may be appreciated.[12,25,26]

Potential disadvantages associated with the endoscopic technique include a loss of binocular three-dimensional (D) vision, a steep initial learning curve, and potential injury to the nasal mucosa that is not under direct visualization on insertion or withdrawal of instruments from the surgical field.[15] Endoscopic techniques are, by necessity, limited by the projection of a 3D image onto a 2D screen, whereas 3D visualization is readily available with the operating microscope. This shortcoming can be partially corrected by the use of large (>50 cm) high-definition video screens and tactile or haptic feedback to help the surgeon gauge surgical depth.[27] Also, the use of a two-surgeon, three-handed technique that allows dynamic movement of the endoscope and comparison between that movement and the motion of the surgical instruments can partially help offset the loss of depth perception.[11] Newer three-dimensional visualization systems are rapidly improving and may, one day, all but obviate this shortcoming associated with endoscopic surgery.[20] The learning curve for neuroendoscopy was initially thought to be prohibitively steep for the procedure to gain widespread acceptance, but recent publications of transitions from microsurgery to endoscopy within large teaching hospitals have reported that the learning curve may not be as steep as originally thought.[27] Also, the endoscopic technique is being introduced widely in residency training programs and more young neurosurgeons are becoming familiar with the endoscopic equipment and instrumentation. Most practicing neurosurgeons, however, were trained with the microsurgical technique and general familiarity with the operating microscope continues to be much greater than that for the endoscope. Finally, compared with endoscopic techniques, the use of a nasal speculum with microsurgery helps to protect the nasal mucosa from injury caused by insertion and withdrawal of instruments.[2] Increased care must be taken by the endoscopic neurosurgeon to recognize that the nasal mucosa not under visualization is subject to injury and must take measures to prevent this.

EQUIPMENT AND SURGICAL INSTRUMENTATION

The continued development and refinement of endoscopic equipment and surgical instrumentation specifically designed for use with neuroendoscopy has greatly contributed to its advancement as a viable procedure for transsphenoidal approaches to the sella and other nearby skull base regions. Basic components of the endoscopic set-up include the rigid-lens endoscope itself, a camera, a fiberoptic cable to connect the endoscope with the monitors, a light source, a large high-definition video monitor, and a video recording system.[22] The most commonly used endoscope is 4 mm in diameter with a length of 18 or 30 cm (**Fig. 2**). Variations in lens angulation are available for specific steps of the operation, including a 0-degree scope, a 30-degree scope, and a 45-degree scope. Larger-angle scopes ranging between 70- to 120-degrees are available for extended approaches, although they are rarely required for most endoscopic skull base operations.

In general, endoscopic instruments are long, rotating tools with a single straight shaft that are equipped with angled tips.[28] The angled tips on the working ends of many surgical instruments permit a wider range of motion than standard instruments. Compared with the microsurgical technique, in which bayoneted instruments are typically used to avoid interference with the light source, the use of straight instruments is preferred with endoscopy. The endoscope is introduced into the nostrils along with a sheath, which is connected to an irrigation system that allows cleaning of the lens without repeated removal and reentry of the

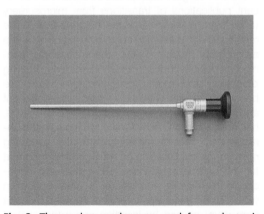

Fig. 2. The modern endoscope used for endoscopic transsphenoidal neurosurgery. (*Courtesy of* Karl Storz, Inc., Tuttlingen, Germany.)

telescope. A three-charge-coupled digital video camera paired with a high definition monitor is used to provide an optimized view of the surgical field. An endoscope holder may be used during the sellar phase of the procedure to stabilize the view of the surgical field, but its use negates the dynamic movement that helps to compensate for loss of depth perception.[11] The use of neuronavigation systems, although not required, can occasionally be helpful in patients with recurrent lesions or abnormal sellar or paranasal sinus anatomy.

PREOPERATIVE ASSESSMENT

A thorough clinical evaluation is necessary for all patients before any operative intervention. In patients with pituitary tumors, this includes formal visual field examination by an ophthalmologist, evaluation for prior endonasal surgery, and a thorough endocrinologic evaluation. A full endocrinologic evaluation for pituitary lesions includes serum levels of thyrotropin, free thyroxine, GH, insulinlike growth factor-1, corticotropin, prolactin, cortisol, luteinizing hormone, follicle-stimulating hormone (in women), and free testosterone (in men). Endocrine dysfunction, especially pertaining to the cortisol and thyroid axes, should be corrected before operative intervention.

Preoperative imaging is imperative for assessing the relevant anatomy that will be encountered during the approach. MRI of the head with and without gadolinium contrast and CT imaging of the head will show the degree of pneumatization of the sphenoid sinuses and the anatomy of the sphenoid septa. Identification of the target lesion, normal pituitary gland, stalk, optic chiasm and optic nerves, and course of the internal carotid arteries should also be assessed, often relying on sagittal and coronal images as the most useful planes to assess relevant neuroanatomic relationships.

The anatomy of the sella turcica, sphenoid sinus, and adjacent anterior and central skull base structures is highly variable. Preoperative imaging, specifically midsagittal MRIs with contrast, must be assessed to identify the morphology of the sellar floor and the configuration of septa within the sphenoid sinus (**Fig. 3**). The sellar angle, defined as the angle between lines drawn tangential to the sellar floor originating at the tuberculum sellae point and the sellar-clival point, can be used to classify the different sellar floor morphologies (**Fig. 4**). Prominent sellar floors (sellar angle <90°) and curved sellar floors (sellar angle between 90° and 150°) can usually be easily located using defined anatomic landmarks intraoperatively. Flat sellar floors (sellar angle >150°) or conchal (no sellar floor) sphenoid phenotypes occur in 11% and 1% of patients,

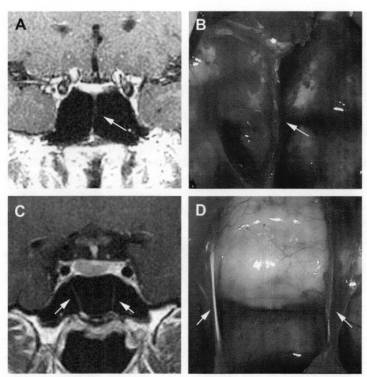

Fig. 3. Correlation of coronal MRI and intraoperative endoscopic views of vertical sphenoid septa in patients with simple sphenoid sinus morphology. The presence of one midline septa (*A* and *B*, *white arrows*) can be used to identify the anatomic midline. The presence of two symmetric septa (*C* and *D*, *white arrows*) can be used to approximate the lateral boundaries of the sella. (*From* Zada G, Agarwalla PK, Mukundan S, et al. The neurosurgical anatomy of the sphenoid sinus and sellar floor in endoscopic transsphenoidal surgery. J Neurosurg 2011;114(5):1319–30; with permission.)

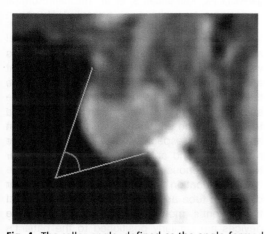

Fig. 4. The sellar angle, defined as the angle formed from lines drawn tangentially to the sella originating at the tuberculum sellae and the sellar-clival junction. (*From* Zada G, Agarwalla PK, Mukundan S, et al. The neurosurgical anatomy of the sphenoid sinus and sellar floor in endoscopic transsphenoidal surgery. J Neurosurg 2011;114(5):1319–30; with permission.)

respectively, and have been shown to be more difficult to identify intraoperatively; neuronavigation systems should, therefore, be strongly considered in these patients (**Figs. 5** and **6**). Additionally, neuronavigation systems are recommended for patients who exhibit complex sphenoid sinus configurations (29% of patients), consisting of two asymmetric septa, three or more septa, or horizontal septa, and patients who have undergone previous transsphenoidal surgery.[29]

SURGICAL TECHNIQUE

The endoscopic transsphenoidal approach to pituitary lesions has been continuously refined since it was first described.[2,22,28,30] Variations to the procedure exist, yet the following represents a general description and the authors' preferred surgical technique used for this approach.

Preparation and Positioning

The video monitor is positioned behind the patient's head and in direct line of sight of the surgeon who, in most cases, stands on the

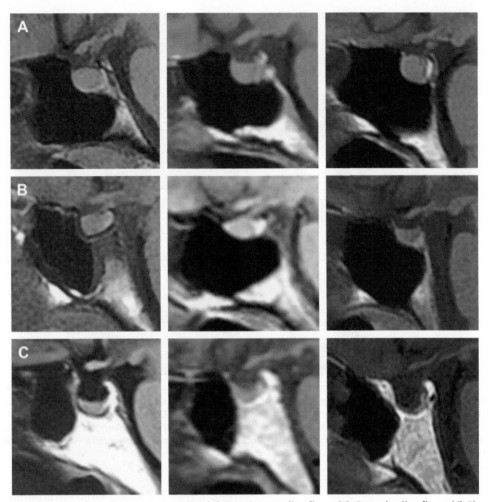

Fig. 5. Variations in sellar phenotypes on MRI. (*A*) Prominent sellar floor. (*B*) Curved sellar floor. (*C*) Flat sellar floor or conchal sphenoid phenotype. (*From* Zada G, Agarwalla PK, Mukundan S, et al. The neurosurgical anatomy of the sphenoid sinus and sellar floor in endoscopic transsphenoidal surgery. J Neurosurg 2011;114(5):1319–30; with permission.)

patient's right side. The anesthesiologist is positioned on the patient's left side. The bed is turned approximately 160° away from the anesthesiologist and the patient is placed in a semirecumbent position with the thorax elevated to 15° to promote venous outflow. If neuronavigation is to be used, the head is placed in rigid three-point fixation. The head is positioned with a slight degree of rotation, approximately 10° toward the surgeon, with the midline of the patient's head parallel to the lateral walls of the operating room and the bridge of the nose parallel to the floor. The degree of flexion and/or extension of the patient's head depends on the location of the lesion. Lesions located primarily in the clivus or sphenoid sinus require slight flexion of the head to permit working space for the endoscope. Lesions located more anteriorly, such as those based in the planum sphenoidale, require the head to be in

a neutral or slightly hyperextended position. As with any operation, all endoscopic equipment and instrumentation should be checked before the operation to ensure proper function. The surgeon must communicate with the anesthesia team before the operation to discuss medication administration, especially with regard to hormone replacement and antibiotics. The authors prefer to use intravenous cefazolin for routine cases.

After intubation, the endotracheal tube and an orogastric tube are positioned to the left side of the patient's mouth. All lines and monitoring devices are similarly positioned to the patient's left side. These maneuvers free the patient's right side for the surgeon. The nasal cavity is then prepared by administration of the nasal decongestant oxymetazoline, followed by intranasal cleansing with an aqueous antiseptic such as chloroxylenol *United States Pharmacopeia* 3%

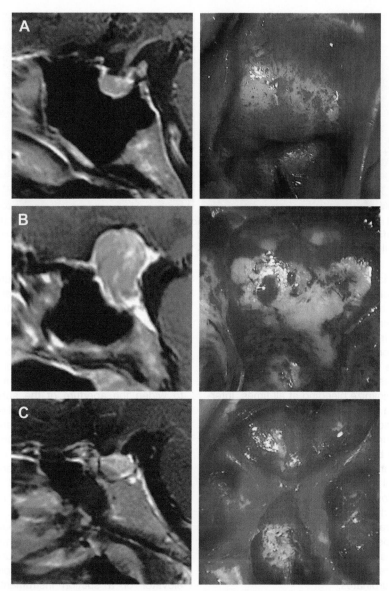

Fig. 6. Sagittal MRI and corresponding intraoperative endoscopic images of the sellar floor. (*A*) Prominent sella phenotype that is easily identifiable intraoperatively. (*B*) Curved sella phenotype. (*C*) Flat sella phenotype that is very difficult to differentiate from the clivus, making neuronavigation extremely important. (*From* Zada G, Agarwalla PK, Mukundan S, et al. The neurosurgical anatomy of the sphenoid sinus and sellar floor in endoscopic transsphenoidal surgery. J Neurosurg 2011;114(5):1319–30; with permission.)

(Techni-Care Solution) or iodine solution. Finally, the nasal region is prepped externally and draped with towels. The abdomen is also prepared under sterile conditions in the event that fat graft harvesting is required during the reconstruction phase. For larger lesions with a high likelihood of intraoperative CSF leakage, a small right-lower-quadrant incision is used so that abdominal fascia can be harvested if necessary. For smaller leaks, or if abdominal cosmesis is an issue, a small (2 cm) subumbilical curvilinear incision is planned.

Nasal Stage

The nasal stage of the operation begins with the surgeon using a short (18 cm) 0° endoscope. The endoscope can be introduced via either nostril, although the right side is used more frequently. On introduction of the endoscope, the landmarks that should be initially identified in the nasal cavity are the inferior turbinate (laterally), the nasal septum (medially), and the choana (posteriorly) (**Fig. 7**A). The surgeon should assess for evidence of prior surgery or any other anatomic variations,

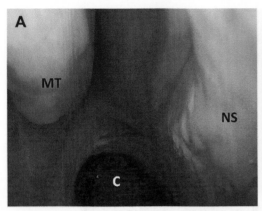 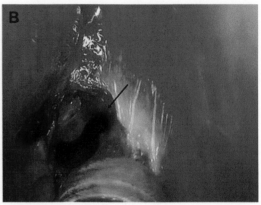

Fig. 7. The nasal stage. (*A*) On entering the nares, the choana (C) is immediately visualized, with the middle turbinate (MT) identified laterally and the nasal septum (NS) medially. (*B*) The sphenoid ostium (*black arrow*) is identified and coagulated in preparation for gaining access to the sphenoid sinus.

including a deviated septum or septal perforation, septal spurs, polyps, or synechiae. Once the choana is identified, maneuvering the endoscope superiorly allows identification of the middle turbinate, which arises from the region of the ethmoid sinuses superiorly. A Freer instrument is used to gently displace the middle turbinate laterally, attempting to preserve the integrity of the overlying mucosa and minimize bleeding at all times. Intermittent packing with lidocaine and/or epinephrine pledgets placed between the middle turbinate and nasal septum helps to maintain the developed working space between the middle turbinate and nasal septum and achieve hemostasis. Following sufficient lateral displacement of the middle turbinate, the endoscope is advanced and angled slightly superiorly, to identify the superior turbinate posteriorly. In rare cases, resection of the middle turbinate will be required to widen the surgical corridor, and is typically reserved for extended skull base operations or patients with acromegaly and enlarged turbinates.

The next landmark that should be identified is the sphenoid ostium, which is usually located just medial to the inferior aspect of the superior turbinate, approximately 1.5 cm superior to the superior edge of the choana. The sphenoid ostium is occasionally concealed by mucosa or a thin layer of bone, in which case attempting to first identify the ostium on the other side may be of benefit. Use of neuronavigation is also helpful in confirming the trajectory into the sphenoid sinus, after which a small dissector instrument, such as a Freer or a fine suction cannula, can be used to probe gently for the ostium and enter the sinus. Once the ostium is identified, its mucosal edges are coagulated using mild monopolar cautery, which can be extended down the medial and inferior surface of the sphenoid rostrum (see **Fig. 7**B).

Avoidance of inferolateral cauterization and dissection helps to prevent arterial bleeding from septal braches of the sphenopalatine artery.

Local anesthesia (lidocaine 1% with epinephrine 1:100,000) is then injected medially into the posterior nasal septum using a spinal needle with the tip bent to 20°. An anterior sphenoidotomy is initialized by using a mushroom (Stammberger) punch to widen the aperture of the sphenoid ostium. The preferred direction of removal of the sphenoid rostrum is in a direction inferior and medial from the ostium. This maneuver is almost always performed on both sides of the nasal cavity, although the approach may be performed entirely from one side, depending on the size and location of the target lesion, and the requirement for using instruments through both nostrils.

A Cottle elevator is used to create a curvilinear incision in the posterior septum immediately over the keel of the sphenoid rostrum (vomer and perpendicular plate of the ethmoid). The Cottle elevator or a suction instrument (ie, suction-Freer) is used to strip the nasal mucosa along a subperiosteal plane on both sides of the vomer, creating two mucosal flaps and exposing the entire bony sphenoid rostrum. Once adequate exposure of the bony keel is achieved, it can be removed using a stout pituitary or Jansen-Middleton rongeur (**Fig. 8**). The remaining superior-most and inferior-most aspects of the bony keel of the vomer serve as useful midline markers during the remainder of the operation (**Fig. 9**). Soft tissue from the posterior septum and elevated superior mucosal flaps can be removed using a sinus microdebrider or Blakesley forceps, ensuring not to resect tissue in the inferolateral aspect of the exposure where the sphenopalatine artery enters the nasal cavity. Arterial bleeding encountered from the sphenopalatine

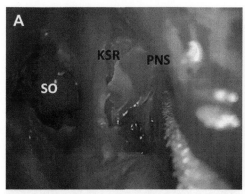
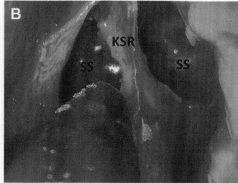

Fig. 8. The nasal stage. (*A*) A posterior septectomy is performed through the posterior nasal septum (PNS) after enlarging the sphenoid ostium (SO). The keel of the sphenoid rostrum (KSR) is identified. (*B*) Removal of the posterior nasal septum allows bimanual access to the sphenoid sinus (SS).

artery at this point requires cauterization or even clipping of the artery and increases the risk for delayed arterial epistaxis despite initial hemostasis. A backbiter instrument may be used to extend the posterior septectomy more anteriorly as required to improve communication between both sides of the nasal cavity. The lateral and superior soft tissue and bony overhang of the sphenoid rostrum and sinus are resected using a Kerrison rongeur, microdebrider, or Blakesley forceps to provide adequate room to dock the endoscope superolaterally for the next stage of the procedure. The bony rostrum is typically removed down to the level of the floor of the sphenoid sinus using a down-biting Kerrison rongeur or high-speed drill, to maximize working space for the endoscope and two instruments (**Fig. 10**). Care should be taken to remove the sphenoid rostrum in pieces and not en bloc because removal of large fragments can cause lacerations to the nasal mucosa.

Sphenoid Stage

On entering the sphenoid sinus, the initial goal is to identify key anatomic landmarks and correlate them with the neuroimaging findings. The surgeon must always study the anatomy of the sphenoid sinus on preoperative imaging, including the morphology and curvature of the sellar floor, the location and course of the carotid arteries, and the configuration of any sphenoid septations that may be present. Septations within the sphenoid sinus should be correlated with the MRI and CT, and often lead directly to the carotid arteries laterally and posteriorly. Careful removal of these septations is performed using a pituitary forceps or Kerrison rongeur. A dehiscent bony covering of the internal carotid artery is identified in up to 10% of the population. The sphenoid mucosa can be stripped and removed using suction and a small-cup forceps.

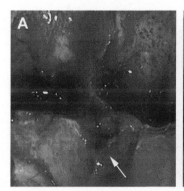
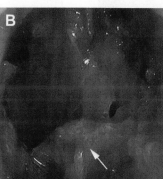
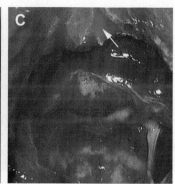

Fig. 9. The nasal stage. Intraoperative endoscopic images of relatively constant midline markers that can often be used even in the presence of complex sphenoid sinus configurations. These markers include the base of the vomer (*A* and *B*, *white arrows*) and the superior rostrum of the sphenoid (*C*, *white arrows*). (*From* Zada G, Agarwalla PK, Mukundan S, et al. The neurosurgical anatomy of the sphenoid sinus and sellar floor in endoscopic transsphenoidal surgery. J Neurosurg 2011;114(5):1319–30; with permission.)

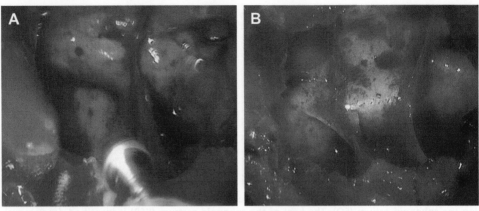

Fig. 10. The nasal stage. (*A*) The bony rostrum is removed to the level of the floor of the sphenoid sinus using a high-speed drill. (*B*) The endoscope and instruments are subsequently advanced through the aperture into the sphenoid sinus.

Once the posterior wall of the sinus is visible, the surgeon should identify the sellar floor, with the tuberculum sphenoidale and planum sphenoidale located above and the clivus located below (**Fig. 11**). Lateral to the sellar floor, the surgeon should identify the bony prominences of the cavernous carotid arteries and the optic nerves, with the opticocarotid recesses between them. The floor of the sella turcica is prominent and thus easily recognizable in most patients; however, a flat, less prominent variety exists in approximately 10% of people.[29] Although neuronavigation is not required for the procedure, it can be extremely beneficial to confirm the identification of key anatomic landmarks in patients with flat sellar subtypes and presellar (conchal)

sphenoid sinuses, and in patients with previous transsphenoidal surgery. Finally, thorough saline irrigation of the sinus using a large bulb syringe is performed to remove blood and bone fragments in preparation for entering the sella.

Sellar Stage

For the sellar phase, the long (30 cm) 0-degree endoscope is used and the operation is converted to a two-surgeon, three-handed technique, so that bimanual microdissection can be performed. Alternatively, the endoscope is fixed with an endoscope holder to permit a single surgeon to work with both hands, although this is not the authors' preference. The floor of the sella, when expanded and thinned by an intrasellar lesion, can usually be fractured open using a pituitary rongeur or blunt nerve hook (**Fig. 12**). In some cases, a thicker

Fig. 11. The sphenoid stage. Anatomic landmarks surrounding the sellar floor (SF) are identified. Paired sphenoid septa (S) can be used as lateral guidelines for dissection if confirmed on preoperative MRI. C, clivus; CP, carotid protuberance; OCR, opticocarotid recess; OP, optic protuberance; PS, planum sphenoidale.

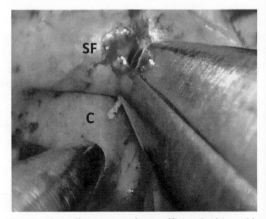

Fig. 12. The sellar stage. When sufficiently thinned by an intrasellar lesion, the sellar floor (SF) can be easily fractured with a pituitary forceps and then removed with a Kerrison rongeur. The clivus (C) aids in localizing the sellar floor.

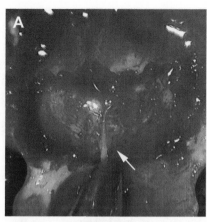
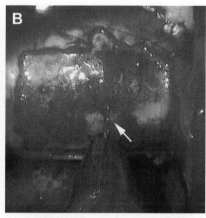

Fig. 13. The sellar stage. Intraoperative endoscopic images following removal of the bony sellar floor. A midline dural filum (*A* and *B*, *white arrows*) can be identified in approximately 50% of patients. (*From* Zada G, Agarwalla PK, Mukundan S, et al. The neurosurgical anatomy of the sphenoid sinus and sellar floor in endoscopic transsphenoidal surgery. J Neurosurg 2011;114(5):1319–30; with permission.)

sellar floor precludes this maneuver, requiring the use of a chisel or drill. A wide sellar exposure is performed, typically from one cavernous sinus to the other, using a 1 or 2 mm Kerrison rongeur (**Fig. 13**). In addition to seeing the cavernous sinuses laterally, the anterior intercavernous sinus is frequently identified in the rostral aspect of the exposure. The preoperative MRI is reviewed at this point to reassess the proximity and location of the internal carotid arteries. A micro-Doppler probe can be used to identify the internal carotid arteries and confirm the location of the planned dural opening. If there is any suspicion of a cystic lesion being an intrasellar aneurysm, a long 25-gauge spinal needle may be inserted through the dura into the sellar midline and aspirated to check for arterial blood. Once this has been ruled out, the dura is incised using a retractable microblade, ensuring penetration of both of its layers (**Fig. 14**). Dural opening is typically performed in a cruciate or x-shaped fashion; however, in cases

where a dural specimen is desired for a pathological testing, a rectangular dural "window" can be resected. Following dural opening, a blunt nerve hook or microdissector is used to develop a subdural, extraglandular, or extracapsular plane around the circumference of the dural opening.

Following exposure of the gland and/or tumor, the target lesion is identified and removed using two-handed microdissection techniques. The surgeon should maintain constant awareness of the normal anterior and posterior pituitary gland, and attempt to identify and preserve them as much as possible. For microadenomas and small intrasellar macroadenomas, angled curettes and Hardy microdissectors are typically used to develop an extracapsular plane around the tumor before delivering it. For larger tumors, angled curettes and small-cup forceps can be used to loosen and deliver the tumor, first inferiorly along the floor of the sella, then laterally to the cavernous sinus on each side, and finally in a superior direction (**Fig. 15**A, B). Removing the

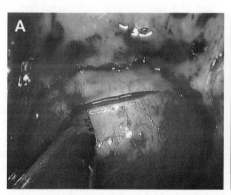
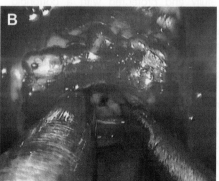

Fig. 14. The sellar stage. Various methods of dural opening. (*A*) A horizontal superior incision is made to create a dural "window" to send dural specimen for pathologic testing to inspect for evidence of dural invasion. (*B*) An x-shaped incision is used to maximize exposure to the gland and tumor.

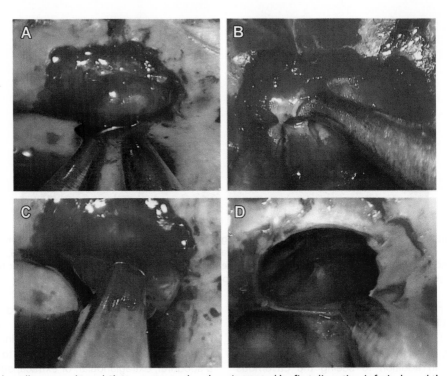

Fig. 15. The sellar stage. (*A* and *B*) An extracapsular plane is created by first dissecting inferiorly and then laterally to aid with tumor delivery. (*C*) Small-cup forceps are then used to remove the lesion. (*D*) The sella is examined for residual tumor before closure.

superior portion of the macroadenoma before the lateral and inferior portions can cause redundant prolapse of the diaphragma sella and arachnoid into the surgical field, obscuring visualization for subsequent tumor resection. Care should be taken to remove as much tumor as possible using a small-cup forceps, and sent for pathologic and/or tissue bank studies (see **Fig. 15**C). Once enough specimen has been collected, curettes and suction can be used to remove the remainder of the tumor (see **Fig. 15**D). The arachnoid may descend into the field of view at this point and should be manipulated carefully and protected with a cottonoid, thereby avoiding direct suctioning on the arachnoid to prevent CSF leakage. Cavernous sinus bleeding is frequently encountered following tumor removal and can be controlled in most settings using temporary gelatin foam packing of the sella and gentle pressure with a cottonoid. A 30° or 45° endoscope can be inserted to look laterally into the cavernous sinuses and superiorly to assess for residual tumor. In cases of macroadenomas with extensive suprasellar extension, the tumor will often descend spontaneously given enough time and gentle curettage. In patients with tumors that have a more firm consistency, a brief Valsalva maneuver, or insertion of saline into a lumbar drain, can be performed to assist with delivery of the tumor. Intrasellar and

cavernous sinus hemostasis can typically be achieved using temporary packing with gelatin sponge, followed by lining the tumor cavity with oxidized cellulose (Surgicel).

Reconstruction and Closure

Once tumor resection is completed, the goal of reconstructing the skull base defect begins. Multiple methods of achieving reconstruction exist, including conventional reconstruction with autologous or artificial grafts, formation and rotation of a vascularized nasoseptal flap, and multilayered closure techniques using dural and bony substitute.[28,31]

The first goal of reconstruction is to assess for a spinal fluid leak, if not already evident. Asking the anesthesiologist to perform a Valsalva maneuver can also be helpful in identifying a subtle CSF leak. In simpler cases where no intraoperative CSF leak is identified, the tumor cavity is lined with cellulose (Surgicel), and additional pieces are used as a dural inlay and onlay. Insertion of a rigid buttress is avoided if no intraoperative CSF leak is observed. If an intraoperative leak is identified, an abdominal fat graft is typically harvested, although for smaller, weeping CSF leaks an allograft or dural substitute in combination with fibrin glue may be sufficient. In extended transsphenoidal cases, fascia lata from the thigh may be harvested, and a pedicled nasoseptal flap may be rotated ahead of time if a large CSF leak is anticipated. Following packing of the sella using any combination of gelatin foam, fat, or fascia lata, an absorbable plate may be tailored for larger sellar defects and inserted as an epidural inlay underneath the lateral edges of the bony sellar face to provide buttressing of the underlying grafts (**Fig. 16**).

Gentle irrigation and hemostasis is then performed. Sphenoid sinus and nasal hemostasis is typically achieved using cautery and absorbable cellulose and/or gelatin sponge. The mucosal margins surrounding the sphenoid rostrum, especially in the location of the sphenopalatine artery, are inspected for any bleeding and appropriately cauterized, preferably with bipolar cautery. The nasal septum is also inspected for any bleeding. The turbinates are medialized to reapproximate their natural position. Nasal packing is not routinely used but may be placed if bleeding persists. The choanae and oropharynx are carefully suctioned.

COMPLICATIONS

Despite the minimally invasive nature of transsphenoidal approaches to the sella turcica, complications can and do arise. Potential complications may occur during any stage of the procedure and can be classified according to where they occur.[32] Complications encountered within the nasal cavity during the approach include saddle nose deformity, anosmia, orbital fracture, cribriform plate injury with subsequent CSF leak, and hemorrhage from the sphenopalatine artery or its branches. Complications arising within the sphenoid sinus include sinusitis, mucoceles, and optic nerve or carotid artery injury from fracture of the sphenoid body. Potential complications

associated with tumor resection and the sellar phase include CSF leak, hypopituitarism, diabetes insipidus, meningitis, postoperative hematoma, carotid artery or other vascular injury, optic nerve injury, ophthalmoplegia, subarachnoid hemorrhage, vasospasm, and tension pneumocephalus.

For both microscopic and endoscopic transsphenoidal surgery, the most common complications are CSF leak, meningitis, and sinusitis.[20,32,33] Recent studies have shown endoscopic techniques to be associated with similar or reduced rates of complications compared with microsurgical techniques.[20,25,32–34] Ciric and colleagues[35] published a widely renowned analysis in 1997 describing the observed rates of complications from microscopic transsphenoidal surgery. In 2002, Cappabianca and colleagues[32] published a large series of pure endoscopic techniques that analyzed the complication rates observed in these procedures and compared them to the complication rates of microsurgical procedures observed in Ciric's study. They found an overall decreased incidence of complications with the endoscopic technique. A recent systematic review performed by Tabaee and colleagues[20] analyzed nine studies with 821 total patients treated with endoscopic transsphenoidal surgery. They found pooled complication rates equal to or less than complication rates for microsurgical techniques reported in the literature. Another recent analysis by Berker and colleagues[33] of 624 endoscopic procedures for pituitary adenomas showed rates of complications to be less than established rates via a microsurgical approach.

POSTOPERATIVE CARE AND FOLLOW-UP

Following endoscopic transsphenoidal procedures, patients must be observed very closely for evidence of visual dysfunction, epistaxis,

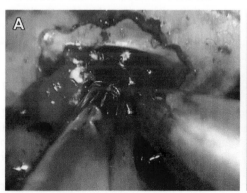
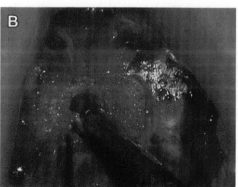

Fig. 16. The reconstruction stage. (*A*) The sella is packed and (*B*) an epidural inlay is placed to aid in buttressing the absorbable graft.

neurologic deterioration, and hormonal deficits, including diabetes insipidus. Most patients are discharged home on postoperative day 2 or 3. In most patients, serum sodium levels and urine output are followed every 6 to 8 hours for the first 48 hours. Patients with any evidence of new hypocortisolemia must be adequately replaced. Patients with functional pituitary adenomas typically undergo basic nonstimulation hormonal testing (serum prolactin, cortisol, or growth hormone) on postoperative days 1 and 2. If nasal packing is used (a minority of cases), it is typically removed on postoperative day 1. Following discharge, patients usually follow-up in clinic 1 week after the operation, with a routine serum sodium level obtained on postoperative day 7 to rule out occult hyponatremia.[36] Routine early postoperative imaging is not performed in most patients. Most patients will undergo standard MRI 3 months following the operation.

SUMMARY

Despite its relatively short existence in the realm of transsphenoidal resection of pituitary lesions, the endoscopic approach has been extensively refined and is quickly becoming the preferred technique over microsurgical transsphenoidal approaches. With increasing exposure to this technique in both residency training programs and within the practicing community, future generations of neurosurgeons will become more adept at this approach and its use will likely become more widespread. Long-term studies with larger numbers of patients will be needed to fully compare endoscopy and microsurgery for pituitary tumor resections; however the current literature is clear that the endoscopic technique leads to equal or improved rates of remission with equal or fewer rates of complications. The future of neuroendoscopy for the resection of pituitary lesions will likely be based on continued miniaturization of the endoscope camera and optical technology, innovation in design of surgical instrumentation, application of 3D cameras and viewing systems to compensate for the loss of depth perception, and introduction of robotics.[1] Combined with increasing surgeon experience and comfort using the endoscopic technique, these advances will likely contribute to improved surgical outcomes in the future.

REFERENCES

1. Zada G, Liu C, Apuzzo ML. "Through the looking glass": optical physics, issues, and the evolution of neuro-endoscopy. World Neurosurg 2012;77(1):92–102.

2. Jane JA Jr, Han J, Prevedello DM, et al. Perspectives on endoscopic transsphenoidal surgery. Neurosurg Focus 2005;19(6):E2.

3. Doglietto F, Prevedello DM, Jane JA Jr, et al. A brief history of endoscopic transsphenoidal surgery—from Philipp Bozzini to the First World Congress of Endoscopic Skull Base Surgery. Neurosurg Focus 2005;19(6):E3.

4. Lindley T, Greenlee JD, Teo C. Minimally invasive surgery (endonasal) for anterior fossa and sellar tumors. Neurosurg Clin N Am 2010;21(4):607–20.

5. Guiot G, Rougerie J, Fourestier M, et al. Intracranial endoscopic explorations. Presse Med 1963;71:1225–8 [in French].

6. Apuzzo ML, Heifetz M, Weiss MH, et al. Neurosurgical endoscopy using the side-viewing telescope: technical note. J Neurosurg 1977;16:398–400.

7. Jankowski R, Auque J, Simon C, et al. Endoscopic pituitary tumor surgery. Laryngoscope 1992;102(2):198–202.

8. Jho HD, Carrau KL. Endoscopy assisted transsphenoidal surgery for pituitary adenoma: technical note. Acta Neurochir (Wien) 1996;138:1416–25.

9. Jho HD, Carrau RL. Endoscopic endonasal transsphenoidal surgery: experience with 50 patients. J Neurosurg 1997;87(1):44–51.

10. Cappabianca P, Alfieri A, de Divitiis E. Endoscopic endonasal transsphenoidal approach to the sell: towards functional endoscopic pituitary surgery (FEPS). Minim Invasive Neurosurg 1998;41:66–73.

11. Prevedello DM, Doglietto F, Jane J Jr, et al. History of endoscopic skull base surgery: its evolution and current reality. J Neurosurg 2007;107:206–13.

12. Goudakos JK, Markou KD, Georgalas C. Endoscopic versus microscopic trans-sphenoidal pituitary surgery: a systematic review and meta-analysis. Clin Otolaryngol 2011;36(3):212–20.

13. Gondim JA, Schops M, de Almeida JP, et al. Endoscopic endonasal transsphenoidal surgery: surgical results of 228 pituitary adenomas treated in a pituitary center. Pituitary 2010;13(1):68–77.

14. Dehdashti AR, Ganna A, Karabatsou K, et al. Pure endoscopic endonasal approach for pituitary adenomas: early surgical results in 200 patients and comparison with previous microsurgical series. Neurosurgery 2008;62(5):1005–15.

15. Zada G, Cappabianca P. Raising the bar in transsphenoidal pituitary surgery. World Neurosurg 2010;74:452–4.

16. D'Haens J, Van Rompaey K, Stadnik T, et al. Fully endoscopic transsphenoidal surgery for functioning pituitary adenomas: a retrospective comparison with traditional transsphenoidal microsurgery in the same institution. Surg Neurol 2009;72(4):336–40.

17. Hofstetter CP, Shin BJ, Mubita L, et al. Endoscopic endonasal transsphenoidal surgery for functional pituitary adenomas. Neurosurg Focus 2011;30(4):E10.

18. Frank G, Pasquini E, Farneti G, et al. The endoscopic versus the traditional approach in pituitary surgery. Neuroendocrinology 2006;83:240–8.

19. Kabil MS, Eby JB, Shahinian HK. Fully endoscopic endonasal vs. transseptal transsphenoidal pituitary surgery. Minim Invasive Neurosurg 2005;48:348–54.

20. Tabaee A, Anand VK, Barron Y, et al. Endoscopic pituitary surgery: a systematic review and meta-analysis. J Neurosurg 2009;111(3):545–54.

21. Doward N. Endocrine outcomes in endoscopic pituitary surgery: a literature review. Acta Neurochir 2010;152(8):1275–9.

22. Cappabianca P, Cavallo LM, de Divitiis E. Endoscopic endonasal transsphenoidal surgery. Neurosurgery 2004;55:933–41.

23. Ceylan S, Koc K, Anik I. Endoscopic endonasal transsphenoidal approach for pituitary adenomas invading the cavernous sinus. J Neurosurg 2010; 112(1):99–107.

24. Zada G, Kelly DF, Cohan P, et al. Endonasal transsphenoidal approach for pituitary adenomas and other sellar lesions: an assessment of efficacy, safety, and patient impressions. J Neurosurg 2003; 98:350–8.

25. Jho HD. Endoscopic transsphenoidal surgery. J Neurooncol 2001;54(2):187–95.

26. Jho HD, Alfieri A. Endoscopic endonasal pituitary surgery: evolution of surgical technique and equipment in 150 operations. Minim Invasive Neurosurg 2001;44(1):1–12.

27. Yang I, Wang MB, Bergsneider M. Making the transition from microsurgery to endoscopic transsphenoidal pituitary neurosurgery. Neurosurg Clin N Am 2010;21(4):643–51.

28. Saeki N, Horiguchi K, Murai H, et al. Endoscopic endonasal pituitary and skull base surgery. Neurol Med Chir 2010;50:756–64.

29. Zada G, Agarwalla PK, Mukundan S, et al. The neurosurgical anatomy of the sphenoid sinus and sellar floor in endoscopic transsphenoidal surgery. J Neurosurg 2011;114(5):1319–30.

30. de Divitiis E, Cappabianca P, Cavallo LM. Endoscopic transsphenoidal approach: adaptability of the procedure to different sellar lesions. Neurosurgery 2002;51:699–707.

31. Cappabianca P, Cavallo LM, Esposito F, et al. Sellar repair in endoscopic endonasal transsphenoidal surgery: results of 170 cases. Neurosurgery 2002; 51:1365–72.

32. Cappabianca P, Cavallo LM, Colao A, et al. Endoscopic endonasal transsphenoidal approach: outcome analysis of 100 consecutive procedures. Minim Invasive Neurosurg 2002;45:1–8.

33. Berker M, Hazer DB, Yucei T, et al. Complications of endoscopic surgery of the pituitary adenomas: analysis of 570 patients and review of the literature. Pituitary 2011. [Epub ahead of print].

34. Graham SM, Iseli TA, Karness LH, et al. Endoscopic approach for pituitary surgery improves rhinologic outcomes. Ann Otol Rhinol Laryngol 2009;118(9): 630–5.

35. Ciric I, Ragin A, Baumgartner C, et al. Complications of transsphenoidal surgery: results of a national survey, review of the literature and personal experience. Neurosurgery 1997;40:225–36.

36. Zada G, Liu CY, Fishback D, et al. Recognition and management of delayed hyponatremia following transsphenoidal surgery. J Neurosurg 2007;106(1):66–71.

External Beam Radiation Therapy and Stereotactic Radiosurgery for Pituitary Adenomas

Jason P. Sheehan, MD, PhD[a,b,]*, Zhiyuan Xu, MD[a],
Mark J. Lobo, MD[b]

KEYWORDS

- Pituitary adenoma • Stereotactic radiosurgery • Radiation therapy

KEY POINTS

- Recurrence of pituitary adenomas after microsurgery is reasonably common.
- Stereotactic radiosurgery (SRS) and radiation therapy provide a high rate of tumor control for recurrent or residual pituitary adenomas.
- After radiosurgery and radiation therapy for patients with functional adenomas, endocrine remission occurs in the majority of patients but the rate is not as high as that observed for tumor control.
- Delayed hypopituitarism is the most common complication after radiosurgery or radiation therapy for pituitary adenoma patients.
- Cranial neuropathies after radiosurgery or radiation therapy are fairly rare.

INTRODUCTION

Pituitary adenomas are found in 10% to 27% of the general population.[1,2] Microadenomas (less than 1 cm in maximum dimension) are usually diagnosed either after being discovered incidentally during MRI or due to hormone hypersecretion. Macroadenomas may be discovered as a result of mass effect leading to hypopituitarism, elevation in prolactin output, or a focal neurologic deficit (eg, cranial nerve dysfunction). As a distribution, microadenomas are divided equally between functioning and nonfunctioning lesions. With regard to macroadenomas, nonfunctioning lesions are more common (approximately 80%).[1] At presentation, pituitary adenoma patients often exhibit symptoms of headache (40%–60%), visual disturbance, hypopituitarism, or rarely apoplexy.[1,2]

Pituitary adenomas are some of the most challenging clinical entities that physicians have dealt with over the past century. It has been more than 100 years since Dr Harvey Cushing published his landmark book, *The Pituitary Body and Its Disorders: Clinical States Produced by Disorders of the Hypophysis Cerebri*.[3] Nevertheless, pituitary adenomas remain difficult to cure with microsurgical techniques alone, and they often require multimodality treatment, which includes surgery, radiation therapy, radiosurgery, and medical management. Cushing recognized the limitations of conventional microsurgical approaches for treating intracranial tumors. Cushing and his colleagues used a device called a radium bomb to deliver a radiation therapy to intracranial tumors.[4,5] Since that time, neurosurgeons and radiation oncologists, in conjunction with medical physicists, have used ionizing radiation to treat patients with recurrent or residual pituitary adenomas.

Great attention and effort in the fields of radiation therapy and SRS have been placed on the

---

[a] Department of Neurological Surgery, University of Virginia, 1240 Lee Street, Box 800212, Charlottesville, VA 22908, USA; [b] Department of Radiation Oncology, University of Virginia, 1240 Lee Street, Box 800383, Charlottesville, VA 22908, USA
* Corresponding author.
E-mail address: jsheehan@virginia.edu

Neurosurg Clin N Am 23 (2012) 571–586
http://dx.doi.org/10.1016/j.nec.2012.06.011
1042-3680/12/$ – see front matter © 2012 Elsevier Inc. All rights reserved.

preservation of surrounding neuronal, vascular, and hormonal structures in an effort to improve the therapeutic ratio. Technical refinements for treating pituitary adenoma patients have been achieved through advances in radiobiology, neuroimaging, medical physics, and biomedical engineering. This article reviews the role of radiation therapy and SRS for pituitary adenomas (**Fig. 1**).

EXTERNAL BEAM RADIATION THERAPY CONCEPT AND TECHNIQUE

Fractionation indicates that the total radiation dose is delivered in several smaller doses over time. Beneficial and adverse outcomes are influenced by the dose per fraction and the total number of fractions. Conventional fractionation uses a dose of 1.8 Gy to 2 Gy per day. Most pituitary adenomas are treated with a total external beam radiation dose of 45 Gy to 54 Gy, which translates to 25 to 30 fractions delivered over a 5-week to 6-week treatment period. Treatment planning uses three-dimensional conformal radiation therapy (3D CRT), and various treatment planning software packages can permit this approach. A minimum of 3 unopposed beams is used in 3D CRT plans to minimize dose inhomogeneity and reduce the risk of nor-

mal tissue toxicity. Alternatively, inverse planned intensity-modulated radiation therapy can be used for challenging cases where the target is in close proximity to a radiation-sensitive normal tissue structure. Intensity-modulated radiation therapy usually divides the primary radiation beam into 5 mm by 5 mm up to 10 mm by 10 mm beamlets of varying intensities to achieve an acceptable dose plan.

STEREOTACTIC RADIOSURGICAL CONCEPT AND TECHNIQUES

In 1951, SRS was described by Lars Leksell[6] as the "closed skull destruction of an intracranial target using ionizing radiation." Leksell treated the first pituitary adenoma patient with the Gamma Knife in 1968. Since that time, SRS has been used to treat thousands of patients with pituitary adenomas.

SRS used focused, high-dose radiation to the target, while sparing surrounding structures of appreciable doses of radiation. Radiosurgery is traditionally delivered in a single session but may be delivered in up to 5 sessions.[7] It is characterized by a steep dose falloff to the surrounding normal tissues. For cobalt-based SRS devices, the gradient index (ie, steepest falloff) is achieved at

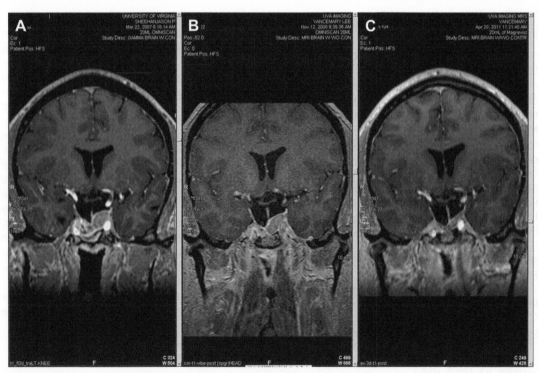

Fig. 1. (*A [left panel]*, *B [middle panel]*, and *C [right panel]*) are postcontrast, coronal MRIs. A 49-year-old man presenting with a recurrent, nonfunctioning pituitary adenoma (*A*). The patient underwent SRS in which 15 Gy was delivered to the tumor margin: 1.5 years later (*B*), the pituitary adenoma had decreased in size, and (*C*) 49 months after radiosurgery, the patient's adenoma continues to regress.

approximately a 50% isodose line, whereas for linear accelerator (LINAC)-based systems, it is usually at the 80% to 90% isodose line. Patients are immobilized using rigid frames fixed to the skull or other immobilization devices (eg, aquaplast masks or bite blocks); each immobilization device has its own stereotactic coordinate system. Radiosurgery is image guided and reliably achieves submillimeter accuracy in intracranial space. Onboard imaging systems may be used to further track and compensate for sources of error (eg, setup error or patient movement).

There are several types of radiosurgical delivery devices, including the Gamma Knife (Elekta AB), modified LINACs, or proton beam units. Single-session radiosurgical margin doses for nonfunctioning adenomas vary from 12 Gy to 18 Gy and 15 Gy to 30 Gy for functioning adenomas. For multisession radiosurgery, these doses may be divided more than 2 to 5 fractions.

Gamma Knife radiosurgery involves the use of multiple isocenters to achieve a dose plan that conforms to the target volume. The number of isocenters varies based on the size, shape, and location of the pituitary adenoma. In the current version of the Gamma Knife Perfexion, each isocenter comprises 8 independent sectors of beams, and each sector comprises no more than 192 simultaneous beams. Beam diameters for the current Gamma Knife Perfexion unit range from 0 mm (ie, blocked) to 16 mm. Other cobalt-based radiosurgical devices are also in use and include the Infini system (MASEP).

LINAC-based radiosurgery (eg, CyberKnife, TrueBeam STx, Trilogy, TomoTherapy, and Axesse) uses multiple radiation arcs to crossfire photon beams at a target.[8] Most systems use nondynamic techniques in which the arc is moved around its radius to deliver radiation that enters from many different vantage points. Technical improvements with LINAC-based radiosurgery include beam shaping, intensity modulation, multileaf collimation, and onboard CT or fluoroscopic imaging.

Proton therapy has been adapted as a radiosurgical tool for intracranial pathology. It takes advantage of the inherently superior dose distribution of protons compared with that of photons because of the Bragg peak phenomenon.[9] Currently, there are just a few centers using proton beam technology to perform radiosurgery (1 session treatment) whereas proton centers perform fractionated stereotactic radiotherapy (FSRT). The number of proton beam centers is increasing as the technology becomes more cost-effective and more compact proton units become available.

CONVENTIONAL FRACTIONATED RADIATION THERAPY VERSUS STEREOTACTIC RADIOSURGERY

For pituitary adenomas, SRS has specific advantages over fractionated external beam radiation therapy (EBRT). It is more convenient for patients and able to better spare normal tissue from appreciable toxicity. As dose is escalated and number of fractions decreased, there is a greater radiobiologic effect on late responding tissues, such as pituitary adenoma cells, compared with early responding tissues. Also, for functioning adenomas, radiosurgery seems to provide a more rapid rate of endocrine remission.[10]

Some patients are not good candidates for SRS secondary to tumor volume, irregular tumor shape, or close proximity of the tumor to radiation-sensitive (ie, critical) structures. In such cases, EBRT may be used to treat such patients. Although each patient must be assessed individually, the advantages and safety of radiosurgery decline when the tumor is greater than 3 cm and when it abuts radiation critical structures, such as the optic apparatus. For pituitary adenomas, the optic apparatus is the most sensitive of the adjacent tissues. Single-session radiosurgical dose to the optic apparatus should generally be kept to below 8 Gy to 10 Gy. Brainstem tolerance for single-session SRS is believed to be 12 Gy to 1 cm^3 or less of tissue.

For EBRT, the 5-year risk of visual deficits is believed to be 5% when 50 Gy is delivered and 50% when 65 Gy is used.[11] Visual complications after EBRT alone, however, have been reported at doses as low as 46 Gy delivered in a 1.8 Gy per fraction scheme. Multimodality treatment, such as patients undergoing treatment with Avastin, can have alteration in the threshold dose of their visual apparatus.

SRS FOR PITUITARY ADENOMAS
SRS and Nonfunctioning Pituitary Adenomas

After a microsurgical resection, control of a pituitary tumor is achieved in 50% to 80% of macroadenomas.[12] SRS provides an excellent treatment approach for patients who have progression or recurrence. It may also be used in cases of residual tumor or presumed tumor progression (eg, patients with silent corticotropin or thyrotropin adenomas). Based on the published literature, radiosurgery affords the vast majority of pituitary adenoma patients with effective, long-term tumor control as well as a low rate of complications.[12]

Table 1 lists the major radiosurgical series since 2002 that detail outcomes in nonfunctioning

Table 1
Summary of the literature review for the radiosurgical management of nonfunctioning pituitary adenomas

Year	Authors	Patients (N)	Mean/Median Follow-Up (Mo)	Mean/Median Margin Dose (Gy)	Radiologic Control of Tumor (%)	Neurologic Deficit (%)	Delayed Hypopituitarism (%)
2002	Feigl et al[14]	61	55.2	15	94	NR	40
2002	Sheehan et al[15]	42	31.2	16	97.6	4.8	0
2002	Wowra and Stummer[16]	30	57.7	16	93.3	0	10
2003	Petrovich et al[17]	52	34	15	100	3	NR
2004	Losa et al[18]	54	41.1	16.6	96.3	0	9.3
2004	Muacevic et al[19]	51	21.7	16.5	95	0	3.9
2005	Kajiwara et al[20]	14	32.1	12.6	92.9	7.1	7.1
2005	Picozzi et al[21]	51	40.6	16.5	96.1	NR	NR
2005	Iwai et al[22]	28	36.4	12.3	93	0	7
2006	Mingione et al[13]	100	46.4	18.5	92.2	0	25
2006	Voges et al[23]	37	56.6	13.4	100	4.2	12.3
2007	Liscak et al[24]	140	60	20	100	0	1.4
2008	Pollock et al[25]	62	64	16	96.8	1.6	27
2009	Höybye & Rähn[12]	23	78	20	100	4.3	0
2009	Kobayashi[26]	71	50.2	NR	96.7	2.8	8.2
2010	Castro et al[27]	14	42	12.5	100	0	0
2010	Hayashi et al[28]	43	36	18.2	100	0	0
2011	Gopalan et al[29]	48	95	18.4	83	6.3	39
2011	Iwata et al[30] (CyberKnife)	100	33	21 Gy/3 Fr 25 Gy/5 Fr	98	1	2
2011	Park et al[31]	125	62	13	90	2.4	24
Total/ average		1146	48.66	15.9	95.7	2.1	12.0

Abbreviations: Fr, fraction; NR, not reported.

adenoma patients (see **Table 1**).[12–31] Single-session radiosurgery margin doses of 12 Gy to 18 Gy are typically used for patients with nonfunctioning adenomas. Tumor control rates range from 83% to 100% (average 95.7%) (see **Table 1**). Neurologic deficits are uncommon (average 2.1%, range 0%–7.1%) as was hypopituitarism (average 12%, range 0%–39%). At the authors' institution, 90% tumor control was reported in a series of 100 patients with nonfunctioning pituitary adenomas.[13] Tumor control was statistically less likely when the margin dose to the adenoma was reduced to below 12 Gy.[13] In a more recent publication from the authors' group, the outcomes of a smaller group of patients with a minimum follow-up of 4 years after radiosurgery were examined. The overall progression-free survival was 83%, with the vast majority of patients (75%) demonstrating marked decrease in the adenoma volume.[29] This same study demonstrated that tumor control was related to adenoma volume and that those patients with an adenoma volume of less than 5 cm^3 were more likely to have tumor control after radiosurgery. This finding underscores the importance of a maximum safe resection prior to radiosurgery.

SRS and Cushing's Disease

In 80% of cases, endogenous Cushing's disease results from overproduction of corticotropin (ACTH), with the vast majority of these secondary to a pituitary adenoma.[32] Although microsurgical resection remains the primary treatment for Cushing's disease, many adenomas show invasion of the surrounding dura and/or cavernous sinus or are difficult to delineate on MRI, thereby making a surgical cure unlikely. Radiosurgery proves an invaluable treatment option for patients with persistent Cushing's disease after a resection.

In **Table 2**, the major radiosurgical series for Cushing patients since 2000 are listed (see **Table 2**).[14,17,20,23,26,28,33–51] Most investigators used 24-hour urinary-free cortisol (UFC) or serum cortisol to define an endocrine remission. In addition, radiosurgical margin doses of 18 Gy to as high as 30 Gy are delivered to the adenomas of patients with persistent Cushing's disease.

Most series demonstrate rates of remission for the majority of patients (ie, >50%) after radiosurgery from 16.7% to 87% (see **Table 2**). Unfortunately, the endocrine remission rates after radiosurgery do not match the excellent rates of radiologic control of purely nonfunctioning adenomas. Based on the authors' experience, endocrine remission of Cushing's disease is achieved on average approximately 12 months after

SRS.[39] In most series, after radiosurgery the rates of newly developed or worsened cranial neuropathies, including visual deterioration, are low (average 3.4%; see **Table 2**). The incidence of hypopituitarism after radiosurgery for Cushing's disease seems slightly higher (average 24.9%; see **Table 2**) compared with that of nonfunctioning adenoma series; this may be due to higher margin doses delivered to the adenoma that results in higher doses to collateral structures, such as the normal pituitary gland and stalk. Long-term radiologic and endocrine follow-up is crucial because late recurrences have been seen in several Cushing's disease series.[39,46]

SRS and Acromegaly

Acromegaly occurs with a prevalence of approximately 60 per million.[52] Uncontrolled acromegaly is associated with significant morbidity and even mortality (hypertension, diabetes, cardiomyopathy, and sleep apnea), conveying a standardized mortality ratio of 1.48.[52] Given its nearly immediate endocrine remission effect if successful, surgical resection remains the first-line therapy. Nevertheless, as in Cushing's disease, those cases in which there is invasion of surrounding structures (eg, the dura or the cavernous sinus) are unlikely to achieve a cure. Also, because many patients with acromegaly have macroadenomas, complete resection is not always feasible because these adenomas tend to be large and infiltrative.

Table 3 delineates the major radiosurgical series for acromegalic patients published since 2000 (see **Table 3**).[14,17,20,23,28,34,35,38,43,45–48,50,51,53–69] Similar margin doses of 18 Gy to 30 Gy are routinely delivered to the adenoma as part of single-session radiosurgery. In published series, endocrine remission after radiosurgery is achieved in 43.6% of acromegalic patients (range 0%–82%; see **Table 3**). Neurologic deficits and hypopituitarism occur after radiosurgery in 1.8% (range 0%–11%) and 15.3% (range 0%–40%) of cases, respectively (see **Table 3**). Temporary cessation of antisecretory medications around the time of the authors' center and other centers.[50] Also, patients who had a low-volume adenoma (<3 cm^3) at the time of radiosurgery were more likely to achieve endocrine remission after radiosurgery.[50] Hence, even if there is clear cavernous sinus invasion of the adenoma, maximum safe resection should be attempted; such a resection will likely yield a greater chance of endocrine remission after radiosurgery.

At the authors' center, the mean time to endocrine remission after radiosurgery for acromegalic patients was 24 months. This is nearly twice as

Table 2
Summary of the literature review for the radiosurgical management of Cushing's disease

Year	Author	Patients (N)	Mean/Median Margin Dose (Gy)	Mean/Median Follow-Up (Mo)	Biochemical Remission (%)	Neurologic Deficit (%)	Hypopituitarism (%)
2000	Izawa et al[38]	12	23.8	26.4	16.7	0	0
2000	Sheehan et al[15]	43	20	39.1	63	2.3	16
2000	Shin et al[45]	7	32.3	88.2	50	6.3	16.7
2001	Hoybye et al[37]	18	NR	16.8	44	0	68.8
2002	Feigl et al[14]	4	15	55.2	60	NR	40
2002	Kobayashi[26]	20	28.7	64	23.3	NR	NR
2002	Laws et al[41]	40	20	NR	74	2.5	24
2002	Pollock et al[51]	9	20	42.4	78	22.2	16
2003	Choi et al[35]	7	28.5	42.5	55.6	0	0
2003	Petrovich et al[17]	3	15	34	NR	3	NR
2003	Wong et al[49]	5	NR	38	100	0	20
2003	Witt[48]	8	24	24	0	0	NR
2004	Devin et al[36]	35	14.7	42	49	0	40
2006	Voges et al[23]	17	16.4	58.7	52.9	4.2	12.3
2007	Castinetti et al[33]	40	29.5	54.7	42.5	5	15
2007	Jagannathan et al[39]	90	23	45	54	5	22
2007	Kajiwara et al[101]	2	26	38.5	50	0	50
2007	Petit et al[42]	33	20	62	52	0	52
2008	Pollock et al[25]	8	20	73	87	0	36
2008	Tinnel et al[46]	12	25	37	50	0	50
2009	Castinetti et al[34]	18	28	94	50	5.3	21
2009	Wan et al[47]	68	23	67.3	27.9	2.9	1.7
2009	Kobayashi[26]	30	28.7	64.1	35	NR	NR
2010	Hayashi et al[28]	13	25.2	36	38	15.4	0
2011	Sheehan et al[50]	82	24	31	54	NR	22
Total/ average		624	23	48.9	49.9	3.4	23.6

Abbreviations: Gy, Gray; GKS, Gamma Knife radiosurgery; NR, Not reported.

Table 3
Summary of the literature review for the radiosurgical management of acromegaly

Year	Authors	Patients (N)	Mean/Median Follow-Up (Mo)	Mean/Median Margin Dose (Gy)	Biochemical Remission (%)	Neurologic Deficit (%)	Hypopituitarism (%)
2000	Izawa et al[38]	29	26.4	23.8	41.4	0	0
2000	Shin et al[45]	6	42.7	34.4	66.7	6.3	0
2000	Zhang et al[64]	68	34	31.3	36.8	2.9	0
2001	Fukuoka et al[55]	9	42	20	50	0	0
2001	Ikeda et al[56]	17	55.8	25	82	0	0
2002	Feigl et al[14]	9	55.2	15	60	NR	40
2002	Pollock et al[51]	26	42.4	20	42	0	16
2003	Attanasio et al[53]	30	46	20	23	0	6.6
2003	Choi et al[35]	9	42.5	28.5	50	0	0
2003	Muramatsu et al[61]	4	30	27.5	50	0	0
2003	Petrovich et al[17]	5	34	15	NR	3	NR
2003	Witt[48]	4	24	24	25	0	NR
2005	Castinetti et al[54]	82	49.5	25	17	0	17.1
2005	Gutt et al[65]	44	22.8	18	47.7	0	NR
2005	Kajiwara et al[20]	2	53.5	13.5	0	0	0
2005	Kobayashi et al[59]	67	63.3	18.9	4.8	11.1	14.6
2006	Jezkova et al[58]	96	53.7	35	50	0	26
2006	Voges et al[23]	64	54.3	16.5	37.5	4.2	12.3
2007	Pollock et al[62]	46	63	20	50	2.2	33
2007	Roberts et al[66]	9	25.4	21	44.4	0	33.3
2007	Vik-Mo et al[63]	61	66	26.5	17	3.3	13.1
2008	Jagannathan et al[57]	95	57	22	53	4.2	34
2008	Losa et al[60]	83	69	21.5	60.2	0	8.5
2008	Pollock et al[25,43]	27	46.9	20	67	0	36
2008	Tinnel et al[46]	9	35	25	44.4	11	22
2009	Castinetti et al[34]	43	102	24	42	5.3	21
2009	Wan et al[47] (MASEP GKS)	103	67.3	21.4	36.9	1	1.7
2009	Ronchi et al[67]	35	120	20	46.0	0	40
2010	Iwai et al[68]	26	84	20	38.0	0	8
2010	Hayashi et al[28]	25	36	25.2	40.0	0	0
2010	Poon et al[69]	40	73.8	20–35	75	0	11.4 (GKS1); 27.3 (repeat GKS)
2011	Sheehan et al[50]	130	31	24	53	NR	34
	Total/average	1303	51.5	22.6	43.6	1.8	14.9

Abbreviation: NR, not reported.

long as the same milestone for Cushing's disease patients. These and similar findings of differential response of secretory pituitary adenomas to radio-surgery warrant further investigation in terms of the underlying radiobiology and ways to enhance the beneficial effects of radiosurgery on subtypes of secretory pituitary adenomas.[43]

SRS and Prolactinomas

Prolactinomas represent one of the more common types of secretory pituitary adenomas. Unlike patients with acromegaly or Cushing's disease, however, those with prolactinomas are managed first and foremost with medical therapy. For those patients with a prolactinoma that cannot be controlled with medical management or for those unable to tolerate the side effects of medical ther-apies, radiosurgery can be used for treatment. Considering that most patients are successfully managed with medications, the prolactinoma patients who undergo radiosurgery are likely atyp-ical in their tumor biology and represent some of the most challenging of this cohort of patients.

The radiologic control rate after radiosurgery for a prolactinoma is high in most series and typically is more than 90%. The endocrine remission rates vary substantially, however, after radiosur-gery (Table 4).[14,17,20,23,26,34,35,38,46,47,51,61,70–76] Biochemical remission off antisecretory medica-tions after radiosurgery ranges from 0% to 83%. In general, biochemical remission for prolactino-mas after radiosurgery tends to be worse than for those with Cushing's disease and acromegaly, even when taking into account preradiosurgical patient and tumor attributes.[43] Some of this varia-tion in endocrine remission rates may be a result of selection bias at respective centers. As with acro-megaly, however, the rates of endocrine remission seem improved in those patients who were treated with radiosurgery while they were off antisecretory medications.[70,72]

SRS-Induced Biochemical Remission and Late Recurrence

SRS yields hormone normalization within a period of time that is longer than that achieved after surgical extirpation.[77] As such, patients are typi-cally bridged with suppressive medications after radiosurgery. Patients are periodically taken off the antisecretory medication and endocrine testing is performed. Antisecretory medications can be halted at the time when a postradiosurgery endocrine remission has been achieved. The time interval in which remission can occur ranges from 3 months to 8 years.[44,45,62] Most series demon-strate endocrine remission in Cushing's disease

and acromegalic patients within 1 to 3 years after radiosurgery.

Several groups have investigated factors that increase the probability of endocrine remission. Castinetti and colleagues[54] demonstrated that preoperative growth hormone (GH) and insulinlike growth factor 1 (IGF-1) levels are significantly asso-ciated with the rate of post-SRS remission. Pollock and colleagues[62] evaluated 46 patients with GH-secreting adenomas and identified 2 significant associations. A preradiosurgical IGF-1 level greater than 2.25 times the upper limit of normal range was significantly associated with a lower rate of endo-crine remission (hazard ratio 2.9; 95% CI, 1.2–6.9). For patients who had IGF-1 levels less than 2.25 times the upper limit of normal and were not taking somatostatin agonists at radiosurgery, the rates of biochemical remission exceeded 80%. A similar finding was reported by Landolt and colleagues,[78] who demonstrated that the post-SRS remission rates fell from 60% to 11% for those using octreotide during the perioperative period. Potential mechanisms underlying this phenom-enon include a decreased radiosensitivity of adenoma cells secondary to decreased cell divi-sion when exposed to somatostatin agonists. Addi-tionally, somatostatin agonists, such as octreotide, may serve as free radical scavengers, thereby reducing the DNA damage after ionizing radiation.

This result is not exclusive to acromegaly. Land-olt and colleagues[78] found a significant trend toward worse outcomes in patients on dopamine agonist who were treated with radiosurgery for prolactinomas. Pouratian and colleagues[72] ana-lyzed 23 patients with refractory prolactinomas and demonstrated a significant increase in the rates of remission in patients who were not taking dopamine agonists at the time of radiosurgery. The authors observed a similar improvement in endocrine remission in acromegalic patients who were systematically taken off pituitary suppressive medications at the time of radiosurgery.[57]

The effect of pituitary suppressive medications on endocrine outcomes after radiosurgery remains controversial. Reports in the literature have not been consistent regarding the importance of a temporary cessation of suppressive medications at the time of radiosurgery.[51,53,54,62,70,78] Two groups analyzed remission rates after radiosur-gery among patients on somatostatin agonists and failed to identify an association between the use of somatostatin agonists and endocrine remis-sion.[53,54] The definition of endocrine remission, however, has not been well defined across series, with GH levels varying from less than 5 ng/mL to (upper limit of remission).[55,79] Second, the follow-up in retrospective series varies widely. Pollock

Table 4
Summary of the literature for the radiosurgical management of prolactinomas

Year	Authors	Patients (N)	Mean/Median Follow-Up (Mo)	Margin Dose (Gy)	Biochemical Remission (%)	Neurologic Deficit (%)	Hypopituitarism (%)
2000	Izawa et al[38]	15	28	22	20	0	NR
2000	Landolt and Lomax[70]	20	29	25	25	0	NR
2000	Pan et al[71]	128	33	32	41	0	NR
2002	Feigl et al[14]	18	55	15	NR	NR	NR
2002	Pollock et al[51]	7	42	20	29	14	16
2003	Choi et al[35]	21	42.5	28.5	24	0	0
2003	Muramatsu et al[61]	1	30	15	0	7.7	0
2003	Petrovich et al[17]	12	41	15	83	0	NR
2005	Kajiwara et al[20]	3	35.3	17.5	33	4.7	9.5
2006	Pouratian et al[72]	23	55	18.6	26	7	28
2006	Voges et al[23]	13	56	20	15.4	4.2	18.3
2006	Ma et al[76]	51	37	26.1	40	NR	17.6
2008	Pollock et al[25,43]	11	48	30	18	2	45
2008	Tinnel et al[46]	2	19.5	30	50	11	22
2009	Castinetti et al[34]	15	85.5	30	46.6	5.3	21
2009	Jezkova et al[73]	35	75.5	49	37.1	0	14.3
2009	Wan et al[47]	176	67.3	35	23.3	1.7	1.7
2009	Kobayashi[26]	27	37.4	18.4	43.5 in 23 pts	0	0
2010	Tanaka et al[74]	22	60	25	17	8	42
2011	Sun et al[75]	1	48	23	0	0	0
Total/average		601			29.4	3.6	15.7

Abbreviations: NR, not reported; pts, patients.

and colleagues[62] demonstrated that remission continued to occur up to 5 years after radiosurgery, whereas in the report by Castinetti and colleagues,[54] 44% of their patient population received the final endocrine evaluation less than 36 months after radiosurgery. At the University of Virginia, the authors discontinue the use of suppressive medication around radiosurgery for 6 to 8 weeks, depending on its pharmacokinetics (ie, the drug's half-life). Most patients can tolerate a brief period off suppressive medications during their radiosurgery.

The rates of biochemical remission vary widely across series. There = seems to be a differential radiosensitivity between specific types of secretory pituitary adenomas.[23,26,43] Overall, Cushing's disease demonstrates the highest rates of biochemical remission, followed by acromegaly, prolactinomas, and Nelson syndrome. This sensitivity discrepancy has been attributed to patient selection, tumor volume, radiation dose, use of suppressive medications, and duration of follow-up.[26,43] Pollock and colleagues[43] reviewed a retrospective series of 46 patients. This case-controlled study demonstrated wide variations in endocrine remission after SRS for various types of secretory adenomas. This study and others suggest that different types of secretory adenomas have different radiosensitivities, but an explanation for this remain obscure.

Overall, few cases of recurrence after SRS-induced biochemical remission have been reported.[39,51] In some SRS series, however, recurrence rates of up to 20% have been reported. This serves to underscore the importance of long-term radiographic and endocrine follow-up after SRS for secretary pituitary adenomas.

Adverse Events After SRS

Fortunately, adverse events after radiosurgery for a pituitary adenoma are uncommon. Delayed onset of hypopituitarism is the most frequently occurring unintended effect of radiosurgery. Retrospective series demonstrate that 30% of patients eventually develop some form of anterior pituitary deficiency after radiosurgery. Hypopituitarism has been correlated to the radiosurgical treatment volume, with those patients having a tumor volume less than or equal to 4.0 cm^3 exhibiting an 18% 5-year risk of hypopituitarism versus 58% for those with larger lesions.[43] The incidence of hypopituitarism after radiosurgery is likely related to the preradiosurgical status of the normal pituitary gland, type and timing of prior treatments, the radiosurgical dose per volume delivered to the normal gland, the dose delivered to the pituitary stalk, and the rigorousness and

length of the follow-up assessment period. A safe radiosurgical dose or dose per volume below which hypopituitarism will not occur probably does not exist. Some investigators have advocated placement of an inert spacer between the residual adenoma and pituitary gland if postoperative radiosurgery is contemplated.[80] A lower dose achieved in part through a steep gradient index, however, is intuitively pleasing in terms of minimizing the risk of hypopituitarism. Nevertheless, delivery of an optimal dose to the target volume should not be compromised when attempting to avoid hypopituitarism. Adenoma progression or persistence of a hypersecretory state is far more of a threat to longevity and quality of life than is delayed hypopituitarism. Hypopituitarism should be managed with hormone replacement under the care of an experienced neuroendocrinologist.

The second most common toxicity is cranial neuropathy. Cranial nerves II, III, IV, V, and VI are located in the parasellar or suprasellar regions and are at risk of injury from radiosurgery. Such neuropathies after radiosurgery occur in 2% or fewer of all patients. Improved conformality, steeper dose gradients, and adequate shielding may help minimize this risk.[77] Rare toxicities include radiation necrosis of the adjacent parenchyma,[23,43,47,51] internal carotid artery stenosis/occlusion,[51,81] and radiation-induced secondary malignancy.[82] No cases of radiation-induced secondary malignancies have been reported to date after SRS for pituitary tumors. Based on the available literature, the risk of serious and irreversible complications after radiosurgery for a pituitary adenoma is low.

EXTERNAL BEAM RADIATION THERAPY

In the current era, most pituitary adenoma patients in the United States are treated with SRS. For those patients with large or diffusely infiltrative adenomas or with suprasellar or brainstem extension, fractionated EBRT should be considered to minimize the risk of late toxicities.[83] The local tumor control rate after conventional fractionated EBRT for nonfunctioning pituitary adenomas is greater than 90% in most series. Similar to that seen with radiosurgery, however, the rate of biochemical normalization of functioning tumors is lower than the rate of tumor control and is dependent on on adenoma subtype.[84–86]

Radiation therapy planning starts with delineation of the target. The gross tumor volume (GTV) is the full extent of the pituitary adenoma based on neuroimaging (MRI and/or CT). Next, the clinical target volume (CTV) is defined as the GTV and areas of presumed disease extension, such as the cavernous sinus or clivus. The planned treatment volume is an expansion of the CTV to accommodate for setup error and patient movement. With sellar-based targets, CTV expansion to create a PTV typically requires expansion of 2 mm to 5 mm, although the expansion may be nonuniform. Unlike in radiosurgery, patient immobilization typically uses a thermoplastic mask, which does not afford the same degree of immobilization and leads to a larger PTV expansion than that achieved using stereotactic approaches. It is the sum of the random errors from intrafractional and interfractional positional variation that requires a larger expansion of the CTV than in radiosurgery. This approach is in marked distinction to radiosurgery in which the PTV is usually equivalent to the GTV. Similar to radiosurgery, however, risk structures, such as the brainstem, optic apparatus, pituitary stalk, hypothalamus, and temporal lobes, are defined. Dosimetric constraints are set for the structures at risk and an optimal radiation dose and fractionation scheme is determined for the PTV. Fractionated radiation doses for pituitary adenomas typically vary from 45 Gy to 54 Gy.

EBRT and Nonfunctioning Adenomas

Conventional fractionated EBRT to a dose of 45 Gy to 54 Gy in 1.8 Gy to 2 Gy fractions has demonstrated effectiveness for patients with recurrent or progressive nonfunctioning pituitary adenomas. A retrospective experience of 2 hospitals in the United Kingdom included 126 patients with nonfunctioning pituitary adenomas. The hospitals had different approaches to management.[87] One hospital chose to treat postoperative patients with radiation therapy (45 Gy in 30–33 fractions) whereas the other did not. The progression-free survival at 15 years significantly favored the cohort who underwent EBRT (93% vs 33%, P<.05). In a similar study, clinicians from the Netherlands evaluated 76 patients who received postoperative EBRT and a group of 28 patients who were conservatively managed.[88] The 10-year tumor control rate was 95% for the EBRT group compared with 22% for the conservatively managed cohort. Although most radiation therapy approaches for pituitary adenomas have used photons, proton beam–based radiation therapy has also been used to treat patients with nonfunctioning adenomas. The Loma Linda group reported its experience using proton beam to treat 24 patients with nonfunctioning adenomas. In a series with a median dose of 54 cobalt Gy equivalents (CGE) and a median follow-up of 47 months, the group noted tumor control achieved in all patients.[89]

If adequate sparing of normal tissue cannot be attained with a single-fraction SRS, FSRT may be used because it combines the precise immobilization of SRS with the radiobiologic benefits of standard fractionation on normal tissue. FSRT has been used by some centers to treat patients with nonfunctioning adenomas. This approach is a blending of the advantages and disadvantages of radiosurgery and EBRT. Colin and colleagues[90] detailed a series of 63 patients with nonfunctioning adenomas who underwent FRST. At a median follow-up of 82 months after FSRT, tumor control was achieved in all patients. In this same series, hypopituitarism was seen in 28.5% of patients at 4 years and 35% of patients at 8 years post-FSRT.

EBRT and Cushing's Disease

EBRT is commonly used for patients with residual or recurrent tumor after an initial transsphenoidal resection or in patients with no radiographic evidence of disease but endocrine evidence of persistent Cushing's disease. Endocrine remission is usually defined as normalization of the 24-hour UFC, salivary cortisol, and serum corticotropin, but significant differences in remission criteria are used, even at leading centers. Both EBRT and SRS seem to achieve biochemical remission rates of 50% to 80%. The latency period between EBRT and endocrine remission is usually a year or more. EBRT tends to be associated with a longer time to achieve endocrine remission in patients with functioning adenomas. In one series comparing time to endocrine remission, patients undergoing radiosurgery achieved endocrine remission at a mean time of 8.5 months, whereas those treated with EBRT achieved remission in 18 months.[83]

In a group of patients with Cushing's disease, Estrada and colleagues[84] reported endocrine remission rates of 44% at 1 year and 83% at 3 years after EBRT. In a group of 40 patients with Cushing's disease treated with doses between 45 Gy and 100 Gy, Hughes and colleagues[91] reported a 10-year endocrine remission rate of 59%.

Early experiences with charged particles from the Lawrence Berkeley National Laboratory demonstrated 85% endocrine remission rates using helium ions, with doses ranging from 30 CGE to 150 CGE in patients with Cushing's disease. The Massachusetts General Hospital proton group noted 52% of radiographic and endocrine remission, with a median dose of 20 CGE at a median follow-up of 62 months.[92]

EBRT and Acromegaly

EBRT has been used to treat patients with persistent acromegaly. Unlike patients with Cushing's disease, where the adenoma may be less apparent on neuroimaging studies, patients with persistent acromegaly after transsphenoidal resection tend to have well-demarcated tumors. Tumor control after EBRT is usually quickly achieved radiographically, but endocrine remission typically takes years to attain. Endocrine remission is usually defined as a normalization of IGF-1 (matched for age and gender) and GH level less than 1 ng/mL after an oral glucose challenge.

The largest experience reported to date was a series of 884 patients reported by 14 different centers in the United Kingdom.[93] GH levels less than 2.5 ng/mL were achieved in 22%, 60%, and 77% at 2, 10, and 20 years, respectively. In that same series, normal IGF-1 levels were found in 63% of patients at a median follow-up of 10 years after EBRT. In another series with a median follow-up of 11.5 years, Barrande and colleagues[94] demonstrated that 66% of 128 patients achieved a GH of less than 2.5 ng/mL at 15 years post-EBRT. In that same series, 79% of patients ultimately achieved a normal IGF-1. In a smaller Dutch series of 36 patients treated with EBRT to a median dose of 40 Gy, IGF-1 normalization rates of 60%, 74%, and 84% were observed at 5, 10, and 15 years, respectively.[95]

In a few institutions, proton beam therapy is used to treat acromegalic patients. The Massachusetts General Hospital group reported a 59% endocrine remission rate in a series of 22 patients with a median follow-up of 6.3 years. The median time to endocrine remission in this series was 3.5 years.[42] The Loma Linda experience with proton beam for 11 acromegalic patients demonstrated a rate of endocrine normalization of 45% at a median follow-up period of 3.9 years.

EBRT and Prolactinomas

As is true for radiosurgery, prolactinomas are seldom treated with EBRT. Most prolactinoma patients are treated medically with dopamine agonists or approached via a transsphenoidal resection. Those prolactinoma patients undergoing EBRT likely represent a selected and poorly behaving cohort of patients.

Biochemical remission is defined as a normal serum prolactin level of less than 20 ng/mL depending on gender. EBRT affords endocrine remission off antisecretory medications in approximately 10% to 30% of patients and the latency of effect is usually achieved over many years.[96,97] In 1991, Littley and colleagues[98] reported their results with EBRT for patients with large prolactinomas. They used standard fractionation schemes of 20 Gy to 42.5 Gy in 8 to 15 fractions and

followed patients for up to 154 months after treatment. In a total of 58 patients, 71% of patients achieved a normal prolactin level while on a dopamine agonist. When off the dopamine agonist, however, only 21% achieved a normal prolactin level after EBRT. Isobe and colleagues[97] reported on their experience with EBRT (48–60 Gy, median 50 Gy) in prolactinoma patients. They noted that patients with a prolactinoma were less likely to achieve local tumor control after EBRT. Although radiation therapy may be used as a salvage approach for prolactinoma patients refractory and/or ineligible for medical therapy, microsurgery, or radiosurgery, its overall chances of achieving endocrine remission seem lower than with Cushing's disease or acromegalic patients.[91]

ADVERSE EVENTS AFTER EBRT

The most common risk associated with EBRT is delayed hypopituitarism. Risks of hypopituitarism after EBRT range from 50% to 100% depending on the length and rigorousness of endocrine follow-up.[84,98] EBRT carries a 1% to 3% risk of optic neuropathy.[86,99] Other more severe complications include a 2.7% risk of radiation-induced neoplasia at 10 years after EBRT and a 4% risk at 5 years of suffering a cerebrovascular accident after EBRT, presumably from radiation-induced carotid stenosis.[100]

EBRT has had a longer track record for use with pituitary adenoma patients. Although the extended follow-up period for EBRT may explain some differences between the frequency and severity of complications associated with EBRT versus SRS, the true differences in the risk profile of EBRT and SRS have yet to be fully defined. Nevertheless, in the United States, contemporary management of pituitary adenoma patients has largely shifted away from EBRT to SRS because of SRS's improved rates of endocrine remission and the perception, at least, of an improved side-effect profile.

SUMMARY

EBRT and SRS play important roles in the management of pituitary adenomas. SRS or EBRT are typically used in patients with substantial residual tumor or recurrence after resection. They are also used for patients with functioning adenomas that fail to achieve endocrine remission after prior resections. Neurologic function after SRS or EBRT is usually preserved or at times improved, even when the treated adenoma extends into the cavernous sinus. Delayed hypopituitarism is the most common complication but is manageable with hormone replacement. Other serious complications are rare. Lifelong follow-up for pituitary adenoma patients is recommended.

REFERENCES

1. Dekkers OM, Pereira AM, Romijn JA. Treatment and follow-up of clinically nonfunctioning pituitary macroadenomas. J Clin Endocrinol Metab 2008; 93(10):3717–26.
2. Vance ML. Treatment of patients with a pituitary adenoma: one clinican's experience. Neurosurg Focus 2004;16(4):1–6.
3. Cushing H. The pituitary body and its disorders: clinical states produced by disorders of the hypophysis cerebri. Philadelphia: J.B. Lippincott; 1912.
4. Seymour ZA, Cohen-Gadol AA. Cushing's lost cases of "radium bomb" brachytherapy for gliomas. J Neurosurg 2010;113(1):141–8.
5. Schulder M, Loeffler JS, Howes AE, et al. Historical vignette: the radium bomb: Harvey Cushing and the interstitial irradiation of gliomas. J Neurosurg 1996;84(3):530–2.
6. Leksell L. The stereotaxic method and radiosurgery of the brain. Acta Chir Scand 1951;102(4): 316–9.
7. Barnett GH, Linskey ME, Adler JR, et al. Stereotactic radiosurgery—an organized neurosurgery-sanctioned definition. J Neurosurg 2007;106(1):1–5.
8. Friedman WA, Foote KD. Linear accelerator radiosurgery in the management of brain tumours. Ann Med 2000;32(1):64–80.
9. Chen CC, Chapman P, Petit J, et al. Proton radiosurgery in neurosurgery. Neurosurg Focus 2007; 23(6):E5.
10. Landolt AM, Haller D, Lomax N, et al. Stereotactic radiosurgery for recurrent surgically treated acromegaly: comparison with fractionated radiotherapy. J Neurosurg 1998;88(6):1002–8.
11. Emami B, Lyman J, Brown A, et al. Tolerance of normal tissue to therapeutic irradiation. Int J Radiat Oncol Biol Phys 1991;21(1):109–22.
12. Höybye C, Rähn T. Adjuvant Gamma Knife radiosurgery in non-functioning pituitary adenomas; low risk of long-term complications in selected patients. Pituitary 2009;12(3):211–6.
13. Mingione V, Yen CP, Vance ML, et al. Gamma surgery in the treatment of nonsecretory pituitary macroadenoma. J Neurosurg 2006;104(6):876–83.
14. Feigl GC, Bonelli CM, Berghold A, et al. Effects of gamma knife radiosurgery of pituitary adenomas on pituitary function. J Neurosurg 2002;97(Suppl 5):415–21.
15. Sheehan JP, Kondziolka D, Flickinger J, et al. Radiosurgery for residual or recurrent nonfunctioning pituitary adenoma. J Neurosurg 2002;97(Suppl 5): 408–14.
16. Wowra B, Stummer W. Efficacy of gamma knife radiosurgery for nonfunctioning pituitary adenomas: a quantitative follow up with magnetic resonance imaging-based volumetric analysis. J Neurosurg 2002;97(Suppl 5):429–32.
17. Petrovich Z, Jozsef G, Yu C, et al. Radiotherapy and stereotactic radiosurgery for pituitary tumors. Neurosurg Clin N Am 2003;14(1):147–66.
18. Losa M, Valle M, Mortini P, et al. Gamma knife surgery for treatment of residual nonfunctioning pituitary adenomas after surgical debulking. J Neurosurg 2004;100(3):438–44.
19. Muacevic A, Uhl E, Wowra B. Gamma knife radiosurgery for nonfunctioning pituitary adenomas. Acta Neurochir Suppl 2004;91:51–4.
20. Kajiwara K, Saito K, Yoshikawa K, et al. Image-guided stereotactic radiosurgery with the CyberKnife for pituitary adenomas. Minim Invasive Neurosurg 2005;48(2):91–6.
21. Picozzi P, Losa M, Mortini P, et al. Radiosurgery and the prevention of regrowth of incompletely removed nonfunctioning pituitary adenomas. J Neurosurg 2005;102(Suppl):71–4.
22. Iwai Y, Yamanaka K, Yoshioka K, et al. The usefulness of adjuvant therapy using gamma knife radiosurgery for the recurrent or residual nonfunctioning pituitary adenomas. No Shinkei Geka 2005;33(8): 777–83.
23. Voges J, Kocher M, Runge M, et al. Linear accelerator radiosurgery for pituitary macroadenomas: a 7-year follow-up study. Cancer 2006;107(6):1355–64.
24. Liscak R, Vladyka V, Marek J, et al. Gamma knife radiosurgery for endocrine-inactive pituitary adenomas. Acta Neurochir (Wien) 2007;149(10): 999–1006 [discussion: 6].
25. Pollock BE, Cochran J, Natt N, et al. Gamma knife radiosurgery for patients with nonfunctioning pituitary adenomas: results from a 15-year experience. Int J Radiat Oncol Biol Phys 2008;70(5):1325–9.
26. Kobayashi T. Long-term results of stereotactic gamma knife radiosurgery for pituitary adenomas. Specific strategies for different types of adenoma. Prog Neurol Surg 2009;22:77–95.
27. Castro DG, Cecilio SA, Canteras MM. Radiosurgery for pituitary adenomas: evaluation of its efficacy and safety. Radiat Oncol 2010;5:109.
28. Hayashi M, Chernov M, Tamura N, et al. Gamma Knife robotic microradiosurgery of pituitary adenomas invading the cavernous sinus: treatment concept and results in 89 cases. J Neurooncol 2010; 98(2):185–94.
29. Gopalan R, Schlesinger D, Vance ML, et al. Long-term outcomes after Gamma Knife radiosurgery for patients with a nonfunctioning pituitary adenoma. Neurosurgery 2011;69(2):284–93.
30. Iwata H, Sato K, Tatewaki K, et al. Hypofractionated stereotactic radiotherapy with CyberKnife for

nonfunctioning pituitary adenoma: high local control with low toxicity. Neuro Oncol 2011;13(8):916–22.

31. Park KJ, Kano H, Parry PV, et al. Long-term outcomes after gamma knife stereotactic radiosurgery for nonfunctional pituitary adenomas. Neurosurgery 2011;69(6):1188–99.

32. Biller BM, Grossman AB, Stewart PM, et al. Treatment of adrenocorticotropin-dependent Cushing's Syndrome: a consensus statement. J Clin Endocrinol Metab 2008;93(7):2454–62.

33. Castinetti F, Nagai M, Dufour H, et al. Gamma knife radiosurgery is a successful adjunctive treatment in Cushing's disease. Eur J Endocrinol 2007; 156(1):91–8.

34. Castinetti F, Nagai M, Morange I, et al. Long-term results of stereotactic radiosurgery in secretory pituitary adenomas. J Clin Endocrinol Metab 2009;94(9):3400–7.

35. Choi JY, Chang JH, Chang JW, et al. Radiological and hormonal responses of functioning pituitary adenomas after gamma knife radiosurgery. Yonsei Med J 2003;44(4):602–7.

36. Devin JK, Allen GS, Cmelak AJ, et al. The efficacy of linear accelerator radiosurgery in the management of patients with Cushing's disease. Stereotact Funct Neurosurg 2004;82(5–6):254–62.

37. Hoybye C, Grenback E, Rahn T, et al. Adrenocorticotropic hormone-producing pituitary tumors: 12- to 22-year follow-up after treatment with stereotactic radiosurgery. Neurosurgery 2001;49(2): 284–91 [discussion: 91–2].

38. Izawa M, Hayashi M, Nakaya K, et al. Gamma knife radiosurgery for pituitary adenomas. J Neurosurg 2000;93(Suppl 3):19–22.

39. Jagannathan J, Sheehan JP, Pouratian N, et al. Gamma Knife surgery for Cushing's disease. J Neurosurg 2007;106(6):980–7.

40. Kobayashi T, Kida Y, Mori Y. Gamma knife radiosurgery in the treatment of Cushing disease: long-term results. J Neurosurg 2002;97(Suppl 5): 422–8.

41. Laws ER, Reitmeyer M, Thapar K, et al. Cushing's disease resulting from pituitary corticotrophic microadenoma. Treatment results from transsphenoidal microsurgery and gamma knife radiosurgery. Neurochirurgie 2002;48(2–3 Pt 2):294–9.

42. Petit JH, Biller BM, Coen JJ, et al. Proton stereotactic radiosurgery in management of persistent acromegaly. Endocr Pract 2007;13(7):726–34.

43. Pollock BE, Brown PD, Nippoldt TB, et al. Pituitary tumor type affects the chance of biochemical remission after radiosurgery of hormone-secreting pituitary adenomas. Neurosurgery 2008;62(6):1271–6 [discussion: 76–8].

44. Sheehan JM, Vance ML, Sheehan JP, et al. Radiosurgery for Cushing's disease after failed transsphenoidal surgery. J Neurosurg 2000;93(5):738–42.

45. Shin M, Kurita H, Sasaki T, et al. Stereotactic radiosurgery for pituitary adenoma invading the cavernous sinus. J Neurosurg 2000;93(Suppl 3):2–5.

46. Tinnel BA, Henderson MA, Witt TC, et al. Endocrine response after gamma knife-based stereotactic radiosurgery for secretory pituitary adenoma. Stereotact Funct Neurosurg 2008;86(5):292–6.

47. Wan H, Chihiro O, Yuan S. MASEP gamma knife radiosurgery for secretory pituitary adenomas: experience in 347 consecutive cases. J Exp Clin Cancer Res 2009;28:36.

48. Witt TC. Stereotactic radiosurgery for pituitary tumors. Neurosurg Focus 2003;14(5):e10.

49. Wong GK, Leung CH, Chiu KW, et al. LINAC radiosurgery in recurrent Cushing's disease after transsphenoidal surgery: a series of 5 cases. Minim Invasive Neurosurg 2003;46(6):327–30.

50. Sheehan JP, Pouratian N, Steiner L, et al. Gamma Knife surgery for pituitary adenomas: factors related to radiological and endocrine outcomes. J Neurosurg 2011;114(2):303–9.

51. Pollock BE, Nippoldt TB, Stafford SL, et al. Results of stereotactic radiosurgery in patients with hormone-producing pituitary adenomas: factors associated with endocrine normalization. J Neurosurg 2002; 97(3):525–30.

52. Melmed S. Acromegaly. N Engl J Med 2006; 355(24):2558–73.

53. Attanasio R, Epaminonda P, Motti E, et al. Gamma-knife radiosurgery in acromegaly: a 4-year follow-up study. J Clin Endocrinol Metab 2003;88(7): 3105–12.

54. Castinetti F, Taieb D, Kuhn JM, et al. Outcome of gamma knife radiosurgery in 82 patients with acromegaly: correlation with initial hypersecretion. J Clin Endocrinol Metab 2005;90(8):4483–8.

55. Fukuoka S, Ito T, Takanashi M, et al. Gamma knife radiosurgery for growth hormone-secreting pituitary adenomas invading the cavernous sinus. Stereotact Funct Neurosurg 2001;76(3–4):213–7.

56. Ikeda H, Jokura H, Yoshimoto T. Transsphenoidal surgery and adjuvant gamma knife treatment for growth hormone-secreting pituitary adenoma. J Neurosurg 2001;95(2):285–91.

57. Jagannathan J, Sheehan JP, Pouratian N, et al. Gamma knife radiosurgery for acromegaly: outcomes after failed transsphenoidal surgery. Neurosurgery 2008;62(6):1262–9 [discussion: 69–70].

58. Jezkova J, Marek J, Hana V, et al. Gamma knife radiosurgery for acromegaly—long-term experience. Clin Endocrinol 2006;64(5):588–95.

59. Kobayashi T, Mori Y, Uchiyama Y, et al. Long-term results of gamma knife surgery for growth hormone-producing pituitary adenoma: is the disease difficult to cure? J Neurosurg 2005;102(Suppl):119–23.

60. Losa M, Gioia L, Picozzi P, et al. The role of stereotactic radiotherapy in patients with growth

hormone-secreting pituitary adenoma [see comment]. J Clin Endocrinol Metab 2008;93(7):2546–52.

61. Muramatsu J, Yoshida M, Shioura H, et al. Clinical results of LINAC-based stereotactic radiosurgery for pituitary adenoma. Nihon Igaku Hoshasen Gakkai Zasshi 2003;63(5):225–30.

62. Pollock BE, Jacob JT, Brown PD, et al. Radiosurgery of growth hormone-producing pituitary adenomas: factors associated with biochemical remission. J Neurosurg 2007;106(5):833–8.

63. Vik-Mo EO, Oksnes M, Pedersen PH, et al. Gamma knife stereotactic radiosurgery for acromegaly. Eur J Endocrinol 2007;157(3):255–63.

64. Zhang N, Pan L, Wang EM, et al. Radiosurgery for growth hormone-producing pituitary adenomas. J Neurosurg 2000;93(Suppl 3):6–9.

65. Gutt B, Wowra B, Alexandrov R, et al. Gamma-knife surgery is effective in normalising plasma insulin-like growth factor I in patients with acromegaly. Exp Clin Endocrinol Diabetes 2005; 113(4):219–24.

66. Roberts BK, Ouyang DL, Lad SP, et al. Efficacy and safety of CyberKnife radiosurgery for acromegaly. Pituitary 2007;10(1):19–25.

67. Ronchi CL, Attanasio R, Verrua E, et al. Efficacy and tolerability of gamma knife radiosurgery in acromegaly: a 10-year follow-up study. Clin Endocrinol (Oxf) 2009;71(6):846–52.

68. Iwai Y, Yamanaka K, Yoshimura M, et al. Gamma knife radiosurgery for growth hormone-producing adenomas. J Clin Neurosci 2010;17(3):299–304.

69. Poon TL, Leung SC, Poon CY, et al. Predictors of outcome following Gamma Knife surgery for acromegaly. J Neurosurg 2010;113(Suppl): 149–52.

70. Landolt AM, Lomax N. Gamma knife radiosurgery for prolactinomas. J Neurosurg 2000;93(Suppl 3): 14–8.

71. Pan L, Zhang N, Wang EM, et al. Gamma knife radiosurgery as a primary treatment for prolactinomas. J Neurosurg 2000;93(Suppl 3):10–3.

72. Pouratian N, Sheehan J, Jagannathan J, et al. Gamma knife radiosurgery for medically and surgically refractory prolactinomas. Neurosurgery 2006; 59(2):255–66 [discussion: 55–66].

73. Jezkova J, Hana V, Krsek M, et al. Use of the Leksell gamma knife in the treatment of prolactinoma patients. Clin Endocrinol (Oxf) 2009;70(5): 732–41.

74. Tanaka S, Link MJ, Brown PD, et al. Gamma knife radiosurgery for patients with prolactin-secreting pituitary adenomas. World Neurosurg 2010;74(1): 147–52.

75. Sun DQ, Cheng JJ, Frazier JL, et al. Treatment of pituitary adenomas using radiosurgery and radiotherapy: a single center experience and review of literature. Neurosurg Rev 2011;34(2):181–9.

76. Ma ZM, Qiu B, Hou YH, et al. Gamma knife treatment for pituitary prolactinomas. Zhong Nan Da Xue Xue Bao Yi Xue Ban 2006;31(5):714–6.

77. Jagannathan J, Yen CP, Pouratian N, et al. Stereotactic radiosurgery for pituitary adenomas: a comprehensive review of indications, techniques and long-term results using the Gamma Knife. J Neurooncol 2009;92(3):345–56.

78. Landolt AM, Haller D, Lomax N, et al. Octreotide may act as a radioprotective agent in acromegaly. J Clin Endocrinol Metab 2000;85(3):1287–9.

79. Morange-Ramos I, Regis J, Dufour H, et al. Gamma-knife surgery for secreting pituitary adenomas. Acta Neurochir 1998;140(5):437–43.

80. Taussky P, Kalra R, Coppens J, et al. Endocrinological outcome after pituitary transposition (hypophysopexy) and adjuvant radiotherapy for tumors involving the cavernous sinus. J Neurosurg 2011;115(1):55–62.

81. Lim YJ, Leem W, Park JT, et al. Cerebral infarction with ICA occlusion after Gamma Knife radiosurgery for pituitary adenoma: a case report. Stereotact Funct Neurosurg 1999;72(Suppl 1):132–9.

82. Loeffler JS, Niemierko A, Chapman PH. Second tumors after radiosurgery: tip of the iceberg or a bump in the road? Neurosurgery 2003;52(6): 1436–40 [discussion: 40–2].

83. Mitsumori M, Shrieve DC, Alexander E 3rd, et al. Initial clinical results of LINAC-based stereotactic radiosurgery and stereotactic radiotherapy for pituitary adenomas. Int J Radiat Oncol Biol Phys 1998; 42(3):573–80.

84. Estrada J, Boronat M, Mielgo M, et al. The long-term outcome of pituitary irradiation after unsuccessful transsphenoidal surgery in Cushing's disease. N Engl J Med 1997;336(3):172–7.

85. Minniti G, Osti M, Jaffrain-Rea ML, et al. Long-term follow-up results of postoperative radiation therapy for Cushing's disease. J Neurooncol 2007;84(1): 79–84.

86. Zierhut D, Flentje M, Adolph J, et al. External radiotherapy of pituitary adenomas. Int J Radiat Oncol Biol Phys 1995;33(2):307–14.

87. Gittoes NJ, Bates AS, Tse W, et al. Radiotherapy for non-function pituitary tumours. Clin Endocrinol (Oxf) 1998;48(3):331–7.

88. van den Bergh AC, van den Berg G, Schoorl MA, et al. Immediate postoperative radiotherapy in residual nonfunctioning pituitary adenoma: beneficial effect on local control without additional negative impact on pituitary function and life expectancy. Int J Radiat Oncol Biol Phys 2007;67(3):863–9.

89. Ronson BB, Schulte RW, Han KP, et al. Fractionated proton beam irradiation of pituitary adenomas. Int J Radiat Oncol Biol Phys 2006;64(2):425–34.

90. Colin P, Jovenin N, Delemer B, et al. Treatment of pituitary adenomas by fractionated stereotactic

radiotherapy: a prospective study of 110 patients. Int J Radiat Oncol Biol Phys 2005; 62(2):333–41.

91. Hughes MN, Llamas KJ, Yelland ME, et al. Pituitary adenomas: long-term results for radiotherapy alone and post-operative radiotherapy. Int J Radiat Oncol Biol Phys 1993;27(5):1035–43.

92. Petit JH, Biller BM, Yock TI, et al. Proton stereotactic radiotherapy for persistent adrenocorticotropin-producing adenomas. J Clin Endocrinol Metab 2008;93(2):393–9.

93. Jenkins PJ, Bates P, Carson MN, et al. Conventional pituitary irradiation is effective in lowering serum growth hormone and insulin-like growth factor-I in patients with acromegaly. J Clin Endocrinol Metab 2006;91(4):1239–45.

94. Barrande G, Pittino-Lungo M, Coste J, et al. Hormonal and metabolic effects of radiotherapy in acromegaly: long-term results in 128 patients followed in a single center. J Clin Endocrinol Metab 2000;85(10):3779–85.

95. Biermasz NR, van Dulken H, Roelfsema F. Long-term follow-up results of postoperative radiotherapy in 36 patients with acromegaly. J Clin Endocrinol Metab 2000;85(7):2476–82.

96. Minniti G, Traish D, Ashley S, et al. Fractionated stereotactic conformal radiotherapy for secreting and nonsecreting pituitary adenomas. Clin Endocrinol (Oxf) 2006;64(5):542–8.

97. Williams M, van Seters AP, Hermans J, et al. Evaluation of the effects of radiotherapy on macroprolactinomas using the decline rate of serum prolactin levels as a dynamic parameter. Clin Oncol (R Coll Radiol) 1994;6(2):102–9.

98. Littley MD, Shalet SM, Reid H, et al. The effect of external pituitary irradiation on elevated serum prolactin levels in patients with pituitary macroadenomas. Q J Med 1991;81(296):985–98.

99. Becker G, Kocher M, Kortmann RD, et al. Radiation therapy in the multimodal treatment approach of pituitary adenoma. Strahlenther Onkol 2002; 178(4):173–86.

100. Brada M, Burchell L, Ashley S, et al. The incidence of cerebrovascular accidents in patients with pituitary adenoma. Int J Radiat Oncol Biol Phys 1999;45(3): 693–8.

101. Kajiwara K, Saito K, Yoshikawa K, et al. Image-guided stereotactic radiosurgery with the Cyber-Knife for pituitary adenomas. Minim Invasive Neurosurg 2005;48(2):91–6.

Management of Large Aggressive Nonfunctional Pituitary Tumors
Experimental Medical Options When Surgery and Radiation Fail

Brandon A. Miller, MD, PhD*, W. Caleb Rutledge, MD, MS,
Adriana G. Ioachimescu, MD, PhD,
Nelson M. Oyesiku, MD, PhD

KEYWORDS

- Pituitary adenoma • Macroadenoma • Nonfunctioning pituitary tumor

KEY POINTS

- Pituitary adenomas are generally considered benign tumors; however, a subset of these tumors displays aggressive behavior and carries a poor prognosis.
- Surgical resection is the mainstay of treatment for nonfunctioning pituitary macroadenomas and functioning tumors that do not respond to medical therapy.
- Radiosurgery is effective in treating tumors that are not completely surgically resected.
- There are several medical therapies being developed for aggressive pituitary adenomas; there are no standard therapy regimens, however, and clinical trials are lacking.

INTRODUCTION

Pituitary adenomas are generally considered benign tumors; however, a subset of these tumors displays aggressive behavior and is not easily cured. These tumors may recur quickly after surgery, grow into the cavernous sinus or skull base, or even metastasize throughout, or outside of, the central nervous system (CNS).[1] In these extreme cases, such tumors would be characterized as pituitary carcinomas. Aggressive pituitary tumors usually carry a poor prognosis. Those that metastasize typically carry with them a mean survival time of less than 5 years.[2]

It is generally believed that pituitary carcinomas originate from transformation of previously benign pituitary adenomas.[3] There is probably a continuum along which pituitary adenomas, atypical pituitary adenomas, and pituitary carcinomas exist, with

mitotic activity, vascularity, and specific genetic changes all contributing to the biologic behavior of specific tumors.[2] World Health Organization (WHO) criteria for atypical pituitary adenomas include high p53 immunoreactivity, MIB-1 proliferative index greater than 3%, and increased mitoses.[4] One recent series showed a significantly higher percentage of atypical pituitary adenomas being silent corticotropin (ACTH)-type tumors (17%) compared with ACTH-negative nonfunctioning adenomas (2%).[4] This supports the concept that silent corticotroph adenomas are more aggressive than other types of pituitary tumors,[5–7] although not every clinical study supports this.[8]

The protocol for nonsurgical treatment of aggressive pituitary lesions is less standardized than that of other CNS tumors. Several options are available for these difficult cases, including

Department of Neurosurgery, Emory University, Atlanta, GA1365 B Clifton Rd NE, Atlanta, GA 30322, USA
* Corresponding author.
E-mail address: brandon.miller@emory.edu

Neurosurg Clin N Am 23 (2012) 587–594
http://dx.doi.org/10.1016/j.nec.2012.06.013

multiple transsphenoidal or transcranial surgeries, radiation therapy, and chemotherapy. The purpose of this article is to summarize recent literature on novel treatments for aggressive pituitary adenomas and analyze recent research that points to new therapeutic strategies for these tumors.

NEW SURGICAL TECHNIQUES

Surgical resection is the mainstay of treatment for nonfunctioning pituitary macroadenomas and functioning tumors that do not respond to medical therapy. Currently, a transsphenoidal approach is the method of choice for resection of pituitary adenomas. While microscopic techniques are still in use, the endoscopic technique is gaining ground.[8,9] Complications after endoscopic surgery are generally low, with transient diabetes insipidus being the most common and still under 5% in recent series.[10,11]

Extended transsphenoidal approaches allow access to pituitary adenomas that previously required a transcranial approach, such as dumbbell-shaped tumors and adenomas with large suprasellar extension. However, these extended approaches may increase the rate of complications.[12,13] Extended transsphenoidal approaches have also improved the ability to access the medial and lateral cavernous sinus, and studies have demonstrated the feasibility and efficacy of this approach for some adenomas with cavernous sinus invasion.[14–16]

Three-dimensional endoscopic pituitary surgery is now being used at some centers. This technique has the advantages of endoscopy in addition to the stereopsis that was previously only available with microscopy. Initial impressions of this technology have been positive, with improved depth perception and no increase in operative time or surgical complications.[17,18] Furthermore, the use of 3-dimensional endoscopy does not appear to increase operative risks.[19] A study examining both subjective and objective performance in 2-dimensional versus 3-dimension endoscopy showed surgeon preference for 3-dimensional endoscopes and a measureable benefit of 3-dimensional visualization when practicing simulated surgical tasks.[18,20]

RADIOTHERAPY

Radiation therapy is not recommended for patients with complete tumor resection.[21] However, since presence of residual tumor postoperatively is a predictor of re-enlargement,[22] accurate assessment of the postoperative magnetic resonance image (MRI) is imperative to determine if radiotherapy is required. Stereotactic radiosurgery and fractionated stereotactic radiation have both been shown to be effective in preventing tumor growth after surgery and are typically well tolerated.[23–25] Stereotactic radiosurgery is the most commonly used technique to deliver radiation to pituitary tumors, although several other modalities are available.[26] Complications after radiosurgery for pituitary adenomas include hypopituitarism and less commonly injury to the visual system.[26] Smaller tumor residuals are more responsive to radiotherapy, and hypopituitarism is less common in these situations.[26]

Outcomes from radiosurgery for nonfunctioning pituitary adenomas are generally favorable, with tumor control rates of greater than 90% being reported in some studies and tumor burden reduction occurring in up to two-thirds of patients.[27] Rates of biochemical response to radiosurgery for ACTH-producing tumors range between 42% and 60%, with most patients exhibiting a response in the first 3 years.[28–31] Rates of biochemical response to radiation for growth hormone (GH)-producing adenomas and prolactinomas are probably near 45% and higher with radiation and medical therapy combined.[26] Radiosurgery has also been used for treatment of pituitary carcinomas with less success.[32]

DOPAMINE AGONISTS

Treatment with dopamine agonists is considered the first line of treatment for prolactinomas.[33] Dopamine receptor agonists exert their effects via activation of the D_2 receptor. The most common dopamine agonists used in clinical trials are bromocriptine and cabergoline.[34] Even large or giant prolactinomas may respond to treatment with dopamine agonists, and therefore in most cases surgery should be deferred until after a trial of medical treatment.[35] However, prolactinomas may be resistant to dopamine agonists either primarily or after an initially positive response. In these cases, surgery, radiation therapy or temozolomide may be of use.[36]

Dopamine agonists have been used for treatment of other types of pituitary adenomas as well. GH-producing adenomas may respond to dopamine agonists, either alone or in combination with somatostatin analogs, although at lower rates than prolactinomas.[34] Response to cabergoline is better in acromegaly patients with mildly elevated insulinlike growth factor 1 (IGF-1) levels and in those with prior radiation treatment, while serum prolactin level and immunohistochemistry for prolactin are less important.[37] Nonfunctioning adenomas may express D_2 receptors, and response to dopamine agonists with reduction in tumor size in some patients has been reported.[38] Corticotroph adenomas may also express D_2 receptors and thus respond to dopamine agonists.[39] Response to dopamine agonists in patients with aggressive pituitary tumors varies from lack of response[40,41] to tumor control or shrinkage, usually with higher doses than the US Food and Drug Administration (FDA)-approved dose for treatment of prolactinomas.[35,42]

SOMATOSTATIN ANALOGS

Somatostatin analogs such as octreotide are used for the treatment of pituitary tumors that produce GH, ACTH, or thyrotropin (TSH). Pasireotide is a new somatostatin agonist with a high affinity for somatostatin receptors that may hold promise for acromegaly, Cushing disease, and silent ACTH clinically nonfunctioning pituitary adenomas.[43] Pasireotide has a high affinity for type 5 somatostatin receptors that are preferentially expressed on corticotroph tumors.[33] A randomized phase 2 trial in patients with acromegaly showed promising results. In this study, patients received octreotide for 28 days followed by 3 different doses of pasireotide in random order, each for 28 days. Twenty seven percent of patients had a biochemical response, and 39% of patients had a 20% or greater reduction in tumor volume after treatment with pasireotide.[44]

Pasireotide has also been used in trials for the treatment of Cushing disease. In a preliminary study with 39 patients, pasireotide was well tolerated, with gastrointestinal symptoms and injection site reactions being the most common adverse effects.[45] Serum cortisol concentrations were reduced in 76% of patients, with 17% of patients having levels that normalized. Given the rigorous inclusion criteria and small sample size of this study, more studies will be needed to determine the efficacy of pasireotide in the treatment of Cushing disease. A phase 3 trial is in progress to assess the efficacy of pasireotide after 7 months of treatment.

TARGETING ANGIOGENESIS

Angiogenesis, the process of new blood vessel growth, is thought to be a key process in tumor growth and has been recognized as a potential therapeutic target for the treatment of neoplasms throughout the body.[46] There are many molecular targets along the angiogenesis pathway, one of the most well studied being vascular endothelial growth factor (VEGF). VEGF is produced by tumor cells and binds to receptors on endothelial cells

stimulating blood vessel proliferation and increased tumor vascularity. Pituitary carcinomas have been shown to exhibit a higher density of microvasculature than adenomas.[2] PTTG, a pituitary tumor oncogene, has been shown to drive increased angiogenesis.[47] There is 1 report of the use of bevacizumab, an anti-VEGF antibody, for treatment of pituitary carcinoma.[48] The patient in this study was initially diagnosed with a silent corticotroph adenoma, a particularly aggressive subtype of pituitary adenoma,[6] that recurred after multiple surgeries and eventually metastasized to the spine. The patient underwent multiple surgeries, treatment with temozolomide, and radiotherapy for the pituitary lesion and spinal metastasis. Because the tumor expressed VEGF, the authors initiated treatment with bevacizumab, with stabilization of tumor growth thereafter. In vitro studies have also shown angiogenesis to be a potential target for treatment of aggressive pituitary tumors, with antibodies against VEGF reducing pituitary tumor size in mouse models.[49,50]

Downstream effectors in the VEGF signaling pathway may also be viable targets for chemotherapy targeting pituitary adenomas. mTOR is a protein kinase in the VEGF signaling pathway that leads to the expression of hypoxia-inducible factor, cell survival, and angiogenesis. One study examining the use of everolimus, an mTOR inhibitor, for treatment of a temozolomide-resistant pituitary carcinoma did not show success.[51] Further studies examining inhibitors of VEGF and its downstream signaling pathways will be needed before antiangiogenic therapy becomes a mainstay of medical treatment for pituitary adenomas.

TEMOZOLOMIDE

Temozolomide is a second-generation oral alkylating agent used primarily in the treatment of glioblastoma. It impairs DNA replication and induces apoptosis by methylating DNA at the O^6 position of guanine.[52] It is useful in the treatment of central nervous system tumors, because it readily crosses the blood–brain barrier. Although the optimal dosing and duration of therapy have not been defined, recent reports suggest that temozolomide is effective in pituitary tumors that are resistant to multimodality therapy.[32,48,53]

Tumors with high levels of O-6-methylguanine-DNA methyltransferase (MGMT) expression are resistant to temozolomide-induced cytotoxicity. The MGMT DNA repair enzyme removes alkyl groups from the O^6 position of guanine, preventing temozolomide-induced cytotoxicity. Epigenetic silencing of the MGMT gene by hypermethylation of its promoter results in accumulation of temozolomide-induced mutations. Low levels of MGMT expression were associated with longer survival in patients with temozolomide-treated glioblastoma.[54] A significant proportion of pituitary tumors exhibit low levels of MGMT expression. Although initial studies suggested that MGMT expression level is inversely correlated with response to temozolomide,[55–59] subsequent studies indicated a poor predictive value of only 53% based on MGMT expression.[58]

Temozolomide has been used for the treatment of pituitary tumors resistant to multimodal therapy. A report from Kovacs and colleagues[60] described a 42 year-old man with a prolactin-producing adenoma refractory to multiple transsphenoidal resections, radiotherapy, and treatment with bromocriptine, pergolide, and cabergoline, who was treated with temozolomide. Morphologic study of the tumor showed evidence of tumor cell injury. Mohammad and colleagues[61] reported marked clinical improvement and radiological evidence of tumor shrinkage in 3 patients with Cushing disease and aggressive macroadenomas treated with temozolomide. Subsequent reports have confirmed the efficacy of temozolomide in aggressive prolactin-producing tumors, corticotroph-producing tumors, GH-producing tumors, gonadotroph-producing tumors, and nonfunctioning adenomas.[53,61]

Temozolomide has also been used successfully in the treatment of patients with pituitary carcinoma. Fadul and colleagues[32] treated a 38-year-old man with a gonadotropin-producing pituitary carcinoma with temozolomide after unsuccessful treatment with octreotide and radiation therapy. The patient's pain and visual field deficits improved, and he was asymptomatic 16 months after completing treatment. More recent reports confirm the efficacy of temozolomide in the treatment of pituitary carcinomas, with patients exhibiting both clinical and radiographic responses.[53,60–65] The authors have used temozolomide in one patient with a pituitary carcinoma; however, the patient exhibited tumor progression and hematological toxicity during the course of her therapy (Ioachimescu and Oyesiku, 2010, personal communication).

Although further research is indicated to clarify the role of temozolomide in treatment of aggressive pituitary tumors, patients who exhibit a progressive course postoperatively should be considered for a trial of temozolomide regardless of MGMT expression.

GLIADEL WAFERS

Gliadel, a bischloroethyl-nitrosourea (BCNU)-impregnated wafer, has been approved by the FDA for treatment of recurrent gliomas. BCNU is a nitrosurea that exerts its effects by alkylating DNA. With the ability to bypass the blood–brain barrier and first pass metabolism by the liver, chemotherapy delivered intraoperatively to brain tumors holds promise as a means to deliver high doses of chemotherapeutics while avoiding systemic adverse effects. In trials for treatment of recurrent gliomas, Gliadel has shown to be effective and well tolerated in patients with gliomas.[66] Only one study has examined the use of Gliadel wafers for the treatment of pituitary tumors. This study demonstrated that Gliadel wafers could be safely implanted in the sella via a transcranial or transsphenoidal approach, with no complications attributed to the wafers.[67] Controlled studies will be necessary to determine if Gliadel wafers are an effective adjunct for the treatment of aggressive pituitary tumors.

PEROXISOME PROLIFERATOR-ACTIVATED RECEPTOR GAMMA AGONISTS

Peroxisome proliferator-activated receptor gamma (PPAR-γ) is a ligand-dependent transcription factor that regulates fat and glucose metabolism and has an pro-apoptotic effect through cell cycle arrest and inhibiting angiogenesis.[68] PPAR-γ activation has shown promise in vitro and in many animal models of malignancy.[69] In 2002, Heaney and colleagues[70] demonstrated PPAR-γ expression in ACTH-secreting cells in normal human pituitary and increased expression of PPAR-γ in ACTH-producing pituitary adenomas. However, in contrast with promising in vitro experiments and animal studies, positive clinical studies supporting the effect of PPAR-γ agonists in patients with pituitary tumors are lacking. A study performed in patients with acromegaly showed no effect of the PPAR-γ agonist rosiglitazone on GH or IGF-1 levels.[71] In another study, patients with Cushing disease and Nelson syndrome showed no response to rosiglitazone.[72]

OTHER TREATMENTS

BIM-23A760 is a chimera of somatostatin and dopamine, and is able to suppress both GH and prolactin. This molecule has gained interest for the treatment of both functional and nonfunctioning pituitary adenomas, as most nonfunctioning pituitary adenomas express dopamine and prolactin receptors.[73–75] In an in vitro study, BIM-23A760 was shown to induce apoptosis of nonfunctioning pituitary adenomas, likely through activation of dopamine receptors.[73] A multicenter study of nonfunctioning pituitary tumors from patients who underwent surgery also showed inhibition of tumor growth by BIM-23A760.[76] A phase 2 clinical study with BIM-23A760 in 11 patients with acromegaly initially showed promising results with a reduction in growth hormone levels; however, subsequent data revealed less impressive somatostatinergic activity, and drug development was halted.[33]

Estrogen receptors are present on pituitary tumors, and high-dose estrogen may increase the growth of some pituitary tumors.[77] In vitro administration of an estrogen antagonist to cultures of human pituitary tumors inhibited the production of pituitary tumor transforming gene, which is involved in pituitary tumorigenesis and angiogenesis.[78] In this same study, estrogen antagonism inhibited rat pituitary tumor growth. Tamoxifen, an estrogen receptor antagonist, has been used in patients with bromocriptine-resistant prolactinomas, with reductions of prolactin levels but without clinical cure.[36]

There are other case reports and smaller studies of novel treatments for aggressive pituitary tumors. Capecitabine, a chemotherapeutic that acts via its conversion to 5-fluorouracil, has been used in combination with temozolomide in 1 case of an aggressive ACTH-producing adenoma. This chemotherapy regimen, which has been used previously for patients with other neuroendocrine tumors, was effective in temporarily reducing tumor burden in the patient.[79]

SUMMARY

The therapy of aggressive pituitary adenomas remains a challenge, and randomized clinical trials are lacking. Even with improved surgical technology and more molecular targets for medical therapy, the prognosis for patients with aggressive pituitary adenomas and carcinomas remains poor. At this time, the authors recommend multimodal therapy, careful evaluation, and individualization of treatment for each patient.

REFERENCES

1. Ono M, Miki N, Amano K, et al. A case of corticotroph carcinoma that caused multiple cranial nerve palsies, destructive petrosal bone invasion, and liver metastasis. Endocr Pathol 2011;22(1):10–7.
2. Kaltsas GA, Nomikos P, Kontogeorgos G, et al. Clinical review: diagnosis and management of pituitary carcinomas. J Clin Endocrinol Metab 2005;90(5):3089–99.
3. Scheithauer BW, Gaffey TA, Lloyd RV, et al. Pathobiology of pituitary adenomas and carcinomas. Neurosurgery 2006;59(2):341–53 [discussion: 53].
4. Zada G, Woodmansee WW, Ramkissoon S, et al. Atypical pituitary adenomas: incidence, clinical characteristics, and implications. J Neurosurg 2011;114(2):336–44.
5. Cho HY, Cho SW, Kim SW, et al. Silent corticotroph adenomas have unique recurrence characteristics compared with other nonfunctioning pituitary adenomas. Clin Endocrinol (Oxf) 2010;72(5):648–53.
6. Scheithauer BW, Jaap AJ, Horvath E, et al. Clinically silent corticotroph tumors of the pituitary gland. Neurosurgery 2000;47(3):723–9 [discussion: 9–30].
7. Bradley KJ, Wass JA, Turner HE. Non-functioning pituitary adenomas with positive immunoreactivity for ACTH behave more aggressively than ACTH immunonegative tumours but do not recur more frequently. Clin Endocrinol (Oxf) 2003;58(1):59–64.
8. Chen L, White WL, Spetzler RF, et al. A prospective study of nonfunctioning pituitary adenomas: presentation, management, and clinical outcome. J Neurooncol 2011;102(1):129–38.
9. Komotar RJ, Starke RM, Raper DM, et al. Endoscopic endonasal compared with microscopic transsphenoidal and open transcranial resection of giant pituitary adenomas. Pituitary 2012;15(2):150–9.
10. Berker M, Hazer DB, Yucel T, et al. Complications of endoscopic surgery of the pituitary adenomas: analysis of 570 patients and review of the literature. Pituitary 2011. [Epub ahead of print].
11. Ciric I, Ragin A, Baumgartner C, et al. Complications of transsphenoidal surgery: results of a national survey, review of the literature, and personal experience. Neurosurgery 1997;40(2):225–36 [discussion: 36–7].
12. Kaptain GJ, Vincent DA, Sheehan JP, et al. Transsphenoidal approaches for the extracapsular resection of midline suprasellar and anterior cranial base lesions. Neurosurgery 2008;62(6 Suppl 3):1264–71.
13. Di Maio S, Cavallo LM, Esposito F, et al. Extended endoscopic endonasal approach for selected pituitary adenomas: early experience. J Neurosurg 2011;114(2):345–53.
14. Kitano M, Taneda M, Shimono T, et al. Extended transsphenoidal approach for surgical management of pituitary adenomas invading the cavernous sinus. J Neurosurg 2008;108(1):26–36.
15. Zhao B, Wei YK, Li GL, et al. Extended transsphenoidal approach for pituitary adenomas invading the anterior cranial base, cavernous sinus, and clivus: a single-center experience with 126 consecutive cases. J Neurosurg 2010;112(1):108–17.
16. Ceylan S, Koc K, Anik I. Extended endoscopic transphenoidal approach for tuberculum sellae meningiomas. Acta Neurochir (Wien) 2011;153(1):1–9.
17. Brown SM, Tabaee A, Singh A, et al. Three-dimensional endoscopic sinus surgery: feasibility and

technical aspects. Otolaryngol Head Neck Surg 2008;138(3):400–2.

18. Kari E, Oyesiku NM, Dadashev V, et al. Comparison of traditional 2-dimensional endoscopic pituitary surgery with new 3-dimensional endoscopic technology: intraoperative and early postoperative factors. Int Forum Allergy Rhinol 2012; 2(1):2–8.

19. Tabaee A, Anand VK, Fraser JF, et al. Three-dimensional endoscopic pituitary surgery. Neurosurgery 2009;64(5 Suppl 2):288–93 [discussion: 94–5].

20. Fraser JF, Allen B, Anand VK, et al. Three-dimensional neurostereoendoscopy: subjective and objective comparison to 2D. Minim Invasive Neurosurg 2009;52(1):25–31.

21. Chang EF, Zada G, Kim S, et al. Long-term recurrence and mortality after surgery and adjuvant radiotherapy for nonfunctional pituitary adenomas. J Neurosurg 2008;108(4):736–45.

22. Greenman Y, Ouaknine G, Veshchev I, et al. Postoperative surveillance of clinically nonfunctioning pituitary macroadenomas: markers of tumour quiescence and regrowth. Clin Endocrinol (Oxf) 2003;58(6):763–9.

23. Molitch ME. Nonfunctioning pituitary tumors and pituitary incidentalomas. Endocrinol Metab Clin North Am 2008;37(1):151–71.

24. Gopalan R, Schlesinger D, Vance ML, et al. Long-term outcomes after gamma knife radiosurgery for patients with a nonfunctioning pituitary adenoma. Neurosurgery 2011;69(2):284–93.

25. Sheehan JP, Pouratian N, Steiner L, et al. Gamma knife surgery for pituitary adenomas: factors related to radiological and endocrine outcomes. J Neurosurg 2011;114(2):303–9.

26. Loeffler JS, Shih HA. Radiation therapy in the management of pituitary adenomas. J Clin Endocrinol Metab 2011;96(7):1992–2003.

27. Mingione V, Yen CP, Vance ML, et al. Gamma surgery in the treatment of nonsecretory pituitary macroadenoma. J Neurosurg 2006;104(6):876–83.

28. Jagannathan J, Sheehan JP, Pouratian N, et al. Gamma knife surgery for Cushing's disease. J Neurosurg 2007;106(6):980–7.

29. Castinetti F, Nagai M, Dufour H, et al. Gamma knife radiosurgery is a successful adjunctive treatment in Cushing's disease. Eur J Endocrinol 2007; 156(1):91–8.

30. Devin JK, Allen GS, Cmelak AJ, et al. The efficacy of linear accelerator radiosurgery in the management of patients with Cushing's disease. Stereotact Funct Neurosurg 2004;82(5–6):254–62.

31. Petit JH, Biller BM, Yock TI, et al. Proton stereotactic radiotherapy for persistent adrenocorticotropin-producing adenomas. J Clin Endocrinol Metab 2008;93(2):393–9.

32. Fadul CE, Kominsky AL, Meyer LP, et al. Long-term response of pituitary carcinoma to temozolomide. Report of two cases. J Neurosurg 2006;105(4):621–6.

33. Gueorguiev M, Grossman AB. Pituitary tumors in 2010: a new therapeutic era for pituitary tumors. Nat Rev Endocrinol 2011;7(2):71–3.

34. Ivan G, Szigeti-Csucs N, Olah M, et al. Treatment of pituitary tumors: dopamine agonists. Endocrine 2005;28(1):101–10.

35. Shimon I, Benbassat C, Hadani M. Effectiveness of long-term cabergoline treatment for giant prolactinoma: study of 12 men. Eur J Endocrinol 2007;156(2): 225–31.

36. Oh MC, Aghi MK. Dopamine agonist-resistant prolactinomas. J Neurosurg 2011;114(5):1369–79.

37. Sandret L, Maison P, Chanson P. Place of cabergoline in acromegaly: a meta-analysis. J Clin Endocrinol Metab 2011;96(5):1327–35.

38. Pivonello R, Matrone C, Filippella M, et al. Dopamine receptor expression and function in clinically nonfunctioning pituitary tumors: comparison with the effectiveness of cabergoline treatment. J Clin Endocrinol Metab 2004;89(4):1674–83.

39. Pivonello R, Ferone D, de Herder WW, et al. Dopamine receptor expression and function in corticotroph pituitary tumors. J Clin Endocrinol Metab 2004;89(5):2452–62.

40. Naves LA, Jaffrain-Rea ML, Vencio SA, et al. Aggressive prolactinoma in a child related to germline mutation in the ARYL hydrocarbon receptor interacting protein (AIP) gene. Arq Bras Endocrinol Metabol 2010;54(8):761–7.

41. Zornitzki T, Knobler H, Nass D, et al. Increased MIB-1/Ki-67 labeling index as a predictor of an aggressive course in a case of prolactinoma. Horm Res 2004;61(3):111–6.

42. Petrossians P, Ronci N, Valdes Socin H, et al. ACTH silent adenoma shrinking under cabergoline. Eur J Endocrinol 2001;144(1):51–7.

43. Colao A, Grasso LF, Pivonello R, et al. Therapy of aggressive pituitary tumors. Expert Opin Pharmacother 2011;12(10):1561–70.

44. Petersenn S, Schopohl J, Barkan A, et al. Pasireotide (SOM230) demonstrates efficacy and safety in patients with acromegaly: a randomized, multicenter, phase II trial. J Clin Endocrinol Metab 2010;95(6):2781–9.

45. Boscaro M, Ludlam WH, Atkinson B, et al. Treatment of pituitary-dependent Cushing's disease with the multireceptor ligand somatostatin analog pasireotide (SOM230): a multicenter, phase II trial. J Clin Endocrinol Metab 2009;94(1):115–22.

46. Folkman J. Angiogenesis: an organizing principle for drug discovery? Nat Rev Drug Discov 2007;6(4): 273–86.

47. Malik MT, Kakar SS. Regulation of angiogenesis and invasion by human pituitary tumor transforming

gene (PTTG) through increased expression and secretion of matrix metalloproteinase-2 (MMP-2). Mol Cancer 2006;5:61.

48. Ortiz LD, Syro LV, Scheithauer BW, et al. Anti-VEGF therapy in pituitary carcinoma. Pituitary 2011. [Epub ahead of print].

49. Korsisaari N, Ross J, Wu X, et al. Blocking vascular endothelial growth factor-A inhibits the growth of pituitary adenomas and lowers serum prolactin level in a mouse model of multiple endocrine neoplasia type 1. Clin Cancer Res 2008;14(1):249–58.

50. Luque GM, Perez-Millan MI, Ornstein AM, et al. Inhibitory effects of antivascular endothelial growth factor strategies in experimental dopamine-resistant prolactinomas. J Pharmacol Exp Ther 2011;337(3):766–74.

51. Jouanneau E, Wierinckx A, Ducray F, et al. New targeted therapies in pituitary carcinoma resistant to temozolomide. Pituitary 2012;15(1):37–43.

52. Stupp R, Mason WP, van den Bent MJ, et al. Radiotherapy plus concomitant and adjuvant temozolomide for glioblastoma. N Engl J Med 2005;352(10): 987–96.

53. Syro LV, Ortiz LD, Scheithauer BW, et al. Treatment of pituitary neoplasms with temozolomide: a review. Cancer 2011;117(3):454–62.

54. Hegi ME, Diserens AC, Gorlia T, et al. MGMT gene silencing and benefit from temozolomide in glioblastoma. N Engl J Med 2005;352(10):997–1003.

55. Annamalai AK, Dean AF, Kandasamy N, et al. Temozolomide responsiveness in aggressive corticotroph tumours: a case report and review of the literature. Pituitary 2011. [Epub ahead of print].

56. Kovacs K, Scheithauer BW, Lombardero M, et al. MGMT immunoexpression predicts responsiveness of pituitary tumors to temozolomide therapy. Acta Neuropathol 2008;115(2):261–2.

57. Salehi F, Scheithauer BW, Kovacs K, et al. MGMT immunohistochemical expression in pituitary corticotroph adenomas. Neurosurgery 2011. [Epub ahead of print].

58. Salehi F, Scheithauer BW, Kros JM, et al. MGMT promoter methylation and immunoexpression in aggressive pituitary adenomas and carcinomas. J Neurooncol 2011;104(3):647–57.

59. Bush ZM, Longtine JA, Cunningham T, et al. Temozolomide treatment for aggressive pituitary tumors: correlation of clinical outcome with O(6)-methylguanine methyltransferase (MGMT) promoter methylation and expression. J Clin Endocrinol Metab 2010;95(11):E280–90.

60. Kovacs K, Horvath E, Syro LV, et al. Temozolomide therapy in a man with an aggressive prolactin-secreting pituitary neoplasm: morphological findings. Hum Pathol 2007;38(1):185–9.

61. Mohammed S, Kovacs K, Mason W, et al. Use of temozolomide in aggressive pituitary tumors: case report. Neurosurgery 2009;64(4):E773–4 [discussion: E4].

62. Lim S, Shahinian H, Maya MM, et al. Temozolomide: a novel treatment for pituitary carcinoma. Lancet Oncol 2006;7(6):518–20.

63. Dillard TH, Gultekin SH, Delashaw JB Jr, et al. Temozolomide for corticotroph pituitary adenomas refractory to standard therapy. Pituitary 2011;14(1):80–91.

64. Raverot G, Sturm N, de Fraipont F, et al. Temozolomide treatment in aggressive pituitary tumors and pituitary carcinomas: a French multicenter experience. J Clin Endocrinol Metab 2010; 95(10):4592–9.

65. Syro LV, Uribe H, Penagos LC, et al. Antitumour effects of temozolomide in a man with a large, invasive prolactin-producing pituitary neoplasm. Clin Endocrinol (Oxf) 2006;65(4):552–3.

66. Brem H, Piantadosi S, Burger PC, et al. Placebo-controlled trial of safety and efficacy of intraoperative controlled delivery by biodegradable polymers of chemotherapy for recurrent gliomas. The Polymer-brain Tumor Treatment Group. Lancet 1995;345(8956):1008–12.

67. Laws ER Jr, Morris AM, Maartens N. Gliadel for pituitary adenomas and craniopharyngiomas. Neurosurgery 2003;53(2):255–69 [discussion: 9–60].

68. Occhi G, Albiger N, Berlucchi S, et al. Peroxisome proliferator-activated receptor gamma in the human pituitary gland: expression and splicing pattern in adenomas versus normal pituitary. J Neuroendocrinol 2007;19(7):552–9.

69. Ondrey F. Peroxisome proliferator-activated receptor gamma pathway targeting in carcinogenesis: implications for chemoprevention. Clin Cancer Res 2009;15(1):2–8.

70. Heaney AP, Fernando M, Yong WH, et al. Functional PPAR-gamma receptor is a novel therapeutic target for ACTH-secreting pituitary adenomas. Nat Med 2002;8(11):1281–7.

71. Bastemir M, Akin F, Yaylali GF. The PPAR-gamma activator rosiglitazone fails to lower plasma growth hormone and insulin-like growth factor-1 levels in patients with acromegaly. Neuroendocrinology 2007;86(2):119–23.

72. Kreutzer J, Jeske I, Hofmann B, et al. No effect of the PPAR-gamma agonist rosiglitazone on ACTH or cortisol secretion in Nelson's syndrome and Cushing's disease in vitro and in vivo. Clin Neuropathol 2009;28(6):430–9.

73. Peverelli E, Olgiati L, Locatelli M, et al. The dopamine–somatostatin chimeric compound BIM-23A760 exerts antiproliferative and cytotoxic effects in human non-functioning pituitary tumors by activating ERK1/2 and p38 pathways. Cancer Lett 2010;288(2):170–6.

74. Jaquet P, Gunz G, Saveanu A, et al. Efficacy of chimeric molecules directed towards multiple somatostatin and dopamine receptors on inhibition of GH and prolactin secretion from GH-secreting

pituitary adenomas classified as partially responsive to somatostatin analog therapy. Eur J Endocrinol 2005;153(1):135–41.

75. Saveanu A, Gunz G, Guillen S, et al. Somatostatin and dopamine-somatostatin multiple ligands directed towards somatostatin and dopamine receptors in pituitary adenomas. Neuroendocrinology 2006;83(3–4):258–63.

76. Florio T, Barbieri F, Spaziante R, et al. Efficacy of a dopamine-somatostatin chimeric molecule, BIM-23A760, in the control of cell growth from primary cultures of human non-functioning pituitary adenomas: a multi-center study. Endocr Relat Cancer 2008;15(2):583–96.

77. Heaney AP. Pituitary tumour pathogenesis. Br Med Bull 2005;75–76:81–97.

78. Heaney AP, Fernando M, Melmed S. Functional role of estrogen in pituitary tumor pathogenesis. J Clin Invest 2002;109(2):277–83.

79. Thearle MS, Freda PU, Bruce JN, et al. Temozolomide (Temodar(R)) and capecitabine (Xeloda(R)) treatment of an aggressive corticotroph pituitary tumor. Pituitary 2011;14(4):418–24.

Clinical Management of Pituitary Carcinomas

Michael C. Oh, MD, PhD[a], Tarik Tihan, MD, PhD[b],
Sandeep Kunwar, MD[a], Lewis Blevins, MD[a],
Manish K. Aghi, MD, PhD[a],*

KEYWORDS

- Pituitary carcinoma • Atypical pituitary adenoma • Invasive pituitary adenoma • Pituitary adenoma
- Temozolomide

KEY POINTS

- Pituitary carcinomas are rare, with one study reporting only 165 cases reported in the English literature as of 2011.[1]
- Pituitary carcinomas make up only 0.1% to 0.2% of all pituitary adenomas.
- Diagnosis of pituitary carcinoma requires presence of metastases distant from the primary tumor in the sella, as local invasion is common (approximately 35%–40% of pituitary adenomas) and cannot be used to diagnose pituitary carcinomas.
- Most patients with pituitary carcinomas present initially with an invasive pituitary adenoma, although rarely, patients can present with primary pituitary carcinomas without a previous history of pituitary tumor.[2,3]
- Studies implementing histology, immunohistochemistry, genetic analysis, and ultrastructural imaging with electron microscopy cannot consistently distinguish pituitary carcinomas from adenomas and should be used only to supplement the diagnosis.

INTRODUCTION

Pituitary tumors represent 10% to 15% of primary intracranial neoplasms[4,5] and the overwhelming majority are benign adenomas. Pituitary carcinomas are very rare and consist of 0.1% to 0.2% of all pituitary tumors.[1,6–8] According to the 2004 World Health Organization (WHO) classification of endocrine tumors, tumors of the adenohypophysis are classified into benign pituitary adenomas, atypical pituitary adenomas, and pituitary carcinomas.[9,10] It is not clear whether pituitary carcinomas arise de novo as distinct malignant tumors or are malignant transformation of typical or atypical pituitary adenomas.

Whether there are clinically useful molecular, genetic or pathologic, differences among the 3 WHO classes of pituitary tumors are not known at this time. The histologic, immunohistochemical, radiographical, and ultrastructural analyses are limited in distinguishing typical and atypical adenomas, and malignant carcinomas.

Pituitary carcinomas portend a poor prognosis. They are mostly endocrine active tumors with very aggressive clinical features and rapid progression, often unresponsive to conventional therapies that are often effective against hormonally active adenomas. Clinical progression includes severe medical morbidities related to hormone overproduction (ie, Cushing's disease) and mass effects from sellar and distant tumor expansion. Current treatment paradigms include multiple surgical resections, although complete resection may be unrealistic given the extent of

[a] Department of Neurological Surgery, California Center for Pituitary Disorders, University of California, San Francisco, 400 Parnassus Avenue, A-808, San Francisco, CA 94143, USA; [b] Department of Pathology, University of California, San Francisco, 505 Parnassus Avenus, M551, San Francisco, CA 94143, USA
* Corresponding author. Department of Neurologic Surgery, University of California at San Francisco, M770, Box0112, 505 Parnassus Avenue, San Francisco, CA 94143.
E-mail address: AghiM@neurosurg.ucsf.edu

Neurosurg Clin N Am 23 (2012) 595–606
http://dx.doi.org/10.1016/j.nec.2012.06.009
1042-3680/12/$ – see front matter © 2012 Elsevier Inc. All rights reserved.

invasion or with multiple metastatic lesions. Other alternatives, such as radiation therapy, systemic chemotherapy, and medical therapies to treat hormone overproduction are also of limited help (ie, dopamine agonist therapy). Despite aggressive treatments, all of these treatments have proven to be palliative at best. Cytotoxic chemotherapies have yielded disappointing results, despite high proliferative index of pituitary carcinomas. Recurrence with rapid tumor growth is often evident following radiation therapy. Recently, however, some strides have been made with the use of temozolomide,[11,12] a methylating alkylator agent commonly used to treat malignant gliomas. Here, we review the histopathologic features of pituitary carcinomas relative to benign and atypical pituitary adenomas, how pituitary carcinomas are best managed in the modern era, and the future directions that will hopefully lead to better treatment for this aggressive malignant disease.

HISTOPATHOLOGIC DEFINITIONS AND FEATURES

Definition of atypical pituitary adenomas is currently made on histologic grounds, while the definition of pituitary carcinoma requires the presence of metastases distant from the primary tumor in the sella.[1,7,8,10,13–15] Atypical pituitary adenomas are defined as pituitary adenomas with elevated mitotic index, Ki-67 labeling index greater than 3%, and excessive p53 immunoreactivity.[10] However, cytologic features of pituitary carcinoma can be quite similar to and often indistinguishable from adenomas (**Fig. 1**).

These WHO definitions focus on histologic evidence of mutations and proliferation (atypical adenomas) or distant metastases (pituitary carcinomas), but they ignore other aspects of pituitary tumor behavior–like invasion. This is because gross evidence of local invasion during surgery is demonstrated in approximately 35% to 40% of pituitary adenomas,[15,16] meaning that the presence of invasion alone is not sufficiently restrictive to be included in the definition of atypical adenoma or carcinoma. Recent studies suggested that atypical pituitary adenomas show higher rates of local invasion by imaging compared with "typical" pituitary adenomas.[17] Thus, local invasion is a feature common to both typical and atypical pituitary adenomas, especially in large macroadenomas, but not enough to

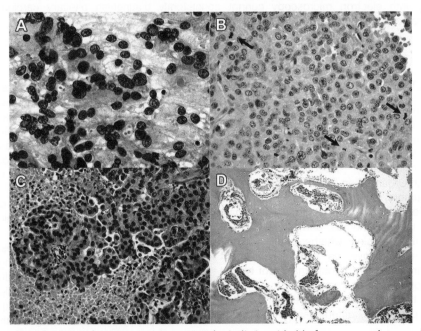

Fig. 1. (*A*) Cytologic features of pituitary carcinoma can be indistinguishable from some adenomas but typically show an increased hyperchromasia and nuclear pleomorphism (hematoxylin-eosin, original magnification ×600). (*B*) Most pituitary adenomas are indistinguishable from other epithelial carcinomas with variable degrees of pleomorphism, increased mitotic figures, and prominent nucleoli (*arrows*). However, these features are neither necessary nor sufficient for the diagnosis of pituitary carcinoma on histologic grounds (hematoxylin-eosin, original magnification ×400). (*C*) Loss of normal acinar architecture along with cytologic anaplasia and necrosis can be seen in most pituitary carcinomas (hematoxylin-eosin, original magnification ×200) (*D*) Bone invasion and invasion of adjacent tissues can be seen in both adenomas and in carcinomas of the pituitary gland. This image demonstrates invasion of the sphenoid bone by a pituitary carcinoma (hematoxylin-eosin, original magnification ×40).

render it diagnostic criteria for atypical adenomas. On the other hand, distant metastases are quite rare and thus represent an extremely restrictive criteria, making pituitary carcinoma a rare diagnostic entity. Some argue that there must be mutation(s) predisposing to metastatic ability, the presence of which might allow widening the diagnostic criteria to include pituitary tumors that look highly aggressive under a microscope without systemic metastases, but no such mutation(s) have been identified to date. Thus, although there is a clear need for well-validated genetic or histologic markers to better distinguish pituitary tumors by clinical aggressiveness, clinicians for the moment must recognize the 3 WHO classes of pituitary tumors defined as described previously.

EPIDEMIOLOGY OF PITUITARY CARCINOMA

Pituitary carcinomas are very rare, with one study reporting only 165 cases reported in the English literature as of 2011.[1] Although the evidence of local invasion is found intraoperative in 35% to 40% of cases,[15,16] pituitary carcinomas make up only 0.1% to 0.2% of all pituitary adenomas. By comparison, atypical pituitary adenomas represent approximately 15% of all pituitary adenomas.[17] Thus, the transformation that allows a pituitary carcinoma to form (ie, metastases) from either a pituitary adenoma, directly from normal pituitary gland tissue, or from an as yet unidentified precursor state is a rare event.

Both genders are equally affected by pituitary carcinomas with a mean age at presentation in the fifth decade. By contrast, pituitary adenomas, especially of prolactinomas, are more common in women,[18,19] possibly because of the ease of detecting endocrine symptoms in women compared with men.

Pituitary carcinoma seems to affect only the adult population, although one case report of pituitary carcinoma in a 9-year-old girl with widespread metastases to the craniospinal axis has been reported.[20] In one study of 15 patients (8 males and 7 females) with pituitary carcinoma,[6] the mean age was 56 with a range of 34 to 71.

Most (88%) pituitary carcinomas are hormonally active tumors.[1,6–8,21] The incidence of nonfunctioning pituitary carcinomas has been very low in recent years.[6,22] According to a study, hormonally active pituitary carcinomas predominantly consist of adrenocorticotropic hormone (ACTH) (42%) and prolactin-secreting (33%) carcinomas, followed by growth hormone (6%), gonadotropic hormones (5%), and thyroid-stimulating hormones (1%).[7] Null-cell pituitary carcinomas represent approximately 12%.[7]

PATHOPHYSIOLOGY OF PITUITARY CARCINOMAS
Etiology of Pituitary Carcinomas: De Novo Versus Malignant Transformation of Invasive Pituitary Adenomas

Whether pituitary carcinomas occur de novo or progress from invasive, typical, or atypical pituitary adenomas is unknown. Pituitary carcinomas without evidence of a prior benign lesion have been reported, suggesting the possibility of de novo occurrences.[2,3] As an entirely speculative possibility, pituitary carcinomas may start out as atypical adenomas that undergo malignant transformation. Typically, histologic features of aggressive pituitary adenomas as well as pituitary carcinomas remain more or less similar throughout the disease course (see **Fig. 1**). Recurrence of pituitary carcinoma is common, and may require repeated surgical resections, more aggressive medical therapy, and radiation therapy. Despite these aggressive measures, most tumors progress and result in the demise of the patient.

Some investigators believe that pituitary carcinomas progress from invasive pituitary adenomas, possibly with the atypical pituitary adenomas being the most likely culprit. Others have speculated dissemination of aggressive adenomas following surgical resection, but this hypothesis has not been adequately supported in the literature. Similarly, malignant transformation caused by radiation therapy has not received a wide support, although there are reports of sarcomatous changes in pituitary adenomas following radiation therapy.[23] A review of 36 cases of pituitary carcinoma in 1989 found that fewer than half (18 of 38) of patients with pituitary carcinomas were previously treated with radiation therapy.[24] The risk of developing secondary brain tumors following external beam radiotherapy for pituitary adenoma is also relatively low at 1.3% at 10 years and 1.9% at 20 years following treatment with a relative risk of 9.38 compared with the normal population.[25] Although these rates seem higher than the progression rates of pituitary adenomas to carcinomas (0.1%–0.2%), in the same study, there were no malignant transformations of pituitary adenomas in 3760 observed patient years.[25] Thus, it appears that radiation treatment does not significantly increase the risk of carcinomatous transformation of pituitary adenomas.

Local Invasion: A Step Toward Metastatic Transformation?

Pituitary adenomas commonly invade through local structures, such as dura, bone, cavernous sinus, and even blood vessels and nerve sheaths (see **Fig. 1**D). Although evidence of local invasion by gross observation during surgery ranges from 35% to 40%,[15,16] microscopic demonstration of dural invasion can be demonstrated in up to 85% of patients with pituitary adenomas.[16] Atypical adenomas have significantly higher rates of local invasion (83%) by imaging compared with "typical" adenomas (45%).[17]

The natural expansion of an adenohypophysial tumor involves the dura mater. Therefore, it is not surprising to find dural invasion increasing in frequency with increasing tumor size. In one study, microadenomas, macroadenomas, and tumors with suprasellar extension had 69%, 88%, and 94% incidence of dural invasion by microscopic evaluation, respectively.[16] In a larger cohort study consisting of 354 patients treated with trans-sphenoidal surgery, percentage of tumors with dural invasion correlated with increasing tumor size: 24% for 10 mm or smaller, 35% for 10 to 20 mm, 55% for 20 to 40 mm, and 70% dural invasion for larger than 40 mm tumor size.[26] Whether dural invasion should be considered similar to invasion of surrounding soft tissues is debatable. There is still much work needed to correlate the extent of dural invasion with evidence of biologic aggressiveness not related to simple tumor growth rate. Currently, there is no evidence to suggest that dural invasion is independent of tumor size or growth rate as a prognostic indicator.

Evidence against this suggestion is the observation that local invasion, including dural invasion, does not confer malignancy or predict future transformation to pituitary carcinomas, as most invasive pituitary adenomas do not metastasize. For example, a recent study found that although dural invasion was significantly more common in the repeated trans-sphenoidal surgery group (69%) compared with the primary surgery group (41%), it is not a predictive factor for recurrence.[26] This study also found that mortality rates were higher in the group with dural invasion (9%) compared with the group with no invasion (0%) at the end of a 6-year follow-up.[26] However, this mortality rate is very small compared with the typical mortality rate in pituitary carcinomas, where 66% of patients with pituitary carcinoma die within the first year of diagnosis.[6] Furthermore, determination of dural invasion does not appear to be independent of tumor size or growth rate. It is still possible that invasive features may predict a more aggressive clinical course and may portend a higher risk, especially in hormonally active tumors. Most importantly, however, invasive features do not consistently predict malignant transformation.

Further evidence suggesting that local invasion does not consistently confer malignancy comes from studies looking at hormonal profiles of pituitary adenomas. For example, dural invasion is most frequently found in the nonfunctioning pituitary adenomas at 54.2%,[26] whereas most pituitary carcinomas are endocrine active.[1,6–8,21] By comparison, only 30% to 35% of endocrine-active tumors have dural invasion.[26] Most of the invasive nonfunctioning pituitary adenomas will never progress to pituitary carcinomas. In another study, 50% of atypical pituitary adenomas were nonfunctioning lesions,[17] suggesting the possibility that only a small percentage of endocrine-active, atypical pituitary adenomas could transform into pituitary carcinomas. The factors that determine which tumors progress to pituitary carcinomas remain elusive at this time, although invasive, atypical macroadenomas that are endocrine active are the most likely candidates.

The evidence for malignant transformation of pituitary adenomas rather than de novo pituitary carcinoma formation include the following:

- Most pituitary carcinomas initially present as aggressive pituitary tumors with multiple recurrences that "escape" medical, surgical, and radiation treatments[1,6–8,13,14,21];
- The latency of transformation from pituitary adenomas to carcinomas usually takes months to years. In the setting of Nelson syndrome, in which ACTH-secreting carcinoma develops following bilateral adrenalectomy for Cushing syndrome, the mean interval between the diagnosis of adenoma and carcinoma is 15.3 years[6];
- There is no histologic distinction between pituitary carcinomas and invasive macroadenomas. The decision of a pituitary carcinoma is made only after a metastatic focus is discovered.

Genetic, Molecular, and Ultrastructural Make-Up of Pituitary Carcinomas

Numerous studies have attempted to distinguish the genetic, molecular, and ultrastructural make-up of pituitary carcinomas from adenomas. Although some trends are important to note, generally the case-to-case variability has been so large that all of these features have failed to consistently distinguish among benign, invasive, and malignant pituitary tumors. Histologic features that define malignancy in other brain tumors, such as necrosis, invasion of surrounding structures, hypercellularity, increased mitotic activity, and pleomorphism, are found in benign and atypical pituitary adenomas, as well as pituitary carcinomas.[14]

Studies indicate that proliferative and mitotic activities are generally higher in carcinomas compared with invasive adenomas. In one study, Ki-67 cell cycle–specific nuclear antigen detected by MIB-1 antibody was increased in the order of invasiveness: mean Ki-67 fractions were 1.37%, 4.66%, and 11.91% for noninvasive adenomas, invasive adenomas, and pituitary carcinomas, respectively.[27] Setting the Ki-67 labeling index threshold at 3% allows one to distinguish noninvasive from invasive tumors with 97% specificity and 73% sensitivity.[27] However, other studies have not found such clear correlation of Ki-67 labeling with the invasive potential of tumors.[28] Evaluation of mitotic figures[29,30] and proliferating cell nuclear antigen[31] have shown increased proliferation index in more invasive, higher grade tumors as well.

Molecular oncogenes that are often altered in other malignancies, such as p53, p27, Ras, retinoblastoma gene, MEN-1, gsp, nm23, and HER-2/neu, are also found to be affected in pituitary carcinomas, but not consistently enough to allow differentiation from benign adenomas.[1,6–8,13,14,21] In one study, p53 was expressed in a larger fraction in higher-grade pituitary tumors with 0%, 15.2%, and 100% expression in noninvasive adenomas, invasive adenomas, and pituitary carcinomas, respectively.[32] Interestingly, a higher fraction of metastatic lesions (83%) expressed p53 compared with primary sellar lesions (57%), suggesting that metastatic lesions may have accumulated more genetic abnormalities that make them able to metastasize.

An ultrastructural study using transmission electron microscopy also confirmed significant cellular atypia and mitotic activity in most pituitary carcinomas, but concluded that pituitary adenomas and carcinomas cannot be distinguished on ultrastructural features alone.[33] A detailed summary of histologic, immunohistochemical, and genetic alternations; proliferation indices; and ultrastructural studies of pituitary carcinomas have been thoroughly reviewed elsewhere.[1,6–8,13–15,21]

CLINICAL PRESENTATION AND PROGRESSION OF PITUITARY CARCINOMA
Clinical Presentation

Most patients with pituitary carcinomas present initially with an invasive pituitary adenoma, although rarely, patients can present with primary pituitary carcinomas without a previous history of pituitary tumor (**Fig. 2**).[2,3] Transformation of pituitary adenomas to pituitary carcinomas usually takes 6 to 8 years.[6,34] Clinical progression includes symptoms related to hormone overproduction (ie, Cushing disease), symptoms of local mass effect from tumor expansion of the sellar and suprasellar space, or symptoms of systemic metastases.

Mass effects near the sellar region consist of symptoms similar to those found in macroadenomas, including visual field deficits and decreased visual acuity owing to compression of optic chiasm; headaches from stretching of the nearby dura or diaphragm sella; cranial neuropathies from compression of cranial nerves in the cavernous sinus; and hypopituitarism owing to compression of portal vessels, pituitary stalk, and/or pituitary gland. The most common presentation of pituitary carcinoma occurs in the setting of a patient with a history of invasive pituitary neoplasm, often with multiple surgical resections or previous radiation therapy, who undergoes rapid recurrence with resistance to medical therapy, as evidenced by rising serum hormone levels. Metastases away from the primary pituitary tumor must be confirmed on imaging.

Patients with functional pituitary carcinomas present with symptoms similar to those in respective functional adenomas,[1,7,13,14,21] but possibly with higher serum hormone levels. Patients with ACTH-secreting carcinomas present with Cushing disease with typical features of hypercortisolism, including round facies, thin skin with delayed wound healing, hirsutism, striae, central obesity, supraclavicular and dorsocervical fat pads, fatigue, muscle atrophy, hypertension, osteoporosis, immunosuppression, and psychiatric problems, including depression and cognitive impairment. Serum ACTH levels ranged from 145 to 280,000 pg/mL (normal 0–60 pg/mL) in one study with 4 of 7 patients presenting in the setting of Nelson syndrome, where patients have previously undergone bilateral adrenalectomy for Cushing syndrome.[6] Extremely high levels of ACTH are common with ACTH-secreting pituitary carcinomas.[35]

Prolactin-secreting carcinomas often release very high levels of prolactin, despite dopamine agonist therapy, ranging from 6 to 21,560 ng/mL (normal <13 ng/mL in men and <27 ng/mL in women; 21,560 ng/mL was obtained in one patient during treatment with bromocriptine).[6] Elevated prolactin levels, however, are often seen in macroadenomas that are unresponsive to dopamine agonists, making the diagnosis based on prolactin levels alone unfeasible. Although patients with prolactin-secreting carcinomas may be responsive to dopamine agonists like bromocriptine or cabergoline initially, their disease eventually becomes unresponsive to medical treatment, and tumors grow despite aggressive therapies. In one study, dopamine D2 receptors (through which the dopamine agonists exert their negative trophic effects) were expressed in initial surgically resected tumor tissues but absent in postmortem

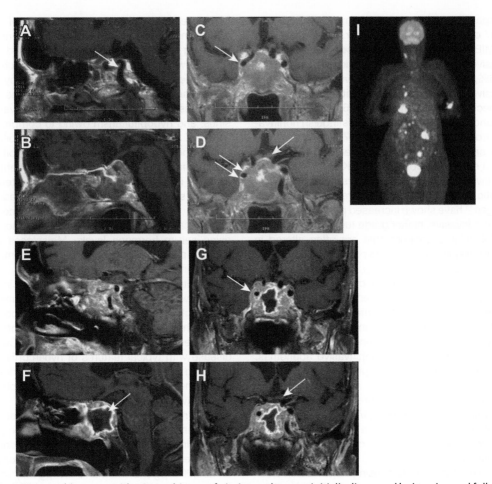

Fig. 2. A 71-year-old woman with a 3-year history of pituitary adenoma, initially diagnosed by imaging and followed with serial images without surgery, presented with 20-pound weight loss, fatigue, right ptosis with third cranial nerve palsy, and right sixth cranial nerve weakness. MRI of the brain was obtained (*A–D*, preoperative images). T1-weighted images with gadolinium enhancement (*A–H*) showed significant expansion of the pituitary tumor encasing the carotid arteries (*A, C, arrows*), a suprasellar extension and the compression of optic chiasm (*D, single arrow*), invasion into sphenoid sinus and clivus (*B*), and invasion of cavernous sinuses, which explains the cranial nerve deficits (*D, double arrows*). The patient underwent trans-sphenoidal decompression with debulking of the tumor, and the MRI obtained about a month following surgery (*E–H*, postoperative images) shows further expansion of the tumor (compare *arrows* in *G* vs *C*) but decompression of the optic chiasm (*H, arrow*). Pathologic specimen revealed MIB-1 (Ki-67) labeling of 54.4%, suggestive of very aggressive tumor. Follow-up whole-body PET scan with 2-(F-18) fluoro-2-deoxy-D-glucose confirmed the diagnosis of pituitary carcinoma with systemic metastases (*I*). Multiple systemic metastases were evident with signals in the right neck (lymph node), right superior mediastinum (hilar lymph nodes), liver, left subdiaphragmatic space, left ovary, left arm, and multiple lymph nodes in the abdomen. The patient succumbed to her disease approximately 3 months after the diagnosis of pituitary carcinoma.

tissues obtained after the diagnosis of metastatic pituitary carcinoma.[36] Thus, loss of dopamine D2 receptor expression could be one potential mechanism of resistance to dopamine agonists in prolactin-secreting carcinomas.

Endocrine symptoms of prolactin-secreting carcinomas are similar to those found in pituitary adenomas, which include decreased libido, galactorrhea, gynecomastia, amenorrhea, and infertility. Growth hormone–secreting tumors present as acromegaly, and gonadotroph and thyroid-stimulating hormone–secreting carcinomas are extremely rare.[1,6–8,13,14,21]

Metastasis can occur in the subarachnoid space, leptomeninges, or parenchyma of the central nervous system including both brain and spinal cord, or systemically with invasion into bone, liver, lymph nodes, ovary, heart, and lung. Patients with systemic metastases are thought to have a worse prognosis compared with those with craniospinal metastases. Most (75%) patients who died within 1 year following the diagnosis of pituitary carcinoma had systemic metastases.[6]

The latency of transformation of invasive pituitary adenoma to pituitary carcinoma can range from months to years. Some studies have reported transformation to pituitary carcinoma after more than a 20-year latency period.[34] In one large series with 15 patients, mean latency period was 6.6 years (median 5.0 years) with a range of 0.3 to 18.0 years.[6] In another large cohort with 15 patients, mean latency period was 7.8 years (median 5 years) with a range of 0 to 24 years.[34] The patients with Nelson syndrome, which is attributable to proliferation of ACTH-secreting tumor following bilateral adrenalectomy for Cushing syndrome, had the longest latency period with a mean of 15.3 years.[6] Interestingly, in the same study, prolactin-secreting tumors transformed to pituitary carcinomas twice as fast compared with ACTH-secreting tumors (4.7 vs 9.5 years, respectively). It is unclear currently what factors determine how quickly pituitary adenomas transform into pituitary carcinomas. It is also unclear what factors allow certain adenomas to transform into pituitary carcinomas, while most other adenomas remain benign. Clinically, patients with long-standing pituitary adenomas who rapidly progress with recurrence and develop new resistance to current therapy warrant a close monitoring for possible malignant transformation.

Diagnosis

According to the 2004 WHO classification of endocrine tumors, the diagnosis of pituitary carcinoma requires primary pituitary tumor with either systemic or craniospinal metastases.[10] Pituitary carcinomas are diagnosed by radiographic imaging with detection of metastases, followed by pathologic confirmation of pituitary origin of the metastases. The pathologic confirmation is critical, because metastatic lesions from elsewhere, including breast, bronchus, kidney, and colon cancers, can metastasize to the sellar region.[21] Thus, other metastatic disease with non-pituitary primary must be considered in the differential.

Imaging Methods

Magnetic resonance imaging (MRI) studies show pituitary carcinomas with characteristics similar to invasive macroadenomas (see **Fig. 2**A–H). T1-weighted images with gadolinium provide the best imaging to evaluate for pituitary carcinomas, which may show suprasellar extension, parasellar cavernous sinus invasion, and/or other intracranial lesions. The primary pituitary tumor

and metastases may have similar imaging characteristics on MRI.[37] In one study, the signal intensity and characteristics of the pituitary tumor and the extra-axial spinal metastatic lesion were found to be the same, suggesting similar vascularity and stroma in the 2 tumor tissues.[37]

Positron emission tomography (PET) scans and radionucleotide scans have been used, although not routinely (see **Fig. 2**I). There are reports of these studies being used for diagnosis and to determine the extent of metastases and response to therapy. In one study, dopamine D2 receptor binding and tumor amino acid metabolism were studied using PET scans. Malignant prolactinoma with high D2 receptor binding and tumor amino acid metabolism initially showed decreased D2 receptor binding, decreased tumor amino acid metabolism, and decreased tumor size in response to bromocriptine.[38] In another case report, malignant prolactinoma was diagnosed with dopamine D2 receptor scintigraphy using [^{123}Iodine]epidepride to detect multiple metastatic lesions in the ribs, femur, and spine in the absence of recurrent pituitary lesion.[39] Growth hormone–secreting pituitary carcinoma has been diagnosed with metastases in the neck without a recurrent pituitary mass using [^{111}Indium]pentetreotide.[40] These studies exemplify the feasibility of PET studies in aiding diagnosis, determining the extent and locations of metastases, and response to therapy in patients with pituitary carcinoma, especially those without a recurrent lesion in the sellar region.[39,40]

Studies implementing histology, immunohistochemistry, genetic analysis, and ultrastructural imaging with electron microscopy cannot consistently distinguish pituitary carcinomas from adenomas and should be used only to supplement the diagnosis. Further studies are needed to determine which targets (ie, histologic features, genetic mutation, oncogene or tumor suppressor gene expression, chromosomal abnormality) provide useful information toward prognosis or predict beneficial response to different treatment modalities.

Prognosis of Pituitary Carcinoma

Pituitary carcinomas portend a poor prognosis with a mean survival of 1.9 years with a range of 3 months to 8 years following the diagnosis of pituitary carcinoma.[6] They are mostly endocrine-active tumors with very aggressive clinical features and rapid progression, typically unresponsive to conventional therapies that are effective for benign adenomas. Despite aggressive multimodal treatment including surgery, radiation therapy, hormonally targeted therapies, and systemic chemotherapy, all of these treatments have proven to be palliative at best. Overall, 66% of patients died within 1 year following diagnosis, with most deaths (75%) in the first year occurring in patients with systemic metastases.[6] Systemic metastases conveys worse prognosis compared with craniospinal metastases, with the median survival with systemic metastases of 1.0 year compared with 2.6 years with craniospinal metastases.[14] Although rare, long-term survivors have been reported.[41] Although no systematic analysis has been performed, negative prognostic factors include loss of response to medical therapies with extremely high serum hormone levels, rapidly expanding tumor despite aggressive treatment, and systemic metastases.

MANAGEMENT OF PITUITARY CARCINOMAS

Because of the rarity of pituitary carcinomas, there are no studies comparing different treatment modalities. The principles applied to treating benign pituitary tumors are also applied to carcinomas. Treatment modalities include surgical resection for the primary pituitary mass and the accessible, symptomatic metastases, medical therapy, radiation therapy, and chemotherapy.

Surgical Resection

First-line therapy for pituitary carcinoma consists of surgical resection, although usually gross-total resection is not achievable because of invasion of pituitary mass into surrounding structures with multiple distant metastases. The most important value of surgical debulking in the sellar region is to decompress the important structures nearby, such as optic chiasm, pituitary stalk, pituitary gland, cranial nerves, and major cerebral blood vessels. Surgical decompression can be critical for metastases to the spine to relieve compression on the spinal cord or nerve roots. Although there are no controlled studies showing long-term benefits of surgery, anecdotal evidence suggests that surgery can provide immediate relief of symptoms.[21] Cases of complete resection of sellar lesion and metastases have been reported previously[42,43]; although the long-term control in these patients has not been followed. In series reported by Pernicone and colleagues,[6] of 15 patients, 14 underwent resection of their pituitary mass with 7 craniotomy, 6 trans-sphenoidal resection, and 1 biopsy with radiation. One patient underwent bilateral adrenalectomy with radiation.

Hormone-Targeted Therapies for Pituitary Carcinomas

The medical therapy for pituitary carcinoma consists of dopamine agonist therapy for prolactinomas and somatostatin analogs for growth hormone–secreting carcinomas. Up to 80% to 95% of prolactinomas can be controlled, both in terms of hormonal normalization and tumor reduction, with either bromocriptine or cabergoline.[44,45] More often, higher doses of drugs are needed to achieve similar results in pituitary carcinomas; however, these drugs are often ineffective for carcinomas, given that most patients are diagnosed once they become unresponsive to medical treatments with increasing serum hormone levels.[14,21,46] Good response to dopamine agonists have been reported for some patients,[38] although effects are temporary in most patients. One case report of growth hormone–secreting carcinoma responsive to bromocriptine has been described as well, in which the patient showed marked improvement in symptoms, including visual field deficits.[24] Despite this symptomatic relief, the patient became unresponsive to treatment and succumbed to the disease about a year later.

Other medical therapies for pituitary carcinomas include somatostatin analog octreotide for growth hormone– and ACTH-secreting carcinomas. Remission rates in benign growth hormone–secreting adenomas are similar for octreotide treatment compared with the surgery group, although 48-week remission rate is slightly higher in the surgery group (39% vs 28%).[47] However, the effects for carcinomas are usually temporary, with a rapid disease progression. There is also a report of thyrotropin-secreting pituitary carcinoma that was temporarily responsive to octreotide.[48] Other drugs used for benign pituitary adenomas, such as ketoconazole and pasireotide (SOM230) for recurrent Cushing disease and pegvisomant for acromegaly, need further testing for pituitary carcinomas.

Radiation Therapy for Pituitary Carcinomas

There are no systemic analyses evaluating the efficacy of radiation therapy to pituitary carcinomas, and the number of reported cases with systemic chemotherapy is low, mostly with poor results.[22] Although fractionated radiotherapy and stereotactic radiosurgery have been generally successful for pituitary adenomas resistant to medical and/or surgical therapies, there are no large series reported for pituitary carcinomas.[14] Most reported cases portray short-term control at best with poor long-term results.[1,7,14]

Systemic Chemotherapy for Pituitary Carcinoma

Despite the high proliferative index of pituitary carcinomas, systemic chemotherapy has yielded disappointing results for pituitary carcinoma, possibly because of the well-differentiated characteristics of pituitary carcinoma cells. Although there are a few reports of short-term stabilization with systemic chemotherapy,[6,24,46,49] most combinations of cytotoxic agents have yielded poor long-term benefits. The most commonly used treatment consists of combination therapy with CCNU and 5-fluorouracil, whereas carboplatin, either alone or in combination with 5-fluorouracil or interferon-α, and dacarbasine have also been used.[22] Recently, temozolomide, a methylating alkylator agent commonly used in malignant gliomas, has shown benefit in some patients with pituitary carcinomas.[11,12]

Temozolomide

Temozolomide (Temodar) is an orally administered agent that readily crosses the blood-brain barrier. It methylates DNA at the O^6 position of guanine, causing mismatch and eventually apoptosis. It is currently used in conjunction with radiation therapy following surgical resection for malignant gliomas,[50] as well as advanced malignant neuroendocrine tumors.[51] The effect of temozolomide is opposed by the expression of O^6-methylguanine DNA methyltransferase (MGMT), which is a DNA repair enzyme. Malignant gliomas that express low levels of MGMT via MGMT promoter methylation[52] are more susceptible to temozolomide-induced tumor suppression and increased survival.[53,54]

The first report of efficacy of temozolomide in 2 patients with pituitary carcinoma was presented in 2006.[55] The first patient had luteinizing hormone–secreting tumor with intradural metastases to the spine, and the second patient had prolactin-secreting macroadenoma that progressed to carcinoma with metastases to the spine, despite dopamine agonist therapy and proton beam radiation therapy. Both patients' symptoms improved shortly after starting therapy with temozolomide with significant improvement in visual field deficits for well over 1 year after the therapy.[55] Temozolomide treatment in prolactinoma has been confirmed to cause necrosis, hemorrhage, focal inflammatory infiltration, marked changes in morphologic features, and reduction in growth potential by histologic, immunohistochemical, and electron microscopic studies.[56]

Since these initial cases reported in 2006, additional studies have reported the use of temozolomide in pituitary carcinomas with encouraging outcomes.[34,56–68] Thus far, 40 patients with aggressive pituitary tumors treated with temozolomide have been reported, consisting of 16 patients with pituitary carcinoma,[11,12,58,65] most recently

reviewed by McCormack and colleagues.[11] Of these 40 patients, 24 (60%) had good outcomes following temozolomide therapy with the highest response rates in prolactinomas (73%), followed by ACTH-secreting tumors (60%) and nonfunctioning tumors (40%).[11] Among the 16 pituitary carcinomas, 11 patients (68.8%) showed good response to temozolomide, whereas 2 patients (12.5%) showed no response and 3 patients (18.8%) showed progressive disease.[11]

Interestingly, patients with low MGMT expression seem to respond better to temozolomide.[11,12,61,63] Approximately 50% to 57% of pituitary carcinomas express low levels of MGMT.[34,69] In a most recent review, 76% of patients with aggressive pituitary tumors with low MGMT expression showed high response to temozolomide, whereas patients with high MGMT expression did not.[11] Among patients with pituitary carcinoma, 5 (62.5%) of 8 patients with absent to intermediate MGMT expression had good response to temozolomide, whereas only 1 (33.3%) of 3 patients with high MGMT expression had good response.[11] However, these results must be interpreted with caution because (1) some studies did not find an association of low MGMT expression with better temozolomide response,[58,65] (2) MGMT promoter methylation status is not correlated with temozolomide response,[11] and (3) the sample size is too small in the current studies. Clearly, further studies with more patients and analysis of MGMT expression and promoter methylation status are needed to make more definitive conclusions. Moreover, studies testing the combination therapies with temozolomide and other drugs, such as dopamine agonists, used for pituitary tumors should be further explored.[57,64,68]

Potential Novel Therapeutic Agents

Although results with the use of temozolomide in pituitary carcinomas and invasive adenomas are encouraging, it is clear that more research is needed to develop novel approaches to treat pituitary tumors resistant to conventional therapeutic modalities, such as surgery, medical therapy, radiation, and chemotherapy. Novel targeted therapies used for other brain and neuroendocrine tumors need further testing to evaluate their efficacy against pituitary carcinomas. One such candidate is the antiangiogenic agent bevacizumab (Avastin), which is a monoclonal antibody that binds and potently blocks vascular endothelial growth factor. As a potent inhibitor of angiogenesis, it is known to delay tumor growth and has been approved for use in metastatic colon cancer, advanced non–small-cell lung cancer, metastatic renal cell carcinoma, and recurrent glioblastoma multiforme.[70] Recently, a 44-year-old man with aggressive silent corticotroph cell pituitary adenoma that progressed to carcinoma despite multiple surgeries, radiation, and temozolomide treatment was treated with bevacizumab. After 16 months of treatment, the disease stabilized with long-term control (26 months) of disease.[71] Another agent that warrants a further review is everolimus (Afinitor), an inhibitor of mammalian target of rapamycin (mTOR). Pituitary adenomas upregulate the PI3 K/Akt/mTOR pathway,[72] and everolimus has been shown to prolong progression-free survival in patients with advanced pancreatic neuroendocrine tumors.[73] A case report of use of everolimus in combination with a somatostatin analog, octreotide, has been presented recently, although the combined therapy failed to control an aggressive ACTH-secreting pituitary carcinoma.[74] More experience with other patients with pituitary carcinomas or invasive adenomas resistant to conventional therapies is needed before any definitive conclusion can be made.

SUMMARY

Pituitary carcinomas are rare malignant pituitary tumors with poor overall survival. Although effective medical, surgical, and radiation therapies are available for pituitary adenomas, such therapies are deemed only palliative for pituitary carcinomas. Although preliminary, results from the use of novel therapeutic agents, such as temozolomide, are encouraging and warrant further investigation for pituitary carcinomas and aggressive, invasive pituitary adenomas that are unresponsive to conventional therapies.

REFERENCES

1. Heaney AP. Pituitary carcinoma: difficult diagnosis and treatment. J Clin Endocrinol Metab 2011; 96(12):3649–60.
2. Luzi P, Miracco C, Lio R, et al. Endocrine inactive pituitary carcinoma metastasizing to cervical lymph nodes: a case report. Hum Pathol 1987;18(1):90–2.
3. Nudleman KL, Choi B, Kusske JA, et al. Primary pituitary carcinoma: a clinical pathological study. Neurosurgery 1985;16(1):90–5.
4. CBTRUS. 2009-2010 CBTRUS statistical report: primary brain and central nervous system tumors diagnosed in the United States in 2004-2006. 2010. Available at: http://www.cbtrus.org. Accessed April 4, 2010.
5. Monson JP. The epidemiology of endocrine tumours. Endocr Relat Cancer 2000;7(1):29–36.
6. Pernicone PJ, Scheithauer BW, Sebo TJ, et al. Pituitary carcinoma: a clinicopathologic study of 15 cases. Cancer 1997;79(4):804–12.
7. Ragel BT, Couldwell WT. Pituitary carcinoma: a review of the literature. Neurosurg Focus 2004;16(4):E7.
8. Scheithauer BW, Kurtkaya-Yapicier O, Kovacs KT, et al. Pituitary carcinoma: a clinicopathological review. Neurosurgery 2005;56(5):1066–74 [discussion: 1066–74].
9. Al-Shraim M, Asa SL. The 2004 World Health Organization classification of pituitary tumors: what is new? Acta Neuropathol 2006;111(1):1–7.
10. DeLellis RA, Lloyd RV, Heitz PU, et al. World Health Organization classification of tumours: tumours of endocrine organs. Lyon (France): IARC; 2004.
11. McCormack AI, Wass JA, Grossman AB, et al. Aggressive pituitary tumours: the role of temozolomide and the assessment of MGMT status. Eur J Clin Invest 2011;41(10):1133–48.
12. Syro LV, Ortiz LD, Scheithauer BW, et al. Treatment of pituitary neoplasms with temozolomide: a review. Cancer 2011;117(3):454–62.
13. Kaltsas GA, Nomikos P, Kontogeorgos G, et al. Clinical review: diagnosis and management of pituitary carcinomas. J Clin Endocrinol Metab 2005;90(5):3089–99.
14. Lopes MB, Scheithauer BW, Schiff D, et al. Pituitary carcinoma: diagnosis and treatment. Endocrine 2005;28(1):115–21.
15. Scheithauer BW, Kovacs KT, Laws ER Jr, et al. Pathology of invasive pituitary tumors with special reference to functional classification. J Neurosurg 1986;65(6):733–44.
16. Selman WR, Laws ER Jr, Scheithauer BW, et al. The occurrence of dural invasion in pituitary adenomas. J Neurosurg 1986;64(3):402–7.
17. Zada G, Woodmansee WW, Ramkissoon S, et al. Atypical pituitary adenomas: incidence, clinical characteristics, and implications. J Neurosurg 2011;114(2):336–44.
18. Casanueva FF, Molitch ME, Schlechte JA, et al. Guidelines of the Pituitary Society for the diagnosis and management of prolactinomas. Clin Endocrinol (Oxf) 2006;65(2):265–73.
19. Daly AF, Rixhon M, Adam C, et al. High prevalence of pituitary adenomas: a cross-sectional study in the province of Liege, Belgium. J Clin Endocrinol Metab 2006;91(12):4769–75.
20. Guzel A, Tatli M, Senturk S, et al. Pituitary carcinoma presenting with multiple metastases: case report. J Child Neurol 2008;23(12):1467–71.
21. Kaltsas GA, Grossman AB. Malignant pituitary tumours. Pituitary 1998;1(1):69–81.
22. Kaltsas GA, Mukherjee JJ, Plowman PN, et al. The role of cytotoxic chemotherapy in the management of aggressive and malignant pituitary tumors. J Clin Endocrinol Metab 1998;83(12):4233–8.

23. Waltz TA, Brownell B. Sarcoma: a possible late result of effective radiation therapy for pituitary adenoma. Report of two cases. J Neurosurg 1966;24(5):901–7.

24. Mountcastle RB, Roof BS, Mayfield RK, et al. Pituitary adenocarcinoma in an acromegalic patient: response to bromocriptine and pituitary testing: a review of the literature on 36 cases of pituitary carcinoma. Am J Med Sci 1989;298(2):109–18.

25. Brada M, Ford D, Ashley S, et al. Risk of second brain tumour after conservative surgery and radiotherapy for pituitary adenoma. BMJ 1992;304(6838):1343–6.

26. Meij BP, Lopes MB, Ellegala DB, et al. The long-term significance of microscopic dural invasion in 354 patients with pituitary adenomas treated with transsphenoidal surgery. J Neurosurg 2002;96(2):195–208.

27. Thapar K, Kovacs K, Scheithauer BW, et al. Proliferative activity and invasiveness among pituitary adenomas and carcinomas: an analysis using the MIB-1 antibody. Neurosurgery 1996;38(1):99–106 [discussion: 106–7].

28. Salehi F, Agur A, Scheithauer BW, et al. Ki-67 in pituitary neoplasms: a review—part I. Neurosurgery 2009;65(3):429–37 [discussion: 437].

29. Scheithauer BW. Surgical pathology of the pituitary: the adenomas. Part II. Pathol Annu 1984;19(Pt 2): 269–329.

30. Thapar K, Yamada Y, Scheithauer BW, et al. Assessment of mitotic activity in pituitary adenomas and carcinomas. Endocr Pathol 1996;7(3):215–21.

31. Hsu DW, Hakim F, Biller BM, et al. Significance of proliferating cell nuclear antigen index in predicting pituitary adenoma recurrence. J Neurosurg 1993; 78(5):753–61.

32. Thapar K, Scheithauer BW, Kovacs K, et al. p53 expression in pituitary adenomas and carcinomas: correlation with invasiveness and tumor growth fractions. Neurosurgery 1996;38(4):765–70 [discussion: 770–1].

33. Scheithauer BW, Fereidooni F, Horvath E, et al. Pituitary carcinoma: an ultrastructural study of eleven cases. Ultrastruct Pathol 2001;25(3):227–42.

34. Lau Q, Scheithauer B, Kovacs K, et al. MGMT immunoexpression in aggressive pituitary adenoma and carcinoma. Pituitary 2010;13(4):367–79.

35. Kaiser FE, Orth DN, Mukai K, et al. A pituitary parasellar tumor with extracranial metastases and high, partially suppressible levels of adrenocorticotropin and related peptides. J Clin Endocrinol Metab 1983;57(3):649–53.

36. Winkelmann J, Pagotto U, Theodoropoulou M, et al. Retention of dopamine 2 receptor mRNA and absence of the protein in craniospinal and extracranial metastasis of a malignant prolactinoma: a case report. Eur J Endocrinol 2002;146(1):81–8.

37. Matsuki M, Kaji Y, Matsuo M, et al. MR findings of subarachnoid dissemination of a pituitary adenoma. J Radiol 2000;73(871):783–5.

38. Muhr C, Bergstrom M, Lundberg PO, et al. Malignant prolactinoma with multiple intracranial metastases studied with positron emission tomography. Neurosurgery 1988;22(2):374–9.

39. Petrossians P, de Herder W, Kwekkeboom D, et al. Malignant prolactinoma discovered by D2 receptor imaging. J Clin Endocrinol Metab 2000; 85(1):398–401.

40. Greenman Y, Woolf P, Coniglio J, et al. Remission of acromegaly caused by pituitary carcinoma after surgical excision of growth hormone-secreting metastasis detected by 111-indium pentetreotide scan. J Clin Endocrinol Metab 1996;81(4):1628–33.

41. Scheithauer BW, Randall RV, Laws ER Jr, et al. Prolactin cell carcinoma of the pituitary. Clinicopathologic, immunohistochemical, and ultrastructural study of a case with cranial and extracranial metastases. Cancer 1985;55(3):598–604.

42. Martin NA, Hales M, Wilson CB, et al. Cerebellar metastasis from a prolactinoma during treatment with bromocriptine. J Neurosurg 1981;55(4):615–9.

43. O'Brien DP, Phillips JP, Rawluk DR, et al. Intracranial metastases from pituitary adenoma. Br J Neurosurg 1995;9(2):211–8.

44. Colao A, di Sarno A, Pivonello R, et al. Dopamine receptor agonists for treating prolactinomas. Expert Opin Investig Drugs 2002;11(6):787–800.

45. Oh MC, Aghi MK. Dopamine agonist-resistant prolactinomas. J Neurosurg 2011;114(5):1369–79.

46. Petterson T, MacFarlane IA, MacKenzie JM, et al. Prolactin secreting pituitary carcinoma. J Neurol Neurosurg Psychiatry 1992;55(12):1205–6.

47. Colao A, Cappabianca P, Caron P, et al. Octreotide LAR vs. surgery in newly diagnosed patients with acromegaly: a randomized, open-label, multicentre study. Clin Endocrinol (Oxf) 2009;70(5):757–68.

48. Mixson AJ, Friedman TC, Katz DA, et al. Thyrotropin-secreting pituitary carcinoma. J Clin Endocrinol Metab 1993;76(2):529–33.

49. McCutcheon IE, Pieper DR, Fuller GN, et al. Pituitary carcinoma containing gonadotropins: treatment by radical excision and cytotoxic chemotherapy: case report. Neurosurgery 2000;46(5):1233–9 [discussion: 1239–40].

50. Stupp R, Hegi ME, Mason WP, et al. Effects of radiotherapy with concomitant and adjuvant temozolomide versus radiotherapy alone on survival in glioblastoma in a randomised phase III study: 5-year analysis of the EORTC-NCIC trial. Lancet Oncol 2009;10(5):459–66.

51. Ekeblad S, Sundin A, Janson ET, et al. Temozolomide as monotherapy is effective in treatment of advanced malignant neuroendocrine tumors. Clin Cancer Res 2007;13(10):2986–91.

52. Esteller M, Hamilton SR, Burger PC, et al. Inactivation of the DNA repair gene O6-methylguanine-DNA methyltransferase by promoter hypermethylation is

a common event in primary human neoplasia. Cancer Res 1999;59(4):793–7.

53. Cao VT, Jung TY, Jung S, et al. The correlation and prognostic significance of MGMT promoter methylation and MGMT protein in glioblastomas. Neurosurgery 2009;65(5):866–75 [discussion: 875].

54. Hegi ME, Diserens AC, Gorlia T, et al. MGMT gene silencing and benefit from temozolomide in glioblastoma. N Engl J Med 2005;352(10):997–1003.

55. Fadul CE, Kominsky AL, Meyer LP, et al. Long-term response of pituitary carcinoma to temozolomide. Report of two cases. J Neurosurg 2006;105(4): 621–6.

56. Kovacs K, Horvath E, Syro LV, et al. Temozolomide therapy in a man with an aggressive prolactin-secreting pituitary neoplasm: morphological findings. Hum Pathol 2007;38(1):185–9.

57. Bode H, Seiz M, Lammert A, et al. SOM230 (pasireotide) and temozolomide achieve sustained control of tumour progression and ACTH secretion in pituitary carcinoma with widespread metastases. Exp Clin Endocrinol Diabetes 2010;118(10):760–3.

58. Bush ZM, Longtine JA, Cunningham T, et al. Temozolomide treatment for aggressive pituitary tumors: correlation of clinical outcome with O(6)-methylguanine methyltransferase (MGMT) promoter methylation and expression. J Clin Endocrinol Metab 2010;95(11):E280–90.

59. Byrne S, Karapetis C, Vrodos N, et al. A novel use of temozolomide in a patient with malignant prolactinoma. J Clin Neurosci 2009;16(12):1694–6.

60. Hagen C, Schroeder HD, Hansen S, et al. Temozolomide treatment of a pituitary carcinoma and two pituitary macroadenomas resistant to conventional therapy. Eur J Endocrinol 2009;161(4):631–7.

61. Kovacs K, Scheithauer BW, Lombardero M, et al. MGMT immunoexpression predicts responsiveness of pituitary tumors to temozolomide therapy. Acta Neuropathol 2008;115(2):261–2.

62. Lim S, Shahinian H, Maya MM, et al. Temozolomide: a novel treatment for pituitary carcinoma. Lancet Oncol 2006;7(6):518–20.

63. McCormack AI, McDonald KL, Gill AJ, et al. Low O6-methylguanine-DNA methyltransferase (MGMT) expression and response to temozolomide in aggressive pituitary tumours. Clin Endocrinol (Oxf) 2009;71(2):226–33.

64. Neff LM, Weil M, Cole A, et al. Temozolomide in the treatment of an invasive prolactinoma resistant to dopamine agonists. Pituitary 2007;10(1):81–6.

65. Raverot G, Sturm N, de Fraipont F, et al. Temozolomide treatment in aggressive pituitary tumors and pituitary carcinomas: a French multicenter experience. J Clin Endocrinol Metab 2010;95(10):4592–9.

66. Syro LV, Scheithauer BW, Ortiz LD, et al. Effect of temozolomide in a patient with recurring oncocytic gonadotrophic pituitary adenoma. Hormones (Athens) 2009;8(4):303–6.

67. Takeshita A, Inoshita N, Taguchi M, et al. High incidence of low O(6)-methylguanine DNA methyltransferase expression in invasive macroadenomas of Cushing's disease. Eur J Endocrinol 2009;161(4): 553–9.

68. Thearle MS, Freda PU, Bruce JN, et al. Temozolomide (Temodar(R)) and capecitabine (Xeloda(R)) treatment of an aggressive corticotroph pituitary tumor. Pituitary 2011;14(4):418–24.

69. Salehi F, Scheithauer BW, Kros JM, et al. MGMT promoter methylation and immunoexpression in aggressive pituitary adenomas and carcinomas. J Neurooncol 2011;104(3):647–57.

70. Norden AD, Drappatz J, Wen PY, et al. Antiangiogenic therapy in malignant gliomas. Curr Opin Oncol 2008;20(6):652–61.

71. Ortiz LD, Syro LV, Scheithauer BW, et al. Anti-VEGF therapy in pituitary carcinoma. Pituitary 2011. [Epub ahead of print].

72. Dworakowska D, Wlodek E, Leontiou CA, et al. Activation of RAF/MEK/ERK and PI3K/AKT/mTOR pathways in pituitary adenomas and their effects on downstream effectors. Endocr Relat Cancer 2009; 16(4):1329–38.

73. Yao JC, Shah MH, Ito T, et al. Everolimus for advanced pancreatic neuroendocrine tumors. N Engl J Med 2011;364(6):514–23.

74. Jouanneau E, Wierinckx A, Ducray F, et al. New targeted therapies in pituitary carcinoma resistant to temozolomide. Pituitary 2012;15(1):37–43.

Visual Outcomes After Treatment of Pituitary Adenomas

Clare Louise Fraser, MBBS, MMed, FRANZCO,
Valérie Biousse, MD, Nancy J. Newman, MD*

KEYWORDS

- Pituitary adenoma • Neuro-ophthalmology • Visual acuity • Visual field • Prognosis

KEY POINTS

- Patients with pituitary adenomas extending above the diaphragm sella should be assessed for visual acuity abnormalities, visual field defects, and ocular motility disturbances.
- Pituitary apoplexy must be considered in the setting of acute vision loss or ocular motor disturbance, especially if associated with headache, even if there is no previously known pituitary tumor or precipitating factor.
- Studies differ regarding the prognostic factors for visual recovery after apoplexy, but early diagnosis and treatment within 1 week will minimize visual morbidity.
- Not all studies are in agreement as to which factors predict a better visual outcome postoperatively; however, the presence of optic disk pallor with associated loss of the retinal nerve fiber layer (as measured by optical coherence tomography) indicates long-standing damage to the optic pathways, which is less likely to recover.
- The overall rate of visual field improvement with transsphenoidal excision of pituitary adenomas is 80%.
- After pituitary surgery, there may be immediate visual improvement secondary to decompression, then early recovery from restoration of axoplasmic flow, and less dramatic delayed recovery over 1 to 4 months because of remyelination and remodeling.
- Neuro-ophthalmic follow-up is required to monitor for recurrence and for complications of therapy, including chiasmal prolapse and radiation optic neuropathy.
- Patients with poor postoperative visual outcome or diplopia should be referred to appropriate low-vision and ophthalmic services for driving assessment and management.

Pituitary adenomas are benign central nervous system tumors; although many are asymptomatic, others can cause significant morbidity because of their mass effect on local structures. Technical advancements have led to the development of noninvasive or minimally invasive therapeutic modalities, with multiple modalities often used for optimal results. A multidisciplinary team approach is commonly chosen, with the preservation of vision a key indication to proceed with treatment.

Funding sources: Dr Fraser: Sydney Eye Hospital Alumni Traveling Fellowship 2010, RANZCO Eye Foundation (Pfizer) Scholarship 2011. Drs Newman and Biousse: unrestricted departmental grant (Department of Ophthalmology) from Research to Prevent Blindness, Inc, New York and by NIH/NEI core grant P30-EY06360 (Department of Ophthalmology). Dr Newman: Research to Prevent Blindness Lew R. Wasserman Merit Award. Conflict of interest: None.
Department of Neuro-Ophthalmology, Emory Eye Center, Emory University School of Medicine, Emory University, 1365 B Clifton Road NE, Atlanta, GA 30322, USA
* Corresponding author.
E-mail address: ophtnjn@emory.edu

NEURO-OPHTHALMIC ANATOMY OF THE PITUITARY REGION

In 1704, in an attempt to explain the phenomenon of perceived singularity of vision derived from the two eyes, it was hypothesized that the optic chiasm was derived from a merger of both optic nerves with partial cross-over of nerve fibers.[1] Today, an understanding of the visual pathways and the normal variants, from optic nerve to the chiasm and optic tracts, is fundamental in understanding the neuro-ophthalmic manifestations of pituitary tumors.

Afferent Visual Pathways

Optic nerves

The optic canal, located superomedially in the sphenoid bone, transmits the optic nerve from the orbit to the intracranial space. The optic canals are separated from the sphenoid sinus by a bony wall, which is only 0.5 mm thick or less in some patients. Therefore, injury to the lateral wall of the sphenoid sinus, such as during forced opening of a transsphenoidal speculum, can result in vision loss (**Fig. 1**).[2]

The falciform process, a reflected leaf of dura mater, covers the optic nerves as they emerge from the optic canals. The length of nerve covered only by dura can vary from 1 mm to 15 mm.[3] Therefore, during any surgical approach, it should not be assumed that bone separates the dura from the proximal portion of the optic nerve.

When there is extensive anterior growth of the pituitary tumor or if the chiasm is postfixed, optic nerve involvement occurs. The *junctional scotoma* is classically seen when a lesion compresses the junction of the posterior optic nerve and chiasm, where the crossed ventral fibers loop anteriorly (Wilbrand knee). The resultant visual field defect is one of a hemianopic or central scotoma in the ipsilateral eye and a superior temporal defect in the contralateral eye (**Fig. 2**).[4] Damage to the anastomotic blood supply to the posterior portion of the nerve can also occur.

Chiasm

The chiasm is usually situated over the diaphragm sella, at the junction of the anterior wall and floor of the third ventricle. The chiasm may, however, be prefixed and overlie the tuberculum sella or postfixed and overlie the dorsum sella (**Fig. 3**). A review of 225 autopsy cases found a normal chiasm in 80%, a prefixed chiasm in 9%, and a postfixed chiasm in 11%.[5] These relationships have a direct bearing on the visual field defect resulting from an enlarging pituitary mass.

Approximately 53% of the axons in each optic nerve decussate in the chiasm.[6] The decussating fibers subserve the nasal retina and, therefore, the temporal hemifield; thus, a bitemporal hemianopic visual field defect localizes a lesion to the optic chiasm (**Fig. 4**). The crossing macular fibers occupy the central and posterior portions of the chiasm and make up the bulk of all crossing fibers. If these fibers are involved early, then a bitemporal hemianopic scotoma will be the first visual field defect seen.

The exact pathophysiological mechanism that produces the bitemporal field defect is debated. The effects of a growing pituitary tumor were simulated using a Foley catheter inserted into an empty sella turcica of adult cadavers.[7,8] As the catheter tip was enlarged, the chiasm elevated, causing nonuniform pressure generation across the chiasm with greater effective stress on the crossing fibers. Another group reported that crossing fibers in the chiasm receive their arterial supply solely from the inferior group of vessels,[9] which are vulnerable to compression by a growing pituitary tumor. However, the vascular theory does not explain why compression from above also causes bitemporal hemianopia. A mathematical model has been proposed that shows adjacent crossing nasal fibers are in contact with each other over a smaller area than adjacent uncrossed fibers, therefore, the compressive force generated at these contact points is greater.[10] This force results in architectural distortion of the nerves, compromising nerve fiber conduction. This theory also explains how transmitted shearing forces across the chiasm in patients with head trauma result in bitemporal hemianopia.

Optic tracts

From the chiasm, the optic tracts diverge anteriorly to the interpeduncular space and continue in

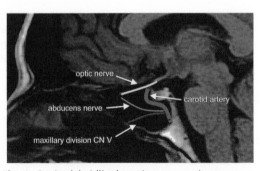

Fig. 1. Sagittal (midline) section magnetic resonance image through the right sphenoid sinus. Note the important neurologic and vascular structures adjacent to the pituitary gland, as indicated by the arrows, and the relative position of each behind the outer wall of the sphenoid sinus.

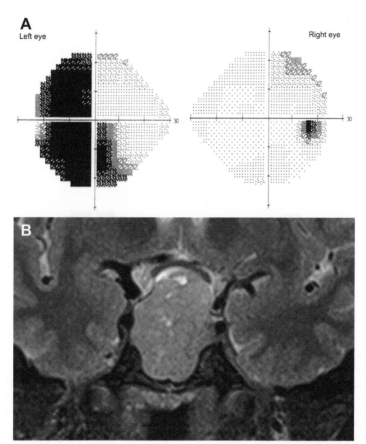

Fig. 2. Junctional scotoma from chiasmal compression. A 54-year-old man presented with visual acuity of 20/20 in the right eye, 20/400 in the left, and a left relative afferent pupillary defect, suggesting a left optic neuropathy. His Humphrey visual fields (*A*) showed a junctional scotoma from distal left optic nerve and chiasmal compression with a dense temporal hemianopic defect (*black shaded area*) in the visual field of the left eye and a small superior temporal defect (*gray shaded area*) in the visual field of the right eye. The coronal magnetic resonance image (*B*) shows chiasmal compression more to the left than the right.

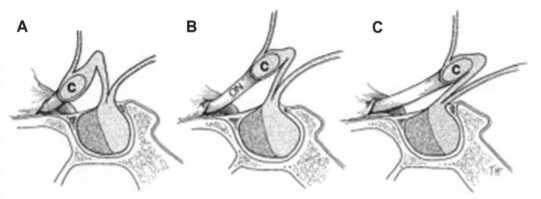

Fig. 3. Three sagittal sections of the optic chiasm and sellar regionshowing the relative positions of the prefixed chiasm (*A*), a normalchiasm (*B*), and a postfixed chiasm (*C*). (*Reproduced from* Rhoton AL Jr, Harrid FS, Renn WH. Microsurgical anatomy of the sellar region and cavernous sinus. In: Glaser JS, editor. Neuroophthalmology symposium of the university of Miami and the Bascon Palmer Eye Institute. St Louis (MO): CV Mosby; 1977. p. 75–105; with permission.)

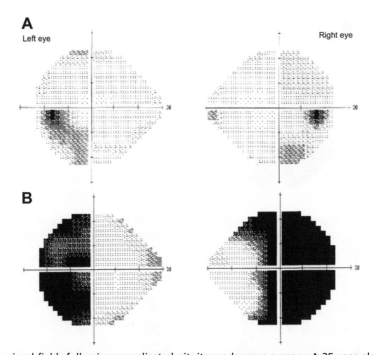

Fig. 4. Change in visual fields following complicated pituitary adenoma surgery. A 35-year-old before and after resection of a large pituitary adenoma. Preoperatively, visual acuity was 20/20 in both eyes with no relative afferent pupillary defect. Visual fields (*A*) showed a mild inferior bitemporal quadrant defect (*gray shading*). Surgery was complicated by hemorrhage in the sella turcica and the patient complained of vision loss in both eyes. Vision postoperatively was reduced to 20/50 in the right and 20/25 in the left, with a right relative afferent pupillary defect. Postoperatively, visual fields showed (*B*) a complete bitemporal hemianopia (*black shading*) with some extension across the vertical midline on the right, suggesting additional right optic nerve involvement.

a posterolateral direction around the cerebral peduncles to enter the middle incisural spaces. The crossed and uncrossed fibers converge, with most of the tract fibers synapsing in the lateral geniculate body. Damage to the optic tracts, as occurs with a prefixed chiasm or a tumor growing posterosuperiorly, will result in an incomplete homonymous visual field defect (see **Fig. 3**).

Efferent Visual Pathways

The cavernous sinuses surround the carotid arteries, lie lateral to the pituitary fossa, and are bound anteriorly and posteriorly by the clinoid processes. A cranial nerve (CN) palsy may occur because of transmission of pressure laterally by the tumor expanding laterally to the wall of the cavernous sinus,[11] compression of the nerve against the interclinoid ligament, direct invasion of the cavernous sinus wall, or surgical trauma (**Figs. 5** and **6**).[12]

Oculomotor nerve: CN III
The oculomotor nerve travels in the lateral wall of the cavernous sinus and enters the superior orbital fissure as 2 divisions. The oculomotor nerve supplies the superior rectus and levator palpebrae muscles in its superior division. The inferior

division controls the medial, inferior rectus and inferior oblique muscles and the parasympathetic fibers for pupillomotor control of the iris sphincter and accommodation via the ciliary muscle.

Trochlear nerve: CN IV
The trochlear nerve enters the lateral wall of the cavernous sinus posterosuperiorly, running parallel

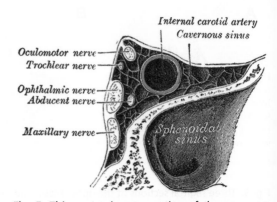

Fig. 5. This anatomic cross section of the cavernous sinus shows the relative positions of the cranial nerves. (*From* Gray H. Anatomy of the human body. Philadelphia: Lea & Febiger, 1918.)

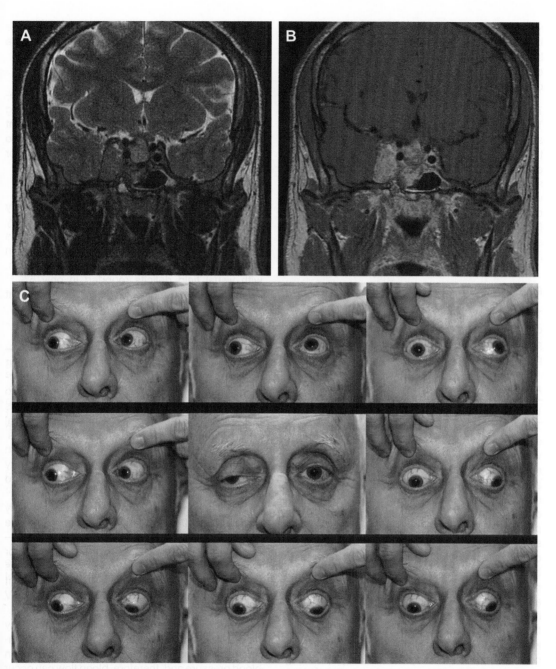

Fig. 6. Right third nerve palsy secondary to a pituitary mass with right cavernous sinus invasion. The coronal magnetic resonance images (*A, B*) show a pituitary mass with extension into the right cavernous sinus and into the right middle cranial fossa despite previous transsphenoidal resection. (*C*) External photography in the 9 cardinal positions of gaze document a partial right oculomotor nerve palsy (third cranial nerve), with partial right ptosis, no elevation or adduction of the right eye, and limited depression of the right eye. The right pupil was poorly reactive to light.

and inferiorly to CN III, then via the superior orbital fissure to control the superior oblique muscle, which is primarily a depressor of the eye in adduction as well as an intorter of the eye.

Abducens nerve: CN VI

The abducens nerve enters the posterior part of the cavernous sinus to run alongside the internal carotid artery, lying freely within the cavernous sinus rather than within the lateral wall. The sympathetic fibers from the carotid plexus join CN VI before traveling with the branches of CN V. The abducens nerve enters the orbit through the superior orbital fissure and innervates the lateral rectus.

Trigeminal nerve: CN V
The trigeminal nerve passes above the petrous apex to enter Meckel cave, which is located lateral to the cavernous sinus. The ophthalmic division enters the cavernous sinus inferiorly and slopes superiorly within the inferior portion of the lateral wall where the sympathetic fibers join for 1 to 2 cm. This division travels via the superior orbital fissure and carries sensory information from the scalp, forehead, upper eyelid, conjunctiva, cornea, nose, frontal sinuses, and parts of the meninges.

PREOPERATIVE ASSESSMENT

The documentation of preoperative neuro-ophthalmic symptoms and signs allows for appropriate counseling of patients and for an objective prediction of the extent of postoperative recovery.

Presenting Symptoms

Visual loss
The time course and description of visual loss associated with pituitary tumors varies, with steady visual failure being the most common (50%), but rapid (27%) or intermittent progression (12.5%) is also reported.[13] A large monocular visual defect may be noticed suddenly on incidental occlusion of the contralateral eye, when in fact it has been present for many months. In cases of genuine sudden vision loss, pituitary apoplexy must be considered (see later discussion). The classic bitemporal defect results in difficulties of depth perception because the residual visual field from each eye does not overlap. Images in the midline beyond the point of fixation fall on the nasal retina, the blind temporal field, for each eye. This condition is referred to as postfixational blindness[14] and may give the impression of objects suddenly appearing centrally when fixation shifts, which is a particular problem when driving.

Diplopia
Diplopia secondary to ocular motor palsy as the presenting symptom is unusual, seen in less than 2% of cases,[15,16] but may be discovered on clinical examination in a larger percentage.[17] Because there are no corresponding retinal points in bitemporal hemianopia to visually link the nasal hemifields, a slight misalignment of the eyes will produce a separation of the visual fields vertically or horizontally,[14] which is often described by patients as double vision. This hemifield slide produces an intermittent diplopia in the absence of ocular muscle paresis.

Unusual symptoms
Other neuro-ophthalmic symptoms have been reported in cases of pituitary tumors, including ocular neuromyotonia[18] after radiation treatment (see later discussion). If the tumor invades into the orbit or cavernous sinus, then proptosis or venous stasis may be seen.[19]

Pediatric
Headache and visual failure, although classically regarded as the presenting signs of pituitary lesions, are uncommon childhood presentations of pituitary adenoma.[20] Presenting symptoms in children primarily reflect endocrine dysfunction, with visual field deficits reported in only 5%.[21] Pubertal boys are more likely than girls to present with headaches and visual impairment.[22]

Emergency Presentation

Pituitary apoplexy is a rare but life-threatening condition caused by sudden hemorrhage or infarction of the pituitary gland, occurring in 0.6% to 10.0% of all cases of pituitary adenoma.[23] It is classically characterized by headache, visual loss, ophthalmoplegia, and altered mental status; however, its presentation is highly variable.[24] In a series of cases of pituitary apoplexy, a pituitary adenoma was previously known in only 14% to 20%.[25,26]

The mean age at presentation with pituitary apoplexy is 50 to 56 years. Symptoms include headache (95%–100%), ocular paresis (56%–78%), and reduced visual fields (45%–64%), or acuities (36%–52%).[25,26] When ophthalmoparesis is present, the majority has CN III involvement (57%), followed by CN VI (30%), and then CN IV (13%).[25]

The many potential factors precipitating apoplexy have been debated. Reduced blood flow in the pituitary gland can precipitate apoplexy. Fluctuations in blood pressure and, therefore, blood flow can occur in the setting of cardiac surgery or hemodialysis. Transient elevations of intracranial pressure with resultant pituitary hypoperfusion causing apoplexy have also been reported. More chronic hypoperfusion may occur after radiation therapy. Alternatively, an acute increase in blood flow in the pituitary gland in conditions, such as malignant hypertension or diabetic ketoacidosis, can also trigger apoplexy. Stimulation of the pituitary gland through increased estrogen states, such as pregnancy, or excessive stimulation of the pituitary gland responding to stress at times of surgery, myocardial infarction, or systemic infections have also been hypothesized as precipitants. Finally, the commencement of anticoagulation was postulated to be a trigger factor in up to 10% of cases in one series.[26] However, in most cases of pituitary apoplexy, there are no identifiable precipitants.

Examination Findings

Visual field defects

Although nearly 75% of patients with pituitary tumors have visual field defects, less than half will complain about vision changes.[16] Therefore, visual field testing should be done in all patients at presentation. The most common types of visual field defects are complete or incomplete bitemporal hemianopia, with the upper temporal quadrant being more frequently and severely affected than the lower temporal quadrant. Other visual field defects seen (in descending frequency) are monocular blindness with temporal defect in the contralateral eye (8.1%), junctional scotoma (5.6%), homonymous hemianopia (4.2%), monocular superior temporal defect (3.3%), and central or temporal scotoma in both eyes (2.7%) or one just eye (1.2%).[16]

Fundoscopic examination

Chiasmal compression can cause the loss of the peripapillary nerve fiber bundle, resulting in optic atrophy.[27] If the decussating fibers are selectively damaged, then band or bow-tie atrophy is seen.[28] This pattern is seen because the decussating fibers originate from the nasal retina and enter the disk both nasally and temporally. However, it takes a minimum of 4 to 8 weeks for optic nerve injury to be reflected in a loss of the retinal nerve fiber layer and optic nerve pallor. Disk pallor is typically maximal at 3 months after injury.[29] Therefore, disk pallor will not be seen early in presentation, even if there is significant optic nerve compromise, unless there was previous longstanding, unrecognized compression.

Papilledema, indicating raised intracranial pressure, is a rare finding with pituitary adenomas.[16] Indeed, other suprasellar lesions, such as craniopharyngioma, are more likely to cause cerebrospinal fluid obstruction and consequent papilledema.

Ocular motility

The prevalence of ocular motor palsy in patients with pituitary adenomas is reported between 1% and 6%.[30] Overall, CN III is the most frequently involved, with the levator palpebrae superioris most commonly affected.[31]

Parasellar lesions, including pituitary tumors, may produce seesaw nystagmus in which elevation and intorsion of one eye is seen with depression and extorsion of the other eye. This phenomenon is not specific to this region or pathologic condition because it also occurs with medullary and pontine lesions affecting the otolithic pathways.[32]

VISUAL PROGNOSIS

Although it is well recognized that visual improvement may occur after surgical excision of a pituitary lesion, this recovery is variable and difficult to predict. A large meta-analysis of transsphenoidal surgery for nonfunctioning pituitary adenomas showed that improvement in visual fields was seen in 78% of cases, with new visual field defects seen postoperatively in 3%.[33] There are several underlying pathophysiological mechanisms that contribute to visual dysfunction that are not associated with significant axonopathy and are, therefore, potentially reversible. Methods of predicting the visual outcomes after surgery would allow for individualized management strategies and more accurate patient counseling regarding their likely visual outcome.

Standard Clinical Assessment

Factors, such as younger age, lack of optic nerve pallor (indicating shorter duration of compression of the anterior visual pathways), and better preoperative visual acuity, have been associated with better postoperative recovery of visual function,[34,35] although not all studies are in agreement. In patients with giant adenomas, postoperative visual outcomes do not seem to be related to preoperative tumor size (<3 cm, 3–4 cm, and >4 cm).[36]

Structural and Functional Measures of the Optic Nerve

Optical coherence tomography

Optical coherence tomography (OCT) allows for the in vivo acquisition of cross-sectional images of the internal microstructure of the retina from which estimates of the neural integrity of the retinal nerve fiber layer (RNFL) can be made. Failure of visual recovery after optic nerve compression is consequent to irreversible damage to the retinal ganglion cell axons. Visual field testing measures defects produced by both dead and damaged retinal ganglion cells, whereas anatomic measurements of the RNFL thinning only reflects axons that have died. Studies of patients with pituitary lesions have shown that a loss of the RNFL thickness at the disk correlates with the severity of visual field loss, occurring diffusely across all sectors.[37] After optic pathway compression is relieved by surgical intervention, the visual field improves for those axons that were damaged but not dead, and the anatomic measurements reflect the surviving axons. In other words, if there is preservation of RNFL thickness in the setting of profound visual loss, then visual recovery is possible. Patients with RNFL loss at the time of surgery for chiasmal compression are less likely to have a return of visual field or visual acuity after surgery.[38] Therefore, OCT is useful when patients have profound visual loss because measurements showing preservation of the RNFL indicate a better potential for recovery (**Fig. 7**).

Electrodiagnostic tests

Even patients with profound decreases in visual evoked potentials (VEP) may show complete recovery within minutes of surgical decompression.[39] Therefore, the VEP is not reliably prognostic.[40] However, the pattern electroretinogram (PERG) provides a functional measure of the integrity of the retinal ganglion cells in the same way that the OCT gives an anatomic measure of integrity. Studies have shown that the chance of visual field improvement in surgery is greater in eyes with a normal PERG.[41] However, in most centers, OCT is more easily obtained than electrophysiology and can be used more reliably for long-term follow-up.

Apoplexy

In about 30% of patients with apoplexy, there will be an identifiable condition associated with the onset, such as anticoagulation, surgical procedures, or cessation of bromocriptine.[26] However, in one study,[26] those patients with apoplexy with a known predisposing event were 5 times more likely to have neuro-ophthalmic sequelae than those with no associated conditions (severe optic neuropathy in 75% and visual field defect in 100% compared with 14.3% and 20.0%, respectively).

The severity of the initial deficit in both visual fields and acuities seems to be unrelated to the final outcome.[42] However, pallor of the optic disk, implying a prolonged period of optic nerve compression before apoplexy, is an important negative prognostic sign. Ocular motor paresis alone is not an absolute indication for surgery because there can still be full improvement with delayed surgery or conservative management.[25] Studies have shown that early decompression of the optic nerves significantly improves visual recovery,[43] with a significant threshold for a worse prognosis if surgery for pituitary apoplexy is delayed by more than 1 week from presentation.[25]

POST-TREATMENT OUTCOMES

A comparison of studies investigating visual outcomes after the management of pituitary adenomas is hampered by the different visual parameters measured and the lack of consistency regarding what constitutes improvement.

Post-Surgical Treatment

Surgical therapies improve visual field defects in almost 80% of patients.[33] Despite individual studies claiming superiority of each available method of surgical treatment over another, a recent meta-analysis of surgical outcomes for nonfunctioning pituitary adenomas[33] concluded that the transsphenoidal approach is safer than the transcranial approach. Overall, transsphenoidal surgery carries a low risk for damage to the visual apparatus and ocular motor cranial nerves.

Most eyes with visual field loss experience an improvement in visual fields after transsphenoidal surgery regardless of the severity of the preoperative defect. The pattern of recovery of visual function after surgical decompression of pituitary adenomas suggests several phases of improvement. Immediate improvement after decompression, as shown by improvement of VEPs within 10 minutes,[39] is likely caused by removal of physiologic conduction block. The early fast phase, within the first week postoperatively, may lead to normalization of visual fields in some individuals. Visual field improvement occurs usually, but not exclusively, within this first week; however, substantial improvement can still occur weeks and even months after surgery.[34] Even eyes that experience worsening of vision in the immediate postoperative period have the potential for visual improvement with time. The early slow phase (1–4 months) is the period of most notable improvement in visual acuity. It is thought that this improvement over weeks to months is caused by a process of restoration of axoplasmic flow and remyelination.[44] A late phase (6 months to 3 years) of mild improvement is usually not significant overall but may still be substantial in rare individuals.[45]

Improvement in deficits of visual acuity, visual fields, and ocular paresis is common in patients decompressed surgically following apoplexy. Indeed, if vision loss has been present for less than 1 day, then 75% to 97% of eyes have been reported to experience improvement in vision (fields and acuity).[23,42] A delay of 2 to 7 days does not seem to result in a worse visual outcome.[23,42] However, those undergoing surgery more than a week after presentation have a poorer visual outcome. The prognosis for ophthalmoplegia following pituitary apoplexy is relatively good in those undergoing surgery as well as those managed conservatively, with less than 20% of patients having residual diplopia.[26]

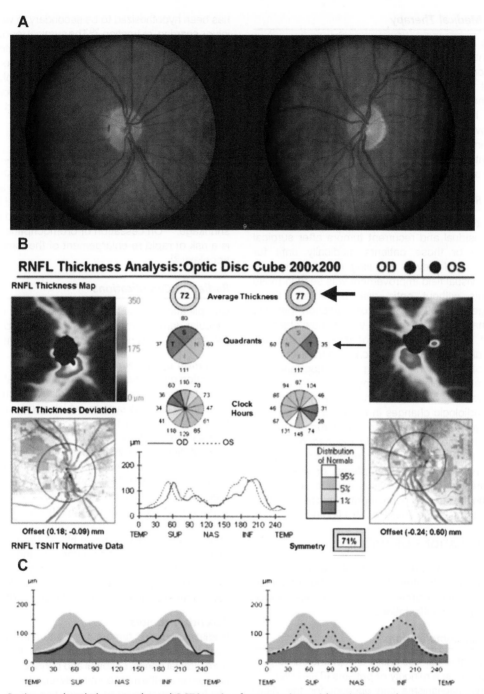

Fig. 7. Optic nerve head photographs and OCT imaging from a patient with a pituitary adenoma compressing the chiasm. (*A*) Fundus photographs of the optic nerve heads show temporal pallor secondary to chronic chiasmal compression. (*B*) RNFL analysis and optic disk scanning obtained with the Cirrus OCT (Carl Zeiss Meditech, California) showing thinning of the RNFL. The normal value for average thickness is 98 μm and 65 μm for the temporal sector. In this patient, the average thickness of the retinal nerve fiber layer is shown as 72 μm in the right and 77 μm in the left (*thick arrow*), suggesting moderate thinning of the RNFL consistent with bilateral chronic optic neuropathies. In addition, the temporal sector (*T*) of the retinal nerve fiber layer (37 μm right and 35 μm left) as shown by the red shading (*thin arrow*) has proportionally greater thinning than the vertical sectors (*S* and *I*). (*C*) The overall cross-sectional result for the patient is drawn as a black line, with the standard population results expected shown in green.

Post-Medical Therapy

There are many reports of visual improvement in patients undergoing medical treatment of hormone-secreting adenomas. Improvement in visual function with bromocriptine therapy is common (90%)[46] and usually occurs within 24 to72 hours of initiation.[47] Bromocriptine also improves ocular dysmotility.[48] When using octreotide, improvement in vision was seen in 75% of patients within hours, with the maximal improvement occurring within 6 to 45 days.[49]

Post-Radiation Therapy

Radiotherapy was historically reserved for patients with residual and recurrent tumors after surgical therapy or those patients medically unfit for surgery.[50] However, following radiation therapy alone, visual field improvement was seen in those patients without optic disk pallor and those younger than 69 years.[51] Post-radiation, patients may have visual complaints with no new objective visual field defect. Many of these patients will have dry eyes,[52] which can cause a transient blurring of vision, highlighting the importance of general ophthalmic assessment.

Worsening of vision does not always correlate with radiologic changes in lesion size. Therefore, it seems that subtle changes in tumor volume not detectable by magnetic resonance imaging (MRI) may be enough to relieve compression and improve patients' symptoms, or exacerbate compression and cause visual defects, again highlighting the need for neuro-ophthalmic assessment rather than relying solely on MRI findings.

COMPLICATIONS OF THERAPY

Aside from the prognostic implications of visual recovery after treatment of a tumor, the prescribed management regimen itself can cause neuro-ophthalmic manifestations.

Surgical Complications

Significant visual loss after transsphenoidal surgery is reported in a minority of patients (0%–11%).[53,54] Various mechanisms can account for the visual loss, including direct injury, vascular compromise, orbital fracture, postoperative hematoma, and chiasmal prolapse. These mechanisms are more frequent in cases of large macroadenoma, a dumbbell-shaped tumor, previous surgery, and previous radiation therapy. Following excision of a pituitary tumor, the suprasellar cistern may extend into the pituitary fossa, with resultant progressive visual impairment if the optic nerves and chiasm prolapse into the empty sella.[55] The associated visual deterioration

has been hypothesized to be secondary to vascular injury, scarring, or traction.[56] The surgical repositioning of the chiasm into a more normal anatomical position, known as chiasmapexy, may be required to restore vision.[57] Packing the sella and sphenoid sinus with fat or muscle is used to try to avoid this complication, but packing itself has caused visual compromise from chiasmal compression.[58]

Medical Complications

Neuro-ophthalmic complications of bromocriptine are very rare, although visual hallucinations are reported in 1% to 2% of patients.[59] Chiasmal herniation has also been reported following rapid tumor shrinkage.[60] On cessation of bromocriptine, there is a risk of rapid re-enlargement of the tumor and apoplexy.[61]

Radiation Complications

Complications of radiotherapy result from neurovascular damage, radionecrosis, and disruption of cellular DNA causing secondary tumor genesis.[62]

Radiation optic neuropathy

Radiation optic neuropathy and chiasmopathy are subsets of the more extensive radiation necrosis of the central nervous system, which occurs with an incidence of 0.25% to 25.0% after radiotherapy and an average time delay of 1 to 2 years.[63] The presentation is usually of an acute unilateral loss of vision, although bitemporal hemianopia has also been reported. MRI acutely reveals enlargement and gadolinium enhancement of the optic nerve and chiasm. In one study, the actuarial rate of optic neuropathy at 10 years after a mean radiation dose of 45 Gy was 0.8%.[64] Potential risk factors for radiation optic neuropathy and chiasmopathy include coincident treatment with chemotherapeutic agents, preexisting vasculopathy, carotid atherosclerosis, and diabetes mellitus.[65]

Secondary tumors

Radiation-induced tumors are a late and very rare complication. They may arise within the brain, dura, cranial bones, or spinal and peripheral nerves. Sarcomas are the most commonly reported intracranial tumors presumed to be radiation induced, followed by gliomas and meningiomas, with a latency period ranging from 1 year to more than 30 years.[66]

Neuromyotonia

Ocular neuromyotonia is a paroxysmal misalignment of the eyes, in the directions of the involved ocular motor nerve (most often CN III), usually triggered by eccentric gaze that can last seconds to minutes. The onset varies between 2 months and 18 years after treatment and has been reported after external beam radiation as well as gamma knife stereotactic radiosurgery.[67] The pathophysiology of neuromyotonia is poorly understood but thought to be caused by alterations in ion channel and neural membrane structures secondary to the radiation effects on the ocular motor nerves.

MANAGEMENT OF POOR POSTOPERATIVE VISUAL FUNCTION

Visual function and diplopia typically improve rapidly after decompression; however, some slow improvement is usually seen up to 6 months to 1 year after treatment. Residual abnormalities may be amenable to symptomatic treatment.

Poor Visual Acuity or Visual Fields

Driving
Although there are strict federal vision standards for commercial driver's licensing, there are no such standards for unrestricted noncommercial passenger vehicle driver's licensing in the United States, and requirements can vary considerably from state to state (listed on the Department of Motor Vehicles website for each state). Restrictions exist based on visual acuity, visual fields, and the presence of double vision. A local ophthalmologist familiar with local requirements should be consulted postoperatively before allowing patients to drive or return to work.

Low-vision services
For patients with poor visual outcomes, services exist to help maximize their visual potential with low-vision aids, home-safety adjustments, and assistance in retraining for work. Low-vision clinics and government services for the visually impaired are essential in the immediate postoperative period.

Double Vision

Patients with persistent double vision postoperatively can be offered monocular occlusion with a simple eye patch or taping of one lens of their glasses to eliminate the second visual image. Although cosmetically this may trouble some patients, it does not delay the recovery process and will allow them to resume normal activities while the ocular motor nerve palsy has an opportunity to resolve. If the strabismus has not resolved and seems stable, then prisms can be fitted into the spectacle correction to compensate for the ocular deviation. After 6 months to 1 year, strabismus surgery can be performed on some patients to realign the eyes and restore binocular vision.

FUTURE DIRECTIONS

Further comparative studies of treatment strategies are needed with adequate bias protection in their methodology.[33] Recent studies have used the Visual Impairment Score, which was originally described as a means to analyze the visual status and surgical outcome of patients with tuberculum sellae and planum sphenoidale meningiomas.[68] Universal use of such a scoring system will allow for better comparison of preoperative and postoperative visual outcomes and among surgical techniques. Such studies would provide stronger evidence to allow patient stratification according to prognostic characteristics, such as tumor size and clinical findings at presentation.

Further ophthalmic studies with respect to structure-function analysis of the retinal nerve fiber layer in relation to visual field defects will also allow for better visual prognostication. Newer OCT machines allow for more selective measurement of the retinal nerve fiber layer distinct from the other retinal layers. Furthermore, objective visual field tests, which avoid much of the bias inherent in repeated standard automated perimetry with its associated learning curve, are becoming more widely available.[69]

Increasing accessibility to 3-T head MRI scans allows for high-resolution anatomic and physiologic images of the optic pathways. Proton MR spectroscopy can provide valuable information on biodistribution of metabolites; if the accuracy improves, it may become possible to accurately distinguish between tumor and scar tissue.[70] Diffusion tensor tractography can depict pathways of the optic nerve fibers and can be combined with treatment-planning images. With pituitary adenomas adjacent to the optic pathways, better surgical and radiotherapy planning is required, and the increased use of these modalities will likely be a topic for future investigation.

REFERENCES

1. Rucker CW. The concept of a semi-decussation of the optic nerves. AMA Arch Ophthalmol 1958; 59(2):159–71.
2. Rhoton AL, Maniscalco JE. Microsurgery of the sellar region. In: Glaser JS, editor. Neuro-ophthalmology. St Louis (MO): C.V. Mosby; 1977. p. 106–27.
3. Renn WH, Rhoton AL Jr. Microsurgical anatomy of the sellar region. J Neurosurg 1975;43(3): 288–98.
4. Lee AG, Siebert KJ, Sanan A. Radiologic-clinical correlation. Junctional visual field loss. AJNR Am J Neuroradiol 1997;18(6):1171–4.

5. Bergland RM, Ray BS, Torack RM. Anatomical variations in the pituitary gland and adjacent structures in 225 human autopsy cases. J Neurosurg 1968; 28(2):93–9.

6. Kupfer C, Chumbley L, Downer JC. Quantitative histology of optic nerve, optic tract and lateral geniculate nucleus of man. J Anat 1967;101(Pt 3):393–401.

7. Hedges TR. Preservation of the upper nasal field in the chiasmal syndrome: an anatomic explanation. Trans Am Ophthalmol Soc 1969;67:131–41.

8. Kosmorsky GS, Dupps WJ Jr, Drake RL. Nonuniform pressure generation in the optic chiasm may explain bitemporal hemianopsia. Ophthalmology 2008; 115(3):560–5.

9. Bergland R. The arterial supply of the human optic chiasm. J Neurosurg 1969;31(3):327–34.

10. McIlwaine GG, Carrim ZI, Lueck CJ, et al. A mechanical theory to account for bitemporal hemianopia from chiasmal compression. J Neuroophthalmol 2005;25(1):40–3.

11. Walsh FB. Bilateral total ophthalmoplegia with adenoma of the pituitary gland; report of two cases; an anatomic study. Arch Ophthalmol 1949;42(5):646–54.

12. Jefferson G. Extrasellar extensions of pituitary adenomas: (section of neurology). Proc R Soc Med 1940;33(7):433–58.

13. Wilson P, Falconer MA. Patterns of visual failure with pituitary tumours. Clinical and radiological correlations. Br J Ophthalmol 1968;52(2):94–110.

14. Kirkham TH. The ocular symptomatology of pituitary tumours. Proc R Soc Med 1972;65(6):517–8.

15. Lyle TK, Clover P. Ocular symptoms and signs in pituitary tumours. Proc R Soc Med 1961;54:611–9.

16. Hollenhorst R, Younge R. Ocular manifestations produced by adenomas of the pituitary gland: 1000 cases. In: Kohler P, Ross G, editors. Diagnosis and treatment of pituitary tumours. Amsterdam: Excerpta Medica; 1973:53.

17. Chen L, White WL, Spetzler RF, et al. A prospective study of nonfunctioning pituitary adenomas: presentation, management, and clinical outcome. J Neurooncol 2011;102(1):129–38.

18. Shults WT, Hoyt WF, Behrens M, et al. Ocular neuromyotonia. A clinical description of six patients. Arch Ophthalmol 1986;104(7):1028–34.

19. Ortiz JM, Stein SC, Nelson P, et al. Pituitary adenoma presenting as unilateral proptosis. Arch Ophthalmol 1992;110(2):282–3.

20. Richmond IL, Wilson CB. Pituitary adenomas in childhood and adolescence. J Neurosurg 1978;49(2):163–8.

21. Partington MD, Davis DH, Laws ER Jr, et al. Pituitary adenomas in childhood and adolescence. Results of transsphenoidal surgery. J Neurosurg 1994;80(2): 209–16.

22. Lafferty AR, Chrousos GP. Pituitary tumors in children and adolescents. J Clin Endocrinol Metab 1999;84(12):4317–23.

23. Turgut M, Ozsunar Y, Basak S, et al. Pituitary apoplexy: an overview of 186 cases published during the last century. Acta Neurochir (Wien) 2010;152(5):749–61.

24. Rolih CA, Ober KP. Pituitary apoplexy. Endocrinol Metab Clin North Am 1993;22(2):291–302.

25. Bills DC, Meyer FB, Laws ER Jr, et al. A retrospective analysis of pituitary apoplexy. Neurosurgery 1993; 33(4):602–8 [discussion: 8–9].

26. Biousse V, Newman NJ, Oyesiku NM. Precipitating factors in pituitary apoplexy. J Neurol Neurosurg Psychiatry 2001;71(4):542–5.

27. Newman NM. Ophthalmoscopic observation of the retinal nerve fiber layer. Trans Sect Ophthalmol Am Acad Ophthalmol Otolaryngol 1977;83(5):786–96.

28. Hoyt CS, Billson FA. Maternal anticonvulsants and optic nerve hypoplasia. Br J Ophthalmol 1978; 62(1):3–6.

29. Lundstrom M, Frisen L. Evolution of descending optic atrophy. A case report. Acta Ophthalmol (Copenh) 1975;53(5):738–46.

30. Anderson D, Faber P, Marcovitz S, et al. Pituitary tumors and the ophthalmologist. Ophthalmology 1983;90(11):1265–70.

31. Robert CM Jr, Feigenbaum JA, Stern EW. Ocular palsy occurring with pituitary tumors. J Neurosurg 1973;38(1):17–9.

32. Daroff RB. See-saw nystagmus. Neurology 1965;15: 874–7.

33. Murad MH, Fernandez-Balsells MM, Barwise A, et al. Outcomes of surgical treatment for nonfunctioning pituitary adenomas: a systematic review and meta-analysis. Clin Endocrinol (Oxf) 2010;73(6):777–91.

34. Marcus M, Vitale S, Calvert PC, et al. Visual parameters in patients with pituitary adenoma before and after transsphenoidal surgery. Aust N Z J Ophthalmol 1991;19(2):111–8.

35. Cohen AR, Cooper PR, Kupersmith MJ, et al. Visual recovery after transsphenoidal removal of pituitary adenomas. Neurosurgery 1985;17(3):446–52.

36. Musluman AM, Cansever T, Yilmaz A, et al. Surgical results of large and giant pituitary adenomas with special consideration of ophthalmologic outcomes. World Neurosurg 2011;76(1–2):141–8 [discussion: 63–6].

37. Danesh-Meyer HV, Carroll SC, Foroozan R, et al. Relationship between retinal nerve fiber layer and visual field sensitivity as measured by optical coherence tomography in chiasmal compression. Invest Ophthalmol Vis Sci 2006;47(11):4827–35.

38. Danesh-Meyer HV, Papchenko T, Savino PJ, et al. In vivo retinal nerve fiber layer thickness measured by optical coherence tomography predicts visual recovery after surgery for parachiasmal tumors. Invest Ophthalmol Vis Sci 2008;49(5):1879–85.

39. Feinsod M, Selhorst JB, Hoyt WF, et al. Monitoring optic nerve function during craniotomy. J Neurosurg 1976;44(1):29–31.

40. Janaky M, Benedek G. Visual evoked potentials during the early phase of optic nerve compression in the orbital cavity. Doc Ophthalmol 1992;81(2): 197–208.

41. Ruther K, Ehlich P, Philipp A, et al. Prognostic value of the pattern electroretinogram in cases of tumors affecting the optic pathway. Graefes Arch Clin Exp Ophthalmol 1998;236(4):259–63.

42. McFadzean RM, Doyle D, Rampling R, et al. Pituitary apoplexy and its effect on vision. Neurosurgery 1991;29(5):669–75.

43. Agrawal D, Mahapatra AK. Visual outcome of blind eyes in pituitary apoplexy after transsphenoidal surgery: a series of 14 eyes. Surg Neurol 2005; 63(1):42–6 [discussion: 6].

44. Kayan A, Earl CJ. Compressive lesions of the optic nerves and chiasm. Pattern of recovery of vision following surgical treatment. Brain 1975; 98(1):13–28.

45. Kerrison JB, Lynn MJ, Baer CA, et al. Stages of improvement in visual fields after pituitary tumor resection. Am J Ophthalmol 2000;130(6):813–20.

46. Moster ML, Savino PJ, Schatz NJ, et al. Visual function in prolactinoma patients treated with bromocriptine. Ophthalmology 1985;92(10):1332–41.

47. Kahn SE, Miller JL. Rapid resolution of visual field defects and reduction in macroprolactinoma size with bromocriptine therapy. A case report. S Afr Med J 1982;62(19):696–9.

48. Landolt AM, Wuthrich R, Fellmann H. Regression of pituitary prolactinoma after treatment with bromocriptine. Lancet 1979;1(8125):1082–3.

49. Warnet A, Timsit J, Chanson P, et al. The effect of somatostatin analogue on chiasmal dysfunction from pituitary macroadenomas. J Neurosurg 1989; 71(5 Pt 1):687–90.

50. Losa M, Picozzi P, Motta M, et al. The role of radiation therapy in the management of non-functioning pituitary adenomas. J Endocrinol Invest 2011; 34(8):623–9.

51. Rush SC, Kupersmith MJ, Lerch I, et al. Neuro-ophthalmological assessment of vision before and after radiation therapy alone for pituitary macroadenomas. J Neurosurg 1990;72(4):594–9.

52. Mackley HB, Reddy CA, Lee SY, et al. Intensity-modulated radiotherapy for pituitary adenomas: the preliminary report of the Cleveland Clinic experience. Int J Radiat Oncol Biol Phys 2007;67(1):232–9.

53. Trautmann JC, Laws ER Jr. Visual status after trans-sphenoidal surgery at the Mayo Clinic, 1971-1982. Am J Ophthalmol 1983;96(2):200–8.

54. Barrow DL, Tindall GT. Loss of vision after trans-sphenoidal surgery. Neurosurgery 1990;27(1):60–8.

55. Lee WM, Adams JE. The empty sella syndrome. J Neurosurg 1968;28(4):351–6.

56. Morello G, Frera C. Visual damage after removal of hypophyseal adenomas: possible importance of vascular disturbances of the optic nerves and chiasma. Acta Neurochir (Wien) 1966;15(1):1–10.

57. Welch K, Stears JC. Chiasmapexy for the correction of traction on the optic nerves and chiasm associated with their descent into an empty sella turcica. Case report. J Neurosurg 1971;35(6):760–4.

58. Slavin ML, Lam BL, Decker RE, et al. Chiasmal compression from fat packing after transsphenoidal resection of intrasellar tumor in two patients. Am J Ophthalmol 1993;115(3):368–71.

59. Fossati P, Dewailly D, Thomas-Desrousseaux P, et al. Medical treatment of hyperprolactinemia. Horm Res 1985;22(3):228–38.

60. Taxel P, Waitzman DM, Harrington JF Jr, et al. Chiasmal herniation as a complication of bromocriptine therapy. J Neuroophthalmol 1996;16(4):252–7.

61. Alhajje A, Lambert M, Crabbe J. Pituitary apoplexy in an acromegalic patient during bromocriptine therapy. Case report. J Neurosurg 1985;63(2):288–92.

62. Stieber VW. Radiation therapy for visual pathway tumors. J Neuroophthalmol 2008;28(3):222–30.

63. Lawrence YR, Li XA, el Naqa I, et al. Radiation dose-volume effects in the brain. Int J Radiat Oncol Biol Phys 2010;76(Suppl 3):S20–7.

64. Erridge SC, Conkey DS, Stockton D, et al. Radiotherapy for pituitary adenomas: long-term efficacy and toxicity. Radiother Oncol 2009;93(3):597–601.

65. Kline LB, Kim JY, Ceballos R. Radiation optic neuropathy. Ophthalmology 1985;92(8):1118–26.

66. Wu-Chen WY, Jacobs DA, Volpe NJ, et al. Intracranial malignancies occurring more than 20 years after radiation therapy for pituitary adenoma. J Neuroophthalmol 2009;29(4):289–95.

67. Much JW, Weber ED, Newman SA. Ocular neuro-myotonia after gamma knife stereotactic radiation therapy. J Neuroophthalmol 2009;29(2):136–9.

68. Fahlbusch R, Schott W. Pterional surgery of meningiomas of the tuberculum sellae and planum sphenoidale: surgical results with special consideration of ophthalmological and endocrinological outcomes. J Neurosurg 2002;96(2):235–43.

69. Horn FK, Kaltwasser C, Junemann AG, et al. Objective perimetry using a four-channel multifocal VEP system: correlation with conventional perimetry and thickness of the retinal nerve fibre layer. Br J Ophthalmol 2012;96(4):554–9.

70. Chernov MF, Kawamata T, Amano K, et al. Possible role of single-voxel (1)H-MRS in differential diagnosis of suprasellar tumors. J Neurooncol 2009;91(2):191–8.

Management Options for Persistent Postoperative Acromegaly

Nestoras Mathioudakis, MD, Roberto Salvatori, MD*

KEYWORDS

- Persistent • Recurrent • Acromegaly • Somatostatin analogues • Dopamine agonists
- Radiotherapy • Growth-hormone adenoma

KEY POINTS

- Control of growth hormone (GH) and insulin-like growth factor I (IGF-I) levels is often not complete after surgery.
- Second surgery may be considered if an anatomic target is evident or to further reduce GH levels.
- Somatostatin analogues (SSAs) are the first line of medical therapy.
- Pegvisomant can be added or switched to if SSAs do not reach control.
- Radiation therapy has good tumor growth control, but hormonal control may require many years.

INTRODUCTION

Nearly one-third of patients with acromegaly will not be cured by initial surgery.[1] This statistic is likely attributable to the fact that growth hormone (GH)-secreting tumors are often large by the time they are discovered, because of the delayed recognition of acromegalic features.[2,3] Recently, the criteria for remission of acromegaly have become more stringent, meaning that an even larger number of individuals may be deemed not cured following surgery. To prevent the morbidity and early mortality associated with uncontrolled acromegaly, treatment options that provide prompt biochemical control while minimizing side effects are essential after unsuccessful surgery.[4] Choosing the appropriate therapy is best done in a multidisciplinary fashion involving close communication between endocrinologists, neurosurgeons, neuro-ophthalmologists, and radiation therapists. This review presents treatment approaches to the patient with persistent or recurrent postoperative acromegaly.

DEFINITIONS

Persistent disease denotes unsuccessful initial treatment, whereas recurrent disease is a return to a state of GH excess following initial remission. Despite advancements in surgical techniques, the cure rate following first-time surgery for acromegaly has not improved significantly over the last 30 years. A recent meta-analysis of 32 surgical series found persistent disease in 39% of patients while the recurrence rate following initial cure was only approximately 3%.[5] Thus, recurrence is much less likely than disease persistence to be encountered. From a management standpoint, the approach to persistent or recurrent disease is generally similar.

Factors Predictive of Tumor Aggressiveness

Tumor size, extrasellar extension, and GH levels are the most important predictors of initial surgical cure.[6] Surprisingly, tumor size and invasiveness

Disclosure statement: N.M. has no relevant financial disclosures. R.S. received research grants support from Ipsen, Novartis, and Pfizer, and sat in the advisory board of Ipsen and Novartis.
Johns Hopkins University School of Medicine, Division of Endocrinology & Metabolism, Department of Medicine, 1830 East Monument Street, Suite 333, Baltimore, MD 21287, USA
* Corresponding author.
E-mail address: salvator@jhmi.edu

Neurosurg Clin N Am 23 (2012) 621–638
http://dx.doi.org/10.1016/j.nec.2012.06.005
1042-3680/12/$ – see front matter © 2012 Elsevier Inc. All rights reserved.

do not appear to predict the likelihood of tumor recurrence after remission.[5] Lower recurrence rate is observed in patients with low postoperative and glucose-suppressed GH levels, while age and gender have no predictive value.[5] The incidence of recurrences appears to peak around 1 to 5 years after surgery, although recurrences have been observed more than 10 years after initial cure.[5]

Even with today's multimodal therapy, which can provide adequate disease control for the majority of patients, there is a subset of individuals (fewer than 10% of those cured surgically) who exhibit treatment-resistant tumor growth.[7] These factors have been associated with more aggressive tumor behavior[7]:

- Younger age at diagnosis
- Larger or extensive and invasive tumors
- Higher pretreatment GH levels
- Molecular and genetic factors
  - gsp, PTTG, GADD45 gene mutations
  - FGF-4 expression
  - MEN-1, AIP gene mutations[8]
- Tumor morphology
  - Sparsely granulated adenomas
  - Dotlike cytokeratin adenoma staining pattern
  - Higher Ki-67 index

Changing Biochemical Definition of Cure

A precise definition of cure has historically been challenging to reach in the absence of clear clinical parameters with which to monitor disease activity. Biochemical markers (insulin-like growth factor I [IGF-I] and GH) have therefore been relied on as the best indicators of disease burden. Higher GH and IGF-I are associated with increased mortality in acromegaly, often because of cardiovascular disease.[9] Thus, goals of therapy include normalization of IGF-I according to age-specific and sex-specific reference ranges, and attainment of GH levels below specific random and oral glucose-suppressed cutoffs. Over the last 50 years, the GH cutoff has been progressively

lowered as GH assays have become more sensitive and specific. In fact, the postoperative basal GH criterion for cure in the 1960s was 10 to 20 times less stringent compared with today.[10] Up until the mid-1990s, GH was measured using polyclonal radioimmunoassay (RIA), and a GH treatment target of less than 2.5 µg/L was chosen as the criterion for cure based on data showing no incremental mortality risk below that level.[9] In 1999, taking into consideration the improved sensitivity of newer monoclonal GH assays (chemiluminescence, immunofluorescence, immunoradiometric, and so forth), a consensus group met in Cortina, Italy to propose criteria for cure. According to these Cortina criteria, a normal IGF-I level and nadir GH level after oral glucose tolerance test (GH_n) of less than 1 µg/L suggested cure.[11] That conference did not specifically mention a cutoff for random GH (GH_r), and several studies have used a cutoff of 2.5 µg/L as a definition of control.

Current Consensus Criteria for Cure

In the years following the publication of the Cortina criteria, significant advancements have been made in the management of acromegaly, particularly with respect to adjunctive medical therapy for persistent disease. The complex, often multimodal treatment in acromegaly, and the development of even more sensitive (ultrasensitive) GH assays led to newer criteria for cure (**Table 1**), published in 2010.[12]

Having only recently been implemented in practice, there are limited long-term outcome data to support the newer targets. The main evidence to date comes from 2 studies showing that mortality risk was similar to that in the reference population in patients whose GH_r was less than 1 µg/L.[13,14] There is a general consensus that using current ultrasensitive GH assays, a GH_r less than 1 µg/L corresponds to the older RIA GH value of 2.5 µg/L, for which a clear mortality benefit has been demonstrated.

Table 1
Biochemical criteria for cure in acromegaly

Consensus Criteria	Random Fasting GH (GH_r) (µg/L)	Nadir GH After OGTT (GH_n) (µg/L)	IGF-I
2000 Cortina criteria	(Not defined)	<1	Age/sex normalized
Current 2010 criteria	<1	<0.4	Age/sex normalized

Abbreviation: OGTT, oral glucose tolerance test.

(Data from Giustina A, Barkan A, Casanueva FF, et al. Criteria for cure of acromegaly: a consensus statement. J Clin Endocrinol Metab 2000;85:526–9; and Giustina A, Chanson P, Bronstein MD, et al. A consensus on criteria for cure of acromegaly. J Clin Endocrinol Metab 2010;95:3141–8.)

Discordant IGF-I and GH

Generally, GH and IGF-I results are concordant following surgery; however, an elevated IGF-I despite normal GH may be seen in up to 24% of surgically treated patients, while high GH despite normal IGF-I is seen in about 10% of patients.[15,16] When there is discordance between IGF-I and GH results, determining the patient's clinical status can be perplexing, and often repeated testing is needed.

The reasons for discordant hormonal results after treatment are not entirely certain, although several possible causes have been identified (**Fig. 1**). The more common scenario of an elevated IGF-I with normal GH may result from inadequate GH sampling to detect elevated GH pulses, testing IGF-I levels too soon after surgery, low but uninterrupted GH secretion, and rare GH-receptor polymorphisms. The less common finding of a normal IGF-I with a high GH can result from any systemic condition that reduces hepatic IGF-I production. It is well known that medical treatment with somatostatin analogues (SSAs) is more likely to be associated with normal IGF-I despite elevated GH. This phenomenon has been attributed to pituitary-independent suppression of hepatic IGF-I production by SSAs.[17] A problem common to both scenarios is the issue of GH and IGF-I interassay variability, which has been discussed extensively in the recent American Association of Clinical Endocrinologists guidelines and current consensus criteria.[18,19]

Timing of Postoperative Biochemical Testing

Given the long biological half-life of IGF-I, accurate assessment of IGF-I status after surgery requires

waiting at least 12 weeks for levels to stabilize.[20] On the other hand, GH has a very short half-life, and elevated values are telling even in the immediate postoperative period. The role of early (1 week postoperative) GH_n as a predictor of long-term remission has been examined in 2 studies.[20,21] Using GH_n cutoffs of 1.0 μg/L, these studies showed a high predictive value for cure based on early postoperative measurements. Although these cutoffs were higher than today's current standard, both studies showed high correlation between early postoperative (1 week) and delayed GH_n testing (12 weeks). This result suggests that an early GH_n by today's standard (<0.4 μg/L) probably predicts long-term remission. However, an early negative response to an oral glucose tolerance test requires follow-up testing at a later time point, because the inadequate sensitivity of this test may initially misclassify a patient in remission as having persistent disease.[20,21]

CLINICAL EVALUATION

In addition to targeting the source of the problem (excess GH), patients should be offered standard of care monitoring (ie, fasting lipid profile, blood pressure control, hemoglobin A_{1C}, and so forth), and treatments for their comorbidities (ie, blood sugar or lipid-lowering agents, osteoarthritis medications, bone-specific therapy, continuous positive airway pressure, and so forth). Worsening of a previously controlled symptom should prompt biochemical investigation for disease recurrence, and persistent symptoms might indicate the need for titration of medical therapy. Hypopituitarism is independently associated with reduced

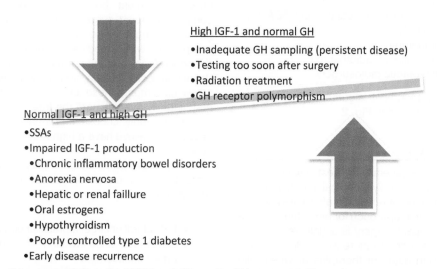

High IGF-1 and normal GH
- Inadequate GH sampling (persistent disease)
- Testing too soon after surgery
- Radiation treatment
- GH receptor polymorphism

Normal IGF-1 and high GH
- SSAs
- Impaired IGF-1 production
  - Chronic inflammatory bowel disorders
  - Anorexia nervosa
  - Hepatic or renal faillure
  - Oral estrogens
  - Hypothyroidism
  - Poorly controlled type 1 diabetes
- Early disease recurrence

Fig. 1. Possible causes of discordant IGF-I and GH results. SSA, somatostatin analogue.

life expectancy, so anterior pituitary deficiencies resulting from the tumor or its treatment should be evaluated and appropriate hormone replacement started for any uncovered deficiencies.[22]

Radiological Evaluation

All patients who are not cured by surgery require follow-up pituitary magnetic resonance imaging (MRI) to determine residual tumor anatomy. It is generally advisable to wait at least 3 months before assessing radiographic response, to avoid misinterpreting postoperative inflammation and edema as tumor remnant. The need for MRI in cured patients is less obvious. When residual tumor is identified, its size, location, invasiveness, and mass effect (optic chiasm compression) are key considerations in determining the next management step. If optic chiasm compression is still present, formal visual field testing is important in establishing a new baseline before other treatment attempts. Repeat surgery is reasonable if the tumor is accessible, regardless of size. Cavernous sinus invasion is associated with a very low likelihood of successful repeat surgery.[23]

TREATMENT OPTIONS

After failed pituitary surgery, treatment options include:

- Repeat surgery
- Medical therapy
  - SSA
  - Dopamine agonist (DA)
  - Growth hormone receptor antagonist (GHRA)
  - Combination medical therapy (SSA ± DA ± GHRA)
- Radiotherapy
  - Conventional radiotherapy
  - Stereotactic radiosurgery

A general treatment algorithm for persistent disease in proposed in **Fig. 2**.

Repeat Surgery

While surgery is generally the best initial treatment choice for acromegaly, medical therapy affords the best chances of remission after failed surgery and is the favored approach for persistent disease. In practice, repeat surgery is usually reserved for debulking purposes to increase the likelihood of remission with adjuvant therapies or when relief of mass effect on the optic chiasm is needed.

Effectiveness of Secondary (Repeat) Surgery

There is scant evidence on the effectiveness of repeat surgery. Among the handful of surgical series that have published outcomes of reoperations, only 5 used Cortina remission criteria (**Table 2**). The mean remission rate for reoperations in these contemporary series is 37%, but there is wide variation among the individual studies (8%–59%). When data from all the studies is combined, 117 of 345 reoperated patients achieved remission (34%), with the same remission rate seen when including only studies that used the Cortina criteria. As a reference, the mean remission rates from primary surgery using Cortina criteria in microadenomas, macroadenomas, and adenomas overall are 80%, 57%, and 64%, respectively.[1,24–26]

One of the major limitations in appraising the value of repeat surgery is the lack of clear inclusion criteria in the studies. When the investigators excluded tumors deemed unresectable on the basis of MRI appearance, the mean remission rate increased in individual studies by 12% to 36%, with an overall increase of 13% among pooled studies using the Cortina criteria.[27–29] For example, in a recent study by Alahmadi and colleagues,[29] when only noninvasive tumors were included in the calculations, 80% of persistent tumors (4 of 5 patients) were successfully cured. By contrast, in a much larger series of 140 reoperated patients by Nomikos and colleagues,[27] the remission rate only increased from 27% to 39% when invasive tumors with very high GH levels before first surgery were excluded.

In pooled data of all resectable tumors using the Cortina criteria, a remission rate of 47% is seen (55 out of 118 reoperations). While this efficacy rate is not significantly inferior to medical therapy (50%–60%), one must be cautious about directly comparing repeat surgery with medical therapy, given the much lower number of reoperated compared with medically treated patients described in the literature, the lack of consistently defined inclusion criteria, and varying durations of follow-up among these studies. Selection bias may actually overestimate the true remission rate if surgeons only choose to reoperate on those cases they believe have a high likelihood of being cured.

As is the case with primary surgery, the following were found to be predictors of unsuccessful repeat surgery:

- Extradural or large suprasellar component[30]
- Cavernous sinus invasion[27,31,32] or carotid artery encasement[28]
- Tumor segmentation[23]

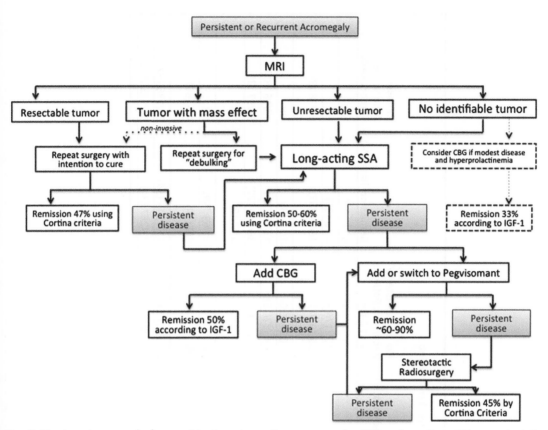

Fig. 2. Treatment approach for persistent postoperative acromegaly. CBG, cabergoline; SSA, somatostatin analogue.

- GH level greater than 40 μg/L before first surgery[23]
- Younger age (<40 years)[23]

Among the combined patients in these series, 79% were persistent tumors while 21% were recurrences. It can therefore be assumed that most invasive tumors at repeat surgery had invasive features before the initial surgery. With the increasing specialization of pituitary surgery, failed initial surgery can more often than not be attributed to larger tumor size and invasiveness rather than lack of surgical expertise; however, if a patient has a residual tumor that appears completely resectable and lacks the aforementioned negative prognostic features (especially if the first surgery was performed by an inexperienced neurosurgeon), it is reasonable to consider repeat surgery by a more experienced pituitary surgeon. The surgeon's experience certainly should weigh heavily in the decision to consider repeat surgery, because several studies have demonstrated higher remission and lower complication rates when surgery is performed by a single experienced surgeon.[18,33,34]

Role of Debulking Surgery

Despite a low prospect of cure, repeated surgery can be used for the purposes of tumor debulking to increase the effectiveness of adjuvant medical therapy.[35,36] In a study of 86 patients poorly responsive to medical treatment with SSAs, partial primary surgical removal improved success rate from 12.8% to 55.5%.[36] Another study of 24 patients taking SSAs found that primary surgery increased the proportion of patients having normal GH and IGF-I from 29% to 54% and 46% to 78%, respectively.[35] Regarding the debulking benefit of secondary surgery, in a recent study of 53 patients whose preoperative GH was greater than 10 μg/L, partial tumor resection resulted in GH reduction below 10, 5, and 2.5 μg/L in 50%, 35%, and 21% of patients, respectively.[37] With respect to IGF-I, 17% of patients had a 30% reduction from preoperative levels while 9% achieved normalization.[37]

Risks of Repeat Surgery

Studies have reported varying incidences of new anterior pituitary hormone deficiencies after repeat transsphenoidal surgery. Yamada and colleagues[23]

Table 2
Outcomes of repeat surgery for persistent or recurrent acromegaly after surgical treatment

Authors,[Ref.] Year	Remission Criteria: Normal IGF-I and		Total No. of Patients	No. of Reoperated Patients	No. of Persistent/ Recurrent Patients (% of Each)	Remission Rate (%)	Remission Rate Among Resectable Tumors Only (%)
	GH_n (µg/L)	GH_r (µg/L)					
Long et al,[30] 1996	<2	<5	212	16	12/1[a] (75/6)	5/16 (31)	NR
Freda et al,[31] 1998	<2	<2	115	12	2/10 (17/83)	4/12 (33)	NR
Abe and Lüdecke,[32] 1998	<2	<4.5	270	28	26/2 (93/7)	16/28 (57)	16/18 (89)
Shimon et al,[74] 2001	<2	<2	103	12	12/0 (100/0)	1/12 (8)	NR
Kurosaki et al,[28] 2003	<1	<2.5	NR	22	18/4 (82/18)	13/22 (59)	13/16 (81)
Nomikos et al,[27] 2005	<1	<2.5	688	140	98/42 (70/30)	38/140 (27)	38/97 (39)
Espinosa de los Monteros,[37] 2009	<1	-	NR	53	53/0 (100/0)	5/53 (9)	NR
Yamada et al,[23] 2010	<1	NR	482	53	NR	31/53 (58)	NR
Alahmadi et al,[29] 2012	<1	<2.5	350	9	NR	4/9 (44)	4/5 (80)
All studies combined				345	221/59 (79/21)	117/345 (34)	71/136 (52)
Combined studies that used Cortina criteria				277	169/46 (79/21)	91/267 (34)	55/118 (47)

Abbreviations: GH_n, post-OGTT GH nadir; GH_r, random fasting GH; NR, not reported.
[a] Indication for surgery was visual impairment for 4 tumors, not specified as persistent or recurrent.

showed that among 31 reoperated patients almost all hormone deficiencies were acquired after the first surgery, with an incidence of new hormone deficiencies of only 1.9% after the second surgery. Recovery of pituitary function was seen in over one-third of patients after second surgery in another study.[32] By contrast, in their study of 53 reoperated patients, Espinosa de los Monteros and colleagues[37] showed nearly the same incidence of individual anterior pituitary hormone deficiencies after primary and secondary surgery. Because the mortality from untreated acromegaly exceeds that of hypopituitarism, and because hormone deficiencies can easily be replaced, the fear of worsening pituitary function should not bear heavily on the decision to consider repeat surgery.[22]

Regarding operative morbidity, in the large study by Nomikos and colleagues[27] of 140 reoperated patients, the complication rates were comparable between primary and secondary surgery. However, the major complication rates from other surgical series (**Table 3**) were higher than expected based on data from first-time surgeries, likely because of the smaller sample size in these studies.[38] For example, meningitis, cerebrospinal fluid (CSF) leak, vascular injury, and ophthalmopathy are reported to occur in 0.7%, 2.2%, 0.6%, and 0.5% of major endoscopic series, respectively.[38] By comparison, in reoperated cases the incidence of meningitis was 1.8% to 6%, CSF leak/fistula 2% to 9%, vascular injury 0.1% to 6%, and ophthalmopathy 6%. There was no reoperative mortality in these series.

Medical Therapy

The 3 main classes of medications used in the treatment of acromegaly each have different receptor target actions:

1. The SSAs work by inhibiting somatotroph cell proliferation and GH secretion by binding to specific somatostatin receptors on GH tumor cells.
2. The DAs work by binding to the dopamine D2 receptor found on both GH and prolactin cells, thereby exerting negative control.
3. The GHRA, pegvisomant, blocks the peripheral target actions of GH.

Which class of medication to use for an individual patient depends on various factors, including the degree of active disease, tumor

Table 3
Complications following repeat surgery

Authors,[Ref.] Year	Operative Mortality Rate, %	Overall Complication Rate, %	Major Complications (Rate, %)
Long et al,[30] 1996	0	19	SAH, intrasellar hemorrhage (6) New bitemporal hemianopsia (resolved) (6) Bacterial meningitis (6) CN III, IV, VI palsies (6)
Abe and Lüdecke,[32] 1998	0	0	
Kurosaki et al,[28] 2002	0	0	
Nomikos et al,[27] 2005	NR	Similar to primary surgery	Overall complications (primary and secondary surgery): Meningitis (1.8) CSF leak (0.8) Carotid artery injury (0.1)
Espinosa de los Monteros et al,[37] 2009	0	21	Arachnoid tear (8) CSF fistula (9) Meningitis (2) CSF fistula + meningitis (2)
Yamada et al,[23] 2010	0	13	CSF leak (3) CN VI palsy (3) Severe nasal bleeding (3) Pituitary abscess (3)

Abbreviations: CN, cranial nerve; CSF, cerebrospinal fluid; NR, not reported; SAH, subarachnoid hemorrhage.

characteristics on MRI, underlying comorbidities, and cost. In general, SSAs are considered first-line medical therapy, as they have a long track record of efficacy as adjuvant therapy following surgery and/or radiotherapy. Because they offer both biochemical and tumor control, they should be used in patients with larger residual tumors. DAs, specifically cabergoline, might be considered in a patient with modest disease or if there is persistent hyperprolactinemia. Pegvisomant is usually reserved as third-line therapy because of its high cost and theoretical concerns about tumor growth, but might be considered in a patient with small tumor burden or persistent symptoms despite normalization of IGF-I.

SOMATOSTATIN ANALOGUES

The presently commercially available SSAs in the United States include octreotide, octreotide long-acting release (LAR) (Sandostatin LAR; Novartis, Basel Switzerland), and lanreotide autogel (ATG) (Somatuline Depot; Ipsen, Basking Ridge, NJ). Oc-treotide has a relatively short half-life of 2 hours after subcutaneous injection, meaning it has to be dosed 3 times daily to achieve therapeutic concentrations. Because of this inconvenient dosing schedule, it has been substituted in prac-tice by the long-acting release form octreotide LAR, which can be administered by intramuscular injection once monthly. Lanreotide SR (sustained release) is an intermediate-acting formulation given every 1 to 2 weeks that is no longer available in the United States. It has been replaced by the longer-acting depot formulation, Lanreotide ATG, administered by deep subcutaneous injection once per month.

Effectiveness as Secondary Therapy

Biochemical control
SSAs have been used as adjunctive therapy following surgery and/or radiotherapy for more than 20 years. The long-acting depot formulations, octreotide LAR and lanreotide ATG, are the 2 widely used medications in practice today. These drugs are conveniently dosed once monthly and show similar efficacy profiles. In recent years, SSAs have increasingly been used as primary therapy or as presurgical treatment to improve chances of surgical cure in macroadenomas. Given their broader uses in clinical practice, it is becoming harder to find studies using modern remission criteria that examine the efficacy of SSAs exclusively in surgically uncured patients. One such study of 68 patients showed that secondary SSA treatment achieved a biochemical remission (using Cortina criteria) in 64% and 78%

of patients taking octreotide LAR and lanreotide ATG, respectively (no statistical difference between groups).[39] A selection bias (unresponsive patients excluded in this retrospective study) has likely contributed to the high percentage of remis-sion. It has been shown that octreotide LAR has similar efficacy in both untreated patients and those who previously received surgery and/or radiotherapy, and that octreotide LAR and lanreo-tide SR are equally effective as secondary treat-ment.[40,41] Therefore, it is reasonable to assume that the efficacy of long-acting SSAs as secondary therapy approximates the overall efficacy among heterogeneous populations of untreated and previously treated patients. Among 32 studies, the long-acting SSAs are 63%, 56%, and 49% effective at normalizing GH, IGF-I, and both GH and IGF-I, respectively (**Table 4**).

Tumor shrinkage
In addition to biochemical control, prevention of tumor growth is an important goal of treatment with SSAs, particularly in the case of larger residual tumors. Octreotide LAR and lanreotide ATG exert pharmacologic effects on tumor growth by targeting distinct somatostatin recep-tors on GH adenomas. It has been suggested that the different receptor affinity profiles of these 2 medications may account for their subtle differ-ences in effect on tumor shrinkage.[42] Most of the data on tumor shrinkage in acromegaly come from studies using either short-acting or long-acting formulations of octreotide and lanreotide SR, with sparse data regarding the effect of lan-reotide ATG.[42]

Two factors may influence the effect of SSAs on tumor shrinkage: (1) whether the SSA is being used as primary or secondary therapy, and (2) tumor size. Although definitions of tumor shrinkage vary across studies, it has generally been shown that the SSAs can achieve greater tumor shrinkage when used as primary therapy. In treatment-naïve patients, 51% of patients treated with SSA had tumor shrinkage as compared with 27% after surgery or radiation.[43] Following noncurative surgery, the mean percentage of tumor-volume reduction has been shown to be similar between octreotide LAR (28.5%) and lanreotide ATG (34.9%).[39] With respect to tumor size, some studies have reported better response to shrinkage in macroadenomas compared with microadeno-mas, although this has not consistently been demonstrated.[42]

Whereas tumor shrinkage and biochemical parameters usually show parallel responses to treatment with SSAs, a dissociation between tumor shrinkage and biochemical response is

Table 4
Biochemical remission rates achieved using long-acting SSAs as both primary and secondary therapy

Authors,[Ref.] Year	% of Patients Achieving GH Criteria for Remission	% of Patients with Normalized IGF-I	% of Patients Achieving Both GH Criteria for Remission and Normalized IGF-I
Octreotide LAR			
Lancranjan and Atkinson,[75] 1999	69.8[a]	63.1	NR
Chanson et al,[76] 2000	68[a]	NR	65
Colao et al,[77] 2001	69.4[a]	61.1	NR
Ayuk et al,[78] 2002	36[b]	67	NR
Ayuk et al,[40] 2004	70[b]	72	NR
Alexopoulou et al,[79] 2004	64[a]	52	NR
Jallad et al,[80] 2005	74[a]	41	NR
Grottoli et al,[81] 2005	64[a]	35.7	28.6
Trepp et al,[82] 2005	NR[a]	NR	65
Cozzi et al,[83] 2006	68.7[a]	70.1	56.7
Colao et al,[84] 2006	NR[a]	NR	55.9
Ronchi et al,[85] 2007	43[a]	35	NR
Maiza et al,[86] 2007	70[b]	67	58
Mercado et al,[87] 2007	42[a]	34	25
Colao et al,[88] 2007	86[a]	84	80
Auriemma et al,[89] 2008	77.7[a,b]	62.9	62.9
Colao et al,[90] 2009	NR[a]	NR	27.5
Baldys-Waligorska et al,[91] 2009	63[a,b]	54.5	NR
Oki et al,[92] 2009	56.7[a]	53.3	36.7
Luque-Ramirez et al,[93] 2010	54[a]	46	NR
Tutuncu et al,[39] 2011	67[c]	67	63.9
Karaca et al,[26] 2011	45[c]	27	27
Octreotide LAR (nonweighted mean ± SD)	63 ± 13	55 ± 15	50 ± 19
Lanreotide Autogel			
Caron et al,[94] 2002	NR[a]	NR	39
Alexopoulou et al,[79] 2004	48[a]	52	NR
Caron et al,[45] 2004	68[a]	NR	43
Caron et al,[95] 2006	77[a]	54	46
Lucas and Astorga,[96] 2006	54[a]	56	40
Ronchi et al,[85] 2007	62[a]	43	NR
Chanson et al,[97] 2008	85[a]	43	38
Melmed et al,[98] 2010	49[a]	54	38
Lombardi et al,[99] 2009	63[a]	37	NR
Attanasio et al,[100] 2008	42[a]	54	38
Salvatori et al,[52] 2010	76.9[c]	84.8	73.1
Tutuncu et al,[39] 2011	78.1[c]	78.1	78.1
Schopohl et al,[101] 2011	71.4[b]	62.9	NR
Lanreotide Autogel (nonweighted mean ± SD)	65 ± 14	56 ± 14	48 ± 16
Both long-acting SSAs (nonweighted mean ± SD)	63 ± 13	56 ± 15	49 ± 17

Abbreviation: NR, not reported.

[a] GH_r <2.5 µg/L.
[b] GH_r <2 µg/L.
[c] GH_n <1 µg/L.

occasionally observed (tumor shrinkage without biochemical control). If a patient who derives benefit from SSAs from the perspective of tumor control fails to achieve biochemical remission, consideration may be given to adding pegvisomant. The theoretical concern about tumor regrowth with pegvisomant would be lessened in the setting of concomitant use of an SSA that has been demonstrated to exert tumoral control.

Symptom control

The SSAs can provide effective symptomatic control after noncurative surgery. In a study of 33 patients with poorly controlled disease requiring multimodal therapy (surgery, radiation therapy, DAs), octreotide LAR resulted in 54% reduction in the prevalence of clinical signs and symptoms at follow-up of nearly 3.5 years.[44] In this cohort of patients, of whom 39% had invasive adenomas, the reductions in acromegalic symptoms were 28%, 38%, 40%, and 70% for arthralgias, perspiration, asthenia, and acral growth, respectively.[44] In a study of 131 patients taking lanreotide ATG, of whom 76% had had prior surgery, there were improvements of 11%, 16%, 14%, 24%, and 16% in sweating, headache, asthenia, edema, and arthralgias, respectively.[45]

Predictors of response

Responsiveness to SSAs is inversely correlated with tumor size and baseline hormonal levels. Smaller, less invasive adenomas with lower GH and IGF-I are more likely to reach biochemical control. Although prior surgery or radiotherapy does not influence the GH response to SSAs, radiotherapy has been associated with a less marked lowering of IGF-I.[46] It has been suggested that the pathologic finding of a densely granulated adenoma and a hypointense T2-weighted MRI signal in acromegalic patients after failed surgery may both predict a better response to SSA treatment.[47,48]

Clinical Considerations

Dose optimization

The response to usual starting doses of SSAs may vary considerably among patients, with respect to both biochemical and symptom control. Doses should be optimized before considering a patient to be a nonresponder. As long as there are no limiting side effects, doses should be increased up to a maximum of 40 mg per month for octreotide LAR (requiring 2 separate injections) and 120 mg per month for lanreotide ATG (maximal doses approved by the Food and Drug Administration). Likewise, the minimal dose required to attain biochemical and symptomatic control should be used.

Recently it has been shown that high-dose or high-frequency treatment with SSAs can improve their efficacy in patients considered refractory to treatment with these drugs.[49] When patients unresponsive to conventional doses of octreotide LAR are switched to high doses (60 mg/mo) or high-frequency dosing (30 mg/3 wk), 27% and 36% achieved control of GH and IGF-I, respectively.[49] There is less experience with high-dose or high-frequency lanreotide ATG; however, a small case series showed 5 of 6 patients achieved GH normalization and 3 of 6 had normalization of IGF-I when lanreotide ATG was sequentially titrated to 180 mg every 3 to 4 weeks.[50]

Side effects

Even at maximal doses, the safety and tolerability of SSAs is generally maintained, with the most common side effects related to gastrointestinal symptoms: abdominal cramps, flatulence, diarrhea, constipation, and nausea.[49,51] Abnormalities of the biliary tract, including gallstones, sediment, sludge, and dilatation occur fairly commonly within the first 2 years of treatment regardless of dose, although they are usually asymptomatic and rarely require surgery. Patients should be questioned about cholelithiasis symptoms at follow-up, but abdominal ultrasound surveillance is not necessary.

Local skin irritation and pain at the injection site may be experienced, but is usually mild and dose dependent. One of the advantages of lanreotide ATG is that, unlike octreotide LAR, the formulation does not have to be reconstituted by a health care professional before administration, and can safely be administered at home by the patient or partner.[52]

With respect to glucose homeostasis, surgery may have a greater effect on reversal of impaired glucose tolerance and type 2 diabetes in comparison with primary therapy with SSAs. This outcome is believed to be due to the negative effects of SSAs on pancreatic β-cell function.[53] However, because GH itself is associated with insulin resistance, SSAs generally have a neutral effect on glycemic control.[54] Also, the addition of GHRA to SSA does not appear to significantly alter glycemic control.[55]

DOPAMINE AGONISTS

The DAs, cabergoline and bromocriptine, are traditionally used in the management of prolactin-secreting pituitary adenomas. Their use in acromegaly is based on the fact that both mixed prolactin-GH and pure GH-secreting adenomas have dopamine receptors on their surfaces.[56] Indeed, even patients without hyperprolactinemia may show a marked biochemical response to cabergoline.[56] The advantages of the DAs are that they are relatively inexpensive compared with other medical therapies and can be taken orally.

In the United States there are 2 commercially available DAs: cabergoline and bromocriptine. Cabergoline is the preferred drug in this class, both for the management of prolactinomas and GH-secreting adenomas, because of its longer half-life, superior efficacy, and better tolerability compared with bromocriptine. Therefore, this review focused mainly on the efficacy of cabergoline in persistent postoperative acromegaly.

Effectiveness as Secondary Therapy

Biochemical control
As monotherapy, cabergoline normalizes IGF-I in less than one-third of patients, and when combined with SSAs, its efficacy increases to about 50%.[56] Therefore, the authors reserve it for those patients who do not completely normalize serum IGF-I with SSA monotherapy (particularly if serum IGF-I levels are less than 2 times normal). As with other treatments in acromegaly, the most significant predictor of responsiveness to cabergoline is the baseline IGF-I level: chances of remission are greatest when IGF-I is less than 150% the upper limit of normal.[56] Prior surgery is not associated with any differences in response to DAs, while prior radiotherapy actually shows an enhanced response to GH reduction.[46] Unfortunately, most of the studies assessing the efficacy of cabergoline as adjuvant or primary therapy did not use the Cortina criteria but rather relied solely on normalization of IGF-I as the indicator of response.[56]

Tumor shrinkage
There is limited prospective data regarding the effect of DAs on tumor shrinkage. Studies differ with respect to the DA used, the proportion of previously operated patients, and definitions of tumor shrinkage.[56] A recent meta-analysis found that cabergoline was shown to reduce tumor volume to varying extents in 17 of 32 patients.[56] Although it cannot predict biochemical response, the presence of hyperprolactinemia may result in a greater degree of tumor shrinkage by cabergoline.[56] Therefore it might be considered in patients with modest disease who have elevated serum prolactin levels.

Dose escalation
The cabergoline dose required for biochemical control in acromegaly can be variable, but averages around 2.5 mg/wk, which is 2 to 5 times higher than doses used to treat prolactinomas.[56] Nonetheless, adverse effects do not appear to be increased as a result of this higher dose.[56] Recently, concerns have been raised about the possibility of cardiac valvular disease in individuals taking high cumulative doses of DAs, as in Parkinson disease. Although this effect has not been clearly demonstrated in patients being treated for prolactinomas, because acromegaly itself confers an increased risk of cardiomyopathy and valvulopathy it may be prudent to monitor patients on higher doses of cabergoline with periodic echocardiograms.[56]

Side effects
Cabergoline is generally well tolerated. The main side effects are nausea and vomiting, followed by headaches, nasal congestion, and dizziness.[56] Bromocriptine causes more pronounced gastrointestinal side effects, with nausea and vomiting occurring in up to one-third of patients.[57] These side effects can be minimized by starting with a low dose and titrating slowly.[57]

PEGVISOMANT

Pegvisomant is a genetically modified GH analogue that acts as a competitive inhibitor at the receptor level to block the action of native GH. Because of its mechanism of action, pegvisomant has no effect on tumor shrinkage. For this reason, and because of its very high cost, pegvisomant is almost never used as monotherapy to treat persistent postoperative disease.[10,58] However, it can play an important role in patients refractory to SSAs or DAs. The medication is administered by subcutaneous injection daily, although less frequent injections in combination with SSAs are also highly effective and offer a financial advantage in patients who might otherwise require high doses of pegvisomant.[59] Average therapeutic doses range from 15 to 20 mg/d, but doses up to 60 mg/d have been used. Because pegvisomant has no effect on GH secretion, serum IGF-I levels serve as a gauge of biochemical remission.

Efficacy as Secondary Therapy

Monotherapy
Initial studies using pegvisomant, which included large numbers of patients who had failed surgery or radiotherapy, found the drug to highly effective at normalizing IGF-I levels (90%–95% of patients) and controlling acromegalic symptoms.[60] Recently, however, this has been brought into question by the results of the large observational Acrostudy of 792

patients, which showed that fewer than 70% of patients had achieved normal IGF-I levels at 5-year follow-up.[61] One of the reasons for this disappointing result may be inadequate dose titration of pegvisomant in study participants, because a large proportion of the patients with high IGF-I were receiving a daily dose of 20 mg or less (which is the highest vial size presently available, but below the maximal dose used in clinical trials of 40 mg/d).[61]

Combination pegvisomant and SSA

In practice, pegvisomant is often considered for the patient who is suboptimally controlled on SSA therapy. A recent study of 27 patients who had previously undergone surgery or radiotherapy and who failed to achieve remission with octreotide LAR found that pegvisomant, whether added onto octreotide LAR or used as monotherapy, was equally effective at normalizing IGF-I (56% as monotherapy, 62% in combination).[62] Similar findings have been observed with lanreotide ATG[63]; however, the lower than expected efficacy seen with the combination of lanreotide ATG and pegvisomant (58%) may be due to the purpose of the study, which focused on the cost-savings benefit of combination therapy. The investigators showed that the dose of pegvisomant could be reduced by the addition of lanreotide ATG, but the full potential of combination therapy may not have been realized because the emphasis was on pegvisomant dose reduction rather than maximization.[64] Indeed, it has been shown that weekly dose reductions of pegvisomant of 80 to 150 mg could be achieved by the addition of lanreotide ATG, with no change in serum IGF-I levels.[64] While this may translate to substantial cost reductions for the patient, it may also come at the expense of inadequate IGF-I control. Therefore, if pegvisomant is to be considered in treatment it should be titrated maximally to guarantee the most effective response.[60] Finally, because of pegvisomant's favorable effects on glucose control, some believe that it should be the first-choice medical therapy in patients with diabetes.[65]

Combination pegvisomant and cabergoline

To date, there is only a single study of 24 patients assessing combination pegvisomant and cabergoline therapy.[66] In this study, 96% of patients had a history of noncurative surgery. As monotherapy, cabergoline normalized IGF-I levels in only 8% of patients, but with the addition of low-dose pegvisomant (10 mg daily) 68% of patients achieved a normal IGF-I. Surprisingly, after being withdrawn from cabergoline treatment, only 26% of patients treated with pegvisomant monotherapy had normal IGF-I levels. This result suggests that the combination of cabergoline and pegvisomant is more effective than either agent alone.

Symptom control

It has been argued by some that normal IGF-I levels alone should not be the sole indicator of clinically controlled acromegaly.[67] A double-blind, placebo-controlled study showed that antagonizing GH action using pegvisomant in patients who had already normalized serum IGF-I levels on SSA improved quality of life.[67] This effect appeared to be mediated by improvement in GH-dependent parameters, such as loss of body weight, reductions in perspiration, and soft-tissue swelling.[67] The concept of extrahepatic acromegaly has been coined to explain this phenomenon: while SSAs, in addition to reducing GH secretion, inhibit the action of GH at the liver (where IGF-I is produced), they do not necessarily target the GH actions in other organs. As a result of the marked improvement in quality-of-life scores, some have questioned whether pegvisomant should only be reserved for patients who fail SSA treatment and should instead be used more liberally.[64]

Risk of tumor growth

Because pegvisomant blocks the negative feedback inhibition of IGF-I on GH cells, there is a theoretical concern that the medication could exacerbate tumor growth. Although there have been case reports of tumor growth in patients taking pegvisomant, it is unclear whether this simply reflects selection bias (ie, more aggressive tumors end up requiring pegvisomant) or whether this may be a rebound effect after withdrawal of SSAs.[68] In the large Acrostudy, the incidence of tumor growth on pegvisomant was 5%, which was slightly higher than the expected 2.2% risk of tumor progression in patients taking SSAs.[69] Given the uncertainty regarding tumor growth, it is advisable not to use pegvisomant as first-line single therapy in patients with large macroadenomas in close proximity to the optic chiasm, and all patients taking pegvisomant should be monitored with serial MRIs at 6-month intervals initially.[18]

Side effects

Pegvisomant is usually well tolerated. A commonly reported adverse effect is elevations in liver transaminases, which is usually asymptomatic and transient even with continuation of the drug. Despite this, regular monitoring of liver function tests is necessary in patients taking pegvisomant. Some patients develop local fat accumulation in the injection areas (lipohypertrophy), believed to be due to the local anti-GH effect on lipolysis. Other uncommon side effects include fatigue, dizziness, headaches, perspiration, and abdominal bloating.[61]

FINANCIAL CONSIDERATIONS WHEN CHOOSING MEDICAL THERAPY

An important factor to consider when choosing adjuvant medical therapy is what financial implications it will have for the patient and society. Although surgery has a high upfront cost, medical treatment is much pricier in the long term.[68] Among the medications, cabergoline is approximately one-fifth the price of a long-acting SSA.[68] If financial constraints pose a barrier to standard treatment, one might consider using the short-acting octreotide, which is appreciably less expensive than the long-acting formulation. Alternatively, in patients with modest disease, a trial of cabergoline monotherapy is a reasonable first option. Pegvisomant can cost $30,000 to $90,000 per year, which is one of the main barriers to its implementation in practice.[10]

EMERGING MEDICAL THERAPIES IN ACROMEGALY

An exciting novel somatostatin analogue is anticipated to join the armamentarium of acromegaly treatments. Unlike octreotide and lanreotide, pasireotide (SOM230) has high affinity for both of the somatostatin receptor subtypes (types 2 and 5) expressed by most GH-secreting adenomas.[70] The durable effect of pasireotide on IGF-I levels suggests a longer half-life compared with octreotide.[71] Preliminary studies have suggested superiority over octreotide; however, results of the phase III randomized trial concluded about 1 year ago are needed to compare the efficacy of this newer agent with that of the existing long-acting SSAs.

RADIATION THERAPY

Radiation therapy (RT) is generally considered the last resort for patients with persistent postoperative acromegaly given the unfavorable side-effect profile and the delayed time to achieve biochemical effect. The indications for its use include uncontrolled GH secretion, tumor growth, or both. Whereas the control of tumor growth can be rapid following pituitary RT, biochemical remission can take years to decades to be achieved. Thus, patients often require continued medical therapy while awaiting the effects of radiation on GH secretion.

Conventional RT

Conventional RT consists of delivery of repeated doses of 160 to 180 cGy several days per week over a 5- to 6-week period for cumulative doses of 4500 to 5000 cGy.[68] The radiation is delivered mainly from 2 to 3 portals while the patient is immobilized wearing a tight-fitting mask, allowing an accuracy of 2 to 5 mm.[68]

Effectiveness

With the evolving biochemical definitions of remission and improved sensitivities of GH assays, the remission rates following RT have declined over the years. In studies that use the Cortina criteria, remission rates of 10% to 60% have been reported.[68] There is an average delay to remission following conventional RT of 10 years, with a predictably longer latency period in patients with high GH and IGF-I levels.[68] Therefore, the majority of patients are continued on medical therapy while awaiting the effect of RT. With respect to tumor control, conventional RT results in tumor shrinkage in 50% and maintains tumor control in up to 90% of patients at 10 years.[68]

Complications

Owing to the unintended radiation exposure to the normal pituitary gland, there is a high incidence of hypopituitarism following fractionated RT. More than half of patients will develop hypopituitarism at 5 to 10 years, with a progressive increase in the incidence over time. This risk appears to be dose dependent. Because hypopituitarism has independently been associated with reduced life expectancy, patients need regular endocrine testing and treatment of any identified hormonal deficiencies.

A rather alarming fact, however, is that even when corrected for hypopituitarism, fractionated RT may be associated with an increased mortality risk. In a study of 501 patients with acromegaly, all-cause mortality in patients who received fractionated RT was increased at 14-year follow-up, with a standardized mortality ratio of 1.58 (95% confidence interval 1.22–2.04).[22] Similar findings have been observed in 2 other large registries of acromegalic patients.[22] The main cause of death in all of these studies is cerebrovascular or cardiovascular disease.[22] Indeed, among patients who received RT for several pituitary conditions, an underlying diagnosis of acromegaly was one of several predictors of a cerebrovascular accident. It appears that prior surgery may also play a role in the mortality after fractionated RT. Although the possibility of selection bias (more aggressive tumors are more likely to require RT) needs to be clarified further, most pituitary centers are shifting away from conventional RT and using radiosurgery when necessary. That being said, the long-term outcome data for radiosurgery remain limited.

In addition to damage to the pituitary gland, patients often fear vision loss caused by optic neuropathy following RT. However, with modern MRI techniques and surgical debulking before RT, this risk is very low.

Stereotactic Radiosurgery

Stereotactic radiosurgery (SRS) encompasses several modalities, including Gamma Knife, Cyber Knife, and Primatom linear accelerator. Most of the experience to date in acromegaly using SRS involves Gamma Knife, which delivers γ-radiation though a hemisphere placed around the patient's head. The increased precision from this modality results from the fact that several beams of radiation must align to target a specific location.

Effectiveness

In a recent meta-analysis of 25 studies of SRS treatment in acromegaly, only 12 used Cortina remission criteria.[72] In these studies the remission rate was 45%, with a mean duration of reported follow-up of 4.6 ± 1.7 years.[72] When all of the studies were included in the analysis, an overall disease control rate of 48% was seen after SRS (without adjuvant medical therapy). The majority of the patients studied were refractory to medical therapy before SRS, but 14% to 17% achieved the defined remission criteria on the same doses of medication after SRS.[72] With respect to tumor control, data from 45 surgical series including 1350 patients showed that SRS is 97% effective at stabilizing or reducing tumor volume.[73] Because the effects of SRS may not be realized for years following treatment, determining the ultimate efficacy of SRS in acromegaly will require review of studies with longer follow-up intervals.

Complications

There is a lack of long-term follow-up data on SRS. As with conventional RT, the main side effect is hypopituitarism, with new-onset anterior pituitary deficiencies reported in as many as 47% of patients.[73] It is difficult to define the true incidence of SRS-induced hypopituitarism because many study patients had received prior conventional RT.[73] Other side effects of SRS include visual complications, cranial neuropathies, seizures, and carotid artery stenosis, although these were relatively uncommon.[73] The low rates of visual complications following SRS has been linked to the lower radiation exposure to the optic apparatus (8–10 Gy).[73]

AREAS OF UNCERTAINTY

At present, the biochemical assessment of disease activity in acromegaly is replete with uncertainty, primarily resulting from the following issues:

- Unacceptable variability in IGF-I and GH assays
- Lack of uniformity in methods of assessment
- Treatment goals based on historical data derived from older hormone assays

Further studies are needed to clarify:

- Clinical implications of GH_n in borderline range (0.1–0.4 µg/L) and normal IGF-I
- Whether GH actions should be targeted even in the context of a normal IGF-I with the use of pegvisomant
- Long-term safety data following SRS
- Efficacy of all currently available treatment modalities using the stringent 2010 remission criteria

SUMMARY

Persistent or recurrent acromegaly after noncurative surgery can be challenging to treat. However, with the various treatment modalities available today, most patients are ultimately able to achieve biochemical remission and control of tumor growth by some means. The SSAs are usually the first-line therapy after noncurative surgery, but repeat surgery might be considered if the tumor is surgically accessible and an experienced pituitary surgeon is available. Surgical debulking may also improve the chances of remission with medical therapy. In cases of SSA resistance, options include the addition of cabergoline or pegvisomant. Radiotherapy, particularly SRS, should be reserved for those patients who are resistant to other treatments, given the uncertainties about long-term risks.

REFERENCES

1. Jane JA Jr, Starke RM, Elzoghby MA, et al. Endoscopic transsphenoidal surgery for acromegaly: remission using modern criteria, complications, and predictors of outcome. J Clin Endocrinol Metab 2011;96:2732–40.
2. Esposito V, Santoro A, Minniti G, et al. Transsphenoidal adenomectomy for GH-, PRL- and ACTH-secreting pituitary tumours: outcome analysis in a series of 125 patients. Neurol Sci 2004;25:251–6.
3. Reid TJ, Post KD, Bruce JN, et al. Features at diagnosis of 324 patients with acromegaly did not change from 1981 to 2006: acromegaly remains

under-recognized and under-diagnosed. Clin Endocrinol (Oxf) 2010;72:203–8.

4. Dekkers OM, Biermasz NR, Pereira AM, et al. Mortality in acromegaly: a metaanalysis. J Clin Endocrinol Metab 2008;93:61–7.

5. Roelfsema F, Biermasz NR, Pereira AM. Clinical factors involved in the recurrence of pituitary adenomas after surgical remission: a structured review and meta-analysis. Pituitary 2012;15(1):71–83.

6. De P, Rees DA, Davies N, et al. Transsphenoidal surgery for acromegaly in Wales: results based on stringent criteria of remission. J Clin Endocrinol Metab 2003;88:3567–72.

7. Besser GM, Burman P, Daly AF. Predictors and rates of treatment-resistant tumor growth in acromegaly. Eur J Endocrinol 2005;153:187–93.

8. Daly AF, Tichomirowa MA, Petrossians P, et al. Clinical characteristics and therapeutic responses in patients with germ-line AIP mutations and pituitary adenomas: an international collaborative study. J Clin Endocrinol Metab 2010;95:E373–83.

9. Holdaway IM, Bolland MJ, Gamble GD. A meta-analysis of the effect of lowering serum levels of GH and IGF-I on mortality in acromegaly. Eur J Endocrinol 2008;159:89–95.

10. Del Porto LA, Liubinas SV, Kaye AH. Treatment of persistent and recurrent acromegaly. J Clin Neurosci 2011;18:181–90.

11. Giustina A, Barkan A, Casanueva FF, et al. Criteria for cure of acromegaly: a consensus statement. J Clin Endocrinol Metab 2000;85:526–9.

12. Giustina A, Chanson P, Bronstein MD, et al. A consensus on criteria for cure of acromegaly. J Clin Endocrinol Metab 2010;95:3141–8.

13. Holdaway IM, Rajasoorya RC, Gamble GD. Factors influencing mortality in acromegaly. J Clin Endocrinol Metab 2004;89:667–74.

14. Wu TE, Lin HD, Lu RA, et al. The role of insulin-like growth factor-1 and growth hormone in the mortality of patients with acromegaly after transsphenoidal surgery. Growth Horm IGF Res 2010; 20:411–5.

15. Boero L, Manavela M, Danilowicz K, et al. Comparison of two immunoassays in the determination of IGF-I levels and its correlation with oral glucose tolerance test (OGTT) and with clinical symptoms in acromegalic patients. Pituitary 2011. [Epub ahead of print].

16. Brzana JA, Yedinak CG, Delashaw JB, et al. Discordant growth hormone and IGF-I levels post pituitary surgery in patients with acromegaly naive to medical therapy and radiation: what to follow, GH or IGF-I values? Pituitary 2011. [Epub ahead of print].

17. Rubeck KZ, Madsen M, Andreasen CM, et al. Conventional and novel biomarkers of treatment outcome in patients with acromegaly: discordant results after somatostatin analog treatment

compared with surgery. Eur J Endocrinol 2010; 163:717–26.

18. Katznelson L, Atkinson JL, Cook DM, et al. American association of clinical endocrinologists medical guidelines for clinical practice for the diagnosis and treatment of acromegaly—2011 update: executive summary. Endocr Pract 2011;17:636–46.

19. Clemmons DR. Consensus statement on the standardization and evaluation of growth hormone and insulin-like growth factor assays. Clin Chem 2011;57:555–9.

20. Feelders RA, Bidlingmaier M, Strasburger CJ, et al. Postoperative evaluation of patients with acromegaly: clinical significance and timing of oral glucose tolerance testing and measurement of (free) insulin-like growth factor I, acid-labile subunit, and growth hormone-binding protein levels. J Clin Endocrinol Metab 2005;90:6480–9.

21. Kim EH, Oh MC, Lee EJ, et al. Predicting long term remission by measuring immediate postoperative growth hormone levels and oral glucose tolerance test in acromegaly. Neurosurgery 2012;70(5): 1106–13.

22. Sherlock M, Ayuk J, Tomlinson JW, et al. Mortality in patients with pituitary disease. Endocr Rev 2010; 31:301–42.

23. Yamada S, Fukuhara N, Oyama K, et al. Repeat transsphenoidal surgery for the treatment of remaining or recurring pituitary tumors in acromegaly. Neurosurgery 2010;67:949–56.

24. Wang YY, Higham C, Kearney T, et al. Acromegaly surgery in Manchester revisited—the impact of reducing surgeon numbers and the 2010 consensus guidelines for disease remission. Clin Endocrinol 2012;76(3):399–406.

25. Dusek T, Kastelan D, Melada A, et al. Clinical features and therapeutic outcomes of patients with acromegaly: single centre experience. J Endocrinol Invest 2011;34(11):e382–5.

26. Karaca Z, Tanriverdi F, Elbuken G, et al. Comparison of primary octreotide-lar and surgical treatment in newly diagnosed patients with acromegaly. Clin Endocrinol 2011;75:678–84.

27. Nomikos P, Buchfelder M, Fahlbusch R. The outcome of surgery in 668 patients with acromegaly using current criteria of biochemical 'cure'. Eur J Endocrinol 2005;152:379–87.

28. Kurosaki M, Luedecke DK, Abe T. Effectiveness of secondary transnasal surgery in GH-secreting pituitary macroadenomas. Endocr J 2003;50:635–42.

29. Alahmadi H, Dehdashti AR, Gentili F. Endoscopic endonasal surgery in recurrent and residual pituitary adenomas after microscopic resection. World Neurosurg 2012;77(3–4):540–7.

30. Long H, Beauregard H, Somma M, et al. Surgical outcome after repeated transsphenoidal surgery in acromegaly. J Neurosurg 1996;85:239–47.

31. Freda PU, Wardlaw SL, Post KD. Long-term endocrinological follow-up evaluation in 115 patients who underwent transsphenoidal surgery for acromegaly. J Neurosurg 1998;89:353–8.

32. Abe T, Ludecke DK. Recent results of secondary transnasal surgery for residual or recurring acromegaly. Neurosurgery 1998;42:1013–21 [discussion: 21–2].

33. Leach P, Abou-Zeid AH, Kearney T, et al. Endoscopic transsphenoidal pituitary surgery: evidence of an operative learning curve. Neurosurgery 2010; 67:1205–12.

34. Erturk E, Tuncel E, Kiyici S, et al. Outcome of surgery for acromegaly performed by different surgeons: importance of surgical experience. Pituitary 2005;8:93–7.

35. Petrossians P, Borges-Martins L, Espinoza C, et al. Gross total resection or debulking of pituitary adenomas improves hormonal control of acromegaly by somatostatin analogs. Eur J Endocrinol 2005;152:61–6.

36. Colao A, Attanasio R, Pivonello R, et al. Partial surgical removal of growth hormone-secreting pituitary tumors enhances the response to somatostatin analogs in acromegaly. J Clin Endocrinol Metab 2006;91:85–92.

37. Espinosa de los Monteros AL, Gonzalez B, Vargas G, et al. Surgical reintervention in acromegaly: is it still worth trying? Endocr Pract 2009; 15:431–7.

38. Berker M, Hazer DB, Yucel T, et al. Complications of endoscopic surgery of the pituitary adenomas: analysis of 570 patients and review of the literature. Pituitary 2011. [Epub ahead of print].

39. Tutuncu Y, Berker D, Isik S, et al. Comparison of octreotide LAR and lanreotide autogel as postoperative medical treatment in acromegaly. Pituitary 2011. [Epub ahead of print].

40. Ayuk J, Stewart SE, Stewart PM, et al. Efficacy of sandostatin LAR (long-acting somatostatin analogue) is similar in patients with untreated acromegaly and in those previously treated with surgery and/or radiotherapy. Clin Endocrinol 2004;60:375–81.

41. Freda PU, Katznelson L, van der Lely AJ, et al. Long-acting somatostatin analog therapy of acromegaly: a meta-analysis. J Clin Endocrinol Metab 2005;90:4465–73.

42. Mazziotti G, Giustina A. Effects of lanreotide SR and Autogel on tumor mass in patients with acromegaly: a systematic review. Pituitary 2010;13:60–7.

43. Colao A, Pivonello R, Di Somma C, et al. Medical therapy of pituitary adenomas: effects on tumor shrinkage. Rev Endocr Metab Disord 2009;10: 111–23.

44. Yetkin DO, Boysan SN, Tiryakioglu O, et al. Forty month follow-up of persistent and difficultly controlled acromegalic patients treated with depot long acting somatostatin analog octreotide. Endocr J 2007;54:459–64.

45. Caron P, Bex M, Cullen DR, et al. One-year follow-up of patients with acromegaly treated with fixed or titrated doses of lanreotide Autogel. Clin Endocrinol 2004;60:734–40.

46. Sherlock M, Fernandez-Rodriguez E, Alonso AA, et al. Medical therapy in patients with acromegaly: predictors of response and comparison of efficacy of dopamine agonists and somatostatin analogues. J Clin Endocrinol Metab 2009;94:1255–63.

47. Puig-Domingo M, Resmini E, Gomez-Anson B, et al. Magnetic resonance imaging as a predictor of response to somatostatin analogs in acromegaly after surgical failure. J Clin Endocrinol Metab 2010; 95:4973–8.

48. Bhayana S, Booth GL, Asa SL, et al. The implication of somatotroph adenoma phenotype to somatostatin analog responsiveness in acromegaly. J Clin Endocrinol Metab 2005;90:6290–5.

49. Fleseriu M. Clinical efficacy and safety results for dose escalation of somatostatin receptor ligands in patients with acromegaly: a literature review. Pituitary 2011;14:184–93.

50. Wuster C, Both S, Cordes U, et al. Primary treatment of acromegaly with high-dose lanreotide: a case series. J Med Case Rep 2010;4:85.

51. Ludlam WH, Anthony L. Safety review: dose optimization of somatostatin analogs in patients with acromegaly and neuroendocrine tumors. Adv Ther 2011;28:825–41.

52. Salvatori R, Nachtigall LB, Cook DM, et al. Effectiveness of self- or partner-administration of an extended-release aqueous-gel formulation of lanreotide in lanreotide-naive patients with acromegaly. Pituitary 2010;13:96–102.

53. Tzanela M, Vassiliadi DA, Gavalas N, et al. Glucose homeostasis in patients with acromegaly treated with surgery or somatostatin analogues. Clin Endocrinol 2011;75:96–102.

54. Mazziotti G, Floriani I, Bonadonna S, et al. Effects of somatostatin analogs on glucose homeostasis: a metaanalysis of acromegaly studies. J Clin Endocrinol Metab 2009;94:1500–8.

55. De Marinis L, Bianchi A, Fusco A, et al. Long-term effects of the combination of pegvisomant with somatostatin analogs (SSA) on glucose homeostasis in non-diabetic patients with active acromegaly partially resistant to SSA. Pituitary 2007; 10:227–32.

56. Sandret L, Maison P, Chanson P. Place of cabergoline in acromegaly: a meta-analysis. J Clin Endocrinol Metab 2011;96:1327–35.

57. Mancini T, Casanueva FF, Giustina A. Hyperprolactinemia and prolactinomas. Endocrinol Metab Clin North Am 2008;37:67–99, viii.

58. Giustina A, Bronstein MD, Casanueva FF, et al. Current management practices for acromegaly: an international survey. Pituitary 2011;14:125–33.

59. Feenstra J, de Herder WW, ten Have SM, et al. Combined therapy with somatostatin analogues and weekly pegvisomant in active acromegaly. Lancet 2005;365:1644–6.

60. van der Lely AJ, Hutson RK, Trainer PJ, et al. Long-term treatment of acromegaly with pegvisomant, a growth hormone receptor antagonist. Lancet 2001;358:1754–9.

61. Trainer PJ. ACROSTUDY: the first 5 years. Eur J Endocrinol 2009;161(Suppl 1):S19–24.

62. Trainer PJ, Ezzat S, D'Souza GA, et al. A randomized, controlled, multicentre trial comparing pegvisomant alone with combination therapy of pegvisomant and long-acting octreotide in patients with acromegaly. Clin Endocrinol 2009; 71:549–57.

63. van der Lely AJ, Bernabeu I, Cap J, et al. Coadministration of lanreotide Autogel and pegvisomant normalizes IGF1 levels and is well tolerated in patients with acromegaly partially controlled by somatostatin analogs alone. Eur J Endocrinol 2011;164:325–33.

64. Neggers SJ, van der Lely AJ. Combination treatment with somatostatin analogues and pegvisomant in acromegaly. Growth Horm IGF Res 2011; 21:129–33.

65. Barkan AL, Burman P, Clemmons DR, et al. Glucose homeostasis and safety in patients with acromegaly converted from long-acting octreotide to pegvisomant. J Clin Endocrinol Metab 2005;90: 5684–91.

66. Higham CE, Atkinson AB, Aylwin S, et al. Effective combination treatment with cabergoline and low-dose pegvisomant in active acromegaly: a prospective clinical trial. J Clin Endocrinol Metab 2012;97(4): 1187–93.

67. Neggers SJ, van Aken MO, de Herder WW, et al. Quality of life in acromegalic patients during long-term somatostatin analog treatment with and without pegvisomant. J Clin Endocrinol Metab 2008;93:3853–9.

68. Katznelson L, Atkinson JL, Cook DM, et al. American Association of Clinical Endocrinologists medical guidelines for clinical practice for the diagnosis and treatment of acromegaly—2011 update. Endocr Pract 2011;17(Suppl 4):1–44.

69. Brue T. ACROSTUDY: status update on 469 patients. Horm Res 2009;71(Suppl 1):34–8.

70. Wilson C. Pharmacotherapy: pasireotide shows promise for the treatment of acromegaly. Nat Rev Endocrinol 2010;6:417.

71. van der Hoek J, de Herder WW, Feelders RA, et al. A single-dose comparison of the acute effects between the new somatostatin analog SOM230 and octreotide in acromegalic patients. J Clin Endocrinol Metab 2004;89:638–45.

72. Yang I, Kim W, De Salles A, et al. A systematic analysis of disease control in acromegaly treated with radiosurgery. Neurosurg Focus 2010;29:E13.

73. Stapleton CJ, Liu CY, Weiss MH. The role of stereotactic radiosurgery in the multimodal management of growth hormone-secreting pituitary adenomas. Neurosurg Focus 2010;29:E11.

74. Shimon I, Cohen ZR, Ram Z, et al. Transsphenoidal surgery for acromegaly: endocrinological follow-up of 98 patients. Neurosurgery 2001;48:1239–43 [discussion: 44–5].

75. Lancranjan I, Atkinson AB. Results of a European multicentre study with Sandostatin LAR in acromegalic patients. Sandostatin LAR Group. Pituitary 1999;1:105–14.

76. Chanson P, Boerlin V, Ajzenberg C, et al. Comparison of octreotide acetate LAR and lanreotide SR in patients with acromegaly. Clin Endocrinol 2000;53: 577–86.

77. Colao A, Ferone D, Marzullo P, et al. Long-term effects of depot long-acting somatostatin analog octreotide on hormone levels and tumor mass in acromegaly. J Clin Endocrinol Metab 2001;86: 2779–86.

78. Ayuk J, Stewart SE, Stewart PM, et al. Long-term safety and efficacy of depot long-acting somatostatin analogs for the treatment of acromegaly. J Clin Endocrinol Metab 2002;87:4142–6.

79. Alexopoulou O, Abrams P, Verhelst J, et al. Efficacy and tolerability of lanreotide Autogel therapy in acromegalic patients previously treated with octreotide LAR. Eur J Endocrinol 2004;151:317–24.

80. Jallad RS, Musolino NR, Salgado LR, et al. Treatment of acromegaly with octreotide-LAR: extensive experience in a Brazilian institution. Clin Endocrinol 2005;63:168–75.

81. Grottoli S, Celleno R, Gasco V, et al. Efficacy and safety of 48 weeks of treatment with octreotide LAR in newly diagnosed acromegalic patients with macroadenomas: an open-label, multicenter, non-comparative study. J Endocrinol Invest 2005; 28:978–83.

82. Trepp R, Stettler C, Zwahlen M, et al. Treatment outcomes and mortality of 94 patients with acromegaly. Acta Neurochir (Wien) 2005;147:243–51 [discussion: 50–1].

83. Cozzi R, Montini M, Attanasio R, et al. Primary treatment of acromegaly with octreotide LAR: a long-term (up to nine years) prospective study of its efficacy in the control of disease activity and tumor shrinkage. J Clin Endocrinol Metab 2006;91:1397–403.

84. Colao A, Pivonello R, Rosato F, et al. First-line octreotide-LAR therapy induces tumour shrinkage and controls hormone excess in patients with

acromegaly: results from an open, prospective, multicentre trial. Clin Endocrinol 2006;64:342–51.

85. Ronchi CL, Boschetti M, Degli Uberti EC, et al. Efficacy of a slow-release formulation of lanreotide (Autogel) 120 mg) in patients with acromegaly previously treated with octreotide long acting release (LAR): an open, multicentre longitudinal study. Clin Endocrinol 2007;67:512–9.

86. Maiza JC, Vezzosi D, Matta M, et al. Long-term (up to 18 years) effects on GH/IGF-I hypersecretion and tumour size of primary somatostatin analogue (SSTa) therapy in patients with GH-secreting pituitary adenoma responsive to SSTa. Clin Endocrinol 2007;67:282–9.

87. Mercado M, Borges F, Bouterfa H, et al. A prospective, multicentre study to investigate the efficacy, safety and tolerability of octreotide LAR (long-acting repeatable octreotide) in the primary therapy of patients with acromegaly. Clin Endocrinol 2007;66:859–68.

88. Colao A, Pivonello R, Auriemma RS, et al. Beneficial effect of dose escalation of octreotide-LAR as first-line therapy in patients with acromegaly. Eur J Endocrinol 2007;157:579–87.

89. Auriemma RS, Pivonello R, Galdiero M, et al. Octreotide-LAR vs lanreotide-SR as first-line therapy for acromegaly: a retrospective, comparative, head-to-head study. J Endocrinol Invest 2008;31:956–65.

90. Colao A, Cappabianca P, Caron P, et al. Octreotide LAR vs. surgery in newly diagnosed patients with acromegaly: a randomized, open-label, multicentre study. Clin Endocrinol 2009;70:757–68.

91. Baldys-Waligorska A, Golkowski F, Krzentowska A, et al. Evaluation of the efficacy of Octreotide LAR in the treatment of acromegaly—a yearly observation. Przegl Lek 2009;66:218–21 [in Polish].

92. Oki Y, Inoue T, Imura M, et al. Investigation into the efficacy and safety of octreotide LAR in Japanese patients with acromegaly: Shizuoka study. Endocr J 2009;56:1095–101.

93. Luque-Ramirez M, Portoles GR, Varela C, et al. The efficacy of octreotide LAR as firstline therapy for

patients with newly diagnosed acromegaly is independent of tumor extension: predictive factors of tumor and biochemical response. Horm Metab Res 2010;42:38–44.

94. Caron P, Beckers A, Cullen DR, et al. Efficacy of the new long-acting formulation of lanreotide (lanreotide Autogel) in the management of acromegaly. J Clin Endocrinol Metab 2002;87:99–104.

95. Caron P, Cogne M, Raingeard I, et al. Effectiveness and tolerability of 3-year lanreotide Autogel treatment in patients with acromegaly. Clin Endocrinol 2006;64:209–14.

96. Lucas T, Astorga R. Efficacy of lanreotide Autogel administered every 4-8 weeks in patients with acromegaly previously responsive to lanreotide microparticles 30 mg: a phase III trial. Clin Endocrinol 2006;65:320–6.

97. Chanson P, Borson-Chazot F, Kuhn JM, et al. Control of IGF-I levels with titrated dosing of lanreotide Autogel over 48 weeks in patients with acromegaly. Clin Endocrinol 2008;69:299–305.

98. Melmed S, Cook D, Schopohl J, et al. Rapid and sustained reduction of serum growth hormone and insulin-like growth factor-1 in patients with acromegaly receiving lanreotide Autogel therapy: a randomized, placebo-controlled, multicenter study with a 52 week open extension. Pituitary 2010;13:18–28.

99. Lombardi G, Minuto F, Tamburrano G, et al. Efficacy of the new long-acting formulation of lanreotide (lanreotide Autogel) in somatostatin analogue-naive patients with acromegaly. J Endocrinol Invest 2009;32:202–9.

100. Attanasio R, Lanzi R, Losa M, et al. Effects of lanreotide Autogel on growth hormone, insulinlike growth factor 1, and tumor size in acromegaly: a 1-year prospective multicenter study. Endocr Pract 2008;14:846–55.

101. Schopohl J, Strasburger CJ, Caird D, et al. Efficacy and acceptability of lanreotide Autogel(R) 120 mg at different dose intervals in patients with acromegaly previously treated with octreotide LAR. Exp Clin Endocrinol Diabetes 2011;119:156–62.

Neurosurgical Treatment of Cushing Disease

Sameer A. Sheth, MD, PhD[a], Sarah K. Bourne, BA[b],
Nicholas A. Tritos, MD, DSc[c], Brooke Swearingen, MD[d],*

KEYWORDS

- Cushing syndrome • Cushing disease • Transsphenoidal surgery • Adrenocorticotropin
- Hypercortisolism

KEY POINTS

- Cushing syndrome (CS) refers to the clinical and metabolic effects of excess systemic glucocorticoids; Cushing disease (CD), or adrenocorticotropin (ACTH) overproduction by an adrenal adenoma or carcinoma, is the most common cause of endogenous CS.
- CD is largely a surgical disease, with microscopic and endoscopic transsphenoidal surgery enjoying similar success rates and relatively low complication rates.
- Remission rates following surgery are 70% to 95%, although the literature demonstrates significant variability in the definition of remission.
- Recurrence following surgery occurs 2% to 20% of the time, after 2 to 10 years.
- Recurrences may be treated with reoperation, radiosurgery, or radiation therapy; interim medical therapy is required in the latter 2 cases.

INTRODUCTION

Cushing syndrome (CS) refers to the constellation of physiologic effects of excess systemic glucocorticoids, including impaired glucose tolerance, skin and bone fragility, compromised immunity, and cardiovascular complications, to name a few. Untreated CS is associated with mortality rates greater than 5 times that of matched controls,[1–4] whereas proper treatment normalizes mortality risk.[5]

Whereas the most common cause of CS is the administration of exogenous steroids, endogenous CS is a consequence of adrenocorticotropin (ACTH) overproduction by a pituitary adenoma or an ectopic tumor, or cortisol overproduction by autonomous adrenal abnormalities. Overproduction of ACTH by a pituitary adenoma (or, rarely,

carcinoma) is the most common of these, and is known as Cushing disease (CD).

DIAGNOSIS

Patients who should be considered for evaluation of possible CS/CD include those with unusual features for their age (including early-onset hypertension, low bone mineral density for age, fractures after minimal trauma, oligomenorrhea in premenopausal-aged women, to name a few), those who manifest multiple features suggestive of cortisol excess over time (including central adiposity, hyperglycemia, spontaneous ecchymoses, wide or darkly pigmented striae, proximal muscle weakness, edema, hypokalemia, thromboembolic events, psychiatric manifestations, and recurrent, opportunistic, or atypical

---

None of the authors has any disclosures or conflicts of interest regarding any of the material in this article.
[a] Department of Neurosurgery, Massachusetts General Hospital, 55 Fruit Street, White 502, Boston, MA 02114, USA; [b] Department of Neurosurgery, Massachusetts General Hospital, 50 Blossom Street, Edwards 410, Boston, MA 02114, USA; [c] Department of Medicine, Neuroendocrine Clinical Center, Massachusetts General Hospital, Zero Emerson Place, Suite 112, E00-112, Boston, MA 02114, USA; [d] Department of Neurosurgery, Massachusetts General Hospital, 15 Parkman Street, WACC 331, Boston, MA 02114, USA
* Corresponding author.
E-mail address: bswearingen@partners.org

infections), children with delay in linear growth, and patients with incidentally found adrenal or pituitary masses.

Once the diagnosis of CS/CD is considered, laboratory testing is aimed at establishing (or refuting) the presence of pathologic hypercortisolism (**Fig. 1**). After the diagnosis of CS is established on a biochemical basis, a thorough, systematic approach is required to identify the underlying cause (pathologic lesion) with the goal of curative resection, if possible.[6,7]

Establishing the Diagnosis of Cushing Syndrome

Laboratory testing is needed to confirm the presence of CS, and distinguish it from other conditions (**Box 1**).[8,9] The physiologic principles underlying laboratory testing for CS include excessive cortisol secretion leading to increased cortisol excretion in the urine (24-hour urine free cortisol [UFC]), blunting of the normal circadian rhythm of cortisol secretion leading to high nocturnal (nadir) cortisol levels (measured in the blood or saliva), and decreased sensitivity of the hypothalamic-pituitary-adrenal axis to negative feedback exerted by glucocorticoids, leading to lack of suppression of early-morning serum cortisol after the oral administration of dexamethasone (dexamethasone suppression testing).[8,9]

Measurement of UFC is optimally performed using liquid chromatography followed by tandem mass spectrometry or high-performance liquid chromatography, and provides a reliable estimate of

---

Box 1
Conditions associated with clinical and/or biochemical evidence of hypercortisolism

Cushing syndrome (endogenous or exogenous)

Pregnancy

Psychiatric conditions (including major depression)

Severe obesity

Poorly controlled diabetes mellitus

Alcohol dependence

Familial glucocorticoid resistance

Physical illness, including trauma or surgery[a]

Strenuous regular exercise[a]

Anorexia nervosa[a]

Excessive serum cortisol binding globulin levels (including women taking oral contraceptives)[a]

[a] Clinical features of Cushing syndrome are generally absent.

---

endogenous cortisol secretion in patients with normal kidney function.[8,10] Several (at least 2–3) specimens should be collected to achieve adequate (95%) sensitivity.[8,10] Measuring urine creatinine excretion in the specimen is recommended to ensure adequacy of collection. In addition, urine volume should be recorded and high fluid intake (>5 L daily) discouraged during collection, as high urine volume is associated with high UFC.[11] A 4-fold or greater UFC above the upper end of the normal range is

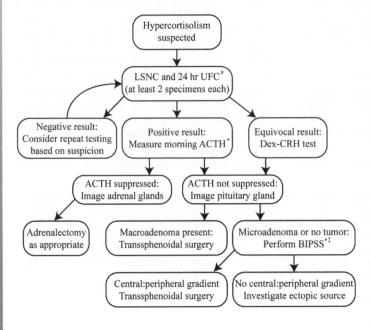

Fig. 1. An approach to the diagnosis of suspected Cushing syndrome and Cushing disease. A flow chart depicting a suggested diagnostic algorithm for determining the etiology of hypercortisolism is presented. # The 1-mg dexamethasone suppression test may also be considered (see text for details). * Testing to be conducted during periods of biochemical hypercortisolism. † Patients whose plasma ACTH levels are not fully suppressed may undergo a (peripheral) CRH stimulation test to fully establish if Cushing syndrome is ACTH dependent. ‡ The 8-mg dexamethasone suppression test and the (peripheral) CRH stimulation test may be helpful in some patients (see text for details). *Abbreviations:* ACTH, adrenocorticotropin; BIPSS, bilateral inferior petrosal sinus sampling; Dex-CRH test, dexamethasone-suppressed corticotropin-releasing hormone stimulation test; LNSC, late-night salivary cortisol; UFC, urine free cortisol.

pathognomonic of CS.[10] However, cortisol excess of lesser magnitude may also occur in other conditions, which need to be distinguished from CS (see **Box 1**).[8,10] Using the upper end of the UFC reference range as the diagnostic cutpoint, the specificity of this test for CS is 81%.[10]

Measurement of late-night (11 PM) salivary cortisol (LNSC) is accurate in the diagnosis of CS.[8,12,13] Collection of at least 2 salivary specimens is advised for adequate test sensitivity (92%–100%).[8,12,13] The specificity of LNSC for CS is 93% to 100% in outpatient populations.[8,12,13] However, there are limited validating data in hospitalized patients.[14] Individuals with altered circadian activities, including third-shift workers, may have falsely elevated LNSC.[8,12,13] Midnight serum cortisol can be measured in sleeping or awake patients, but is cumbersome and has not been validated in the acutely ill.[8]

Dexamethasone suppression tests (DST) in common use include the overnight, 1-mg DST and the 2-day, 2 mg/d DST.[7,8,10] Using a cutpoint of 1.8 μg/dL for early morning (8–9 AM) serum cortisol, the overnight, 1-mg DST has sensitivity exceeding 95% with specificity of 80%. Falsely elevated results may occur in patients with any of the conditions in **Box 1**, or among individuals taking medications that can accelerate dexamethasone clearance.[8] Measuring serum dexamethasone is advised to ensure sufficient exposure to dexamethasone. Using serum cortisol end points, the 2-day, 2-mg/d DST has comparable sensitivity with the overnight, 1-mg DST, but is cumbersome and requires adequate patient instruction.[7,8,10]

The dexamethasone-suppressed, corticotropin-releasing hormone (CRH) stimulation test may help distinguish between CS and other conditions (pseudo–Cushing states) associated with cortisol excess (see **Box 1**). This test is cumbersome, but can be helpful in patients whose prior laboratory investigations for hypercortisolism have yielded inconsistent results, or patients suspected of having other conditions associated with hypercortisolism (including major depression). Initial reports suggested that this test has 100% sensitivity and specificity in the diagnosis of CS, using a cortisol cutpoint of 1.4 μg/dL at 15 minutes after CRH administration.[15] However, more recent findings suggested that the diagnostic performance of this test is less than perfect, especially in patients taking medications that increase dexamethasone clearance.[16]

Distinguishing Between Causes of Cushing Syndrome

Once CS is confirmed, additional testing is needed to identify the underlying cause (**Box 2**).[7,9,10,12]

> **Box 2**
> **Etiology of Cushing syndrome**
>
> *ACTH-Dependent Cushing Syndrome*
>
> Pituitary tumor (adenoma, or rarely carcinoma); Cushing disease (70%)
>
> Ectopic ACTH secretion (10%)
>
> Ectopic CRH secretion (rare)
>
> *ACTH-Independent Cushing Syndrome*
>
> Adrenal adenoma (10%)
>
> Adrenal carcinoma (5%)
>
> Macronodular adrenal hyperplasia (1%–2%)
>
> Primary pigmented nodular adrenal disease (1%–2%)
>
> McCune-Albright syndrome (1%–2%)

Measuring plasma ACTH in early-morning specimens distinguishes between ACTH-dependent and ACTH-independent causes in most patients, as plasma ACTH levels usually exceed 20 pg/mL in the former group and are usually less than 5 pg/mL in the latter.[9,10] Patients with intermediate ACTH levels may undergo a (peripheral) CRH stimulation test to fully establish if CS is ACTH dependent.

Patients with ACTH-dependent CS most often have an underlying pituitary corticotroph adenoma or, very rarely, carcinoma (CD), but may sometimes have an ectopic tumor secreting either ACTH or, rarely, CRH (see **Box 2**).[7,10,17]

Pituitary corticotroph tumors are microadenomas in the vast majority (90%) of patients with CD. High-resolution magnetic resonance imaging (MRI) using a pituitary protocol detects a sellar mass in 60% to 70% of CD patients.[10,12,18] However, it should be noted that incidental sellar hypodensities of small size (<10 mm) are present in approximately 10% of individuals in the general population.[19] Therefore, the presence of a presumed microadenoma does not assure that it is the source of ACTH excess.

Two dynamic tests proposed to distinguish between pituitary and ectopic sources of ACTH excess include the high-dose (8-mg) DST and the (peripheral) CRH stimulation test, and can be helpful in some patients.[7] The 8-mg DST has 81% to 82% sensitivity and 67% to 79% specificity for CD.[9,10] The CRH stimulation test has 70% to 93% sensitivity and 88% specificity for CD.[9,10,20] As the pretest probability of CD exceeds 85% among patients with ACTH-dependent CS, neither test has adequate diagnostic accuracy, when performed alone.[9] Of note, patients with concordant positive results on 8-mg DST and the (peripheral) CRH stimulation test have an approximately 98% probability of having a corticotroph tumor, but likely represent a minority (35%) among patients with ACTH-dependent CS.[10,21]

Bilateral inferior petrosal sinus sampling (BIPSS) with measurement of plasma ACTH levels before and after CRH administration has a 94% sensitivity and specificity, using a cutpoint (peak central/peripheral ACTH ratio) of 2:1 before CRH or 3:1 after CRH administration.[10,22,23] This test is considered the gold standard for distinguishing between pituitary and ectopic sources.[10,22,23] However, the test requires considerable expertise to be performed reliably and safely, and has been rarely associated with thrombotic or neurologic complications.[10] As anomalous venous drainage or incorrect sampling may mitigate the diagnostic performance of this test, it is imperative that both the venous anatomy and accurate catheter positioning in the inferior petrosal sinuses be verified before and after specimen collection to ensure appropriate sampling. Measuring serum prolactin level in specimens may also help improve the diagnostic accuracy of this test.[24–26]

Patients with ACTH-dependent CS who are suspected of having an ectopic source should undergo imaging studies, including computed tomography (CT) and MRI examinations of the neck, chest, abdomen, and pelvis, whole-body scintigraphy using indium-111–labeled pentetreotide, or positron emission tomography in combination with CT. Tumors associated with ectopic ACTH-dependent CS lesions are frequently small (**Box 3**), and may not be detected despite extensive imaging examinations in up to 19% of patients.[17]

Additional laboratory tests may be helpful in localizing an occult ectopic tumor, including tests for serum CRH, calcitonin, chromogranin A, fractionated plasma metanephrines, and 24-hour urine 5-hydroxyindoleacetic acid.[17] A recommended approach to the diagnosis of CS/CD is outlined in **Fig. 1**.

SURGICAL OPTIONS

CD is a surgical disease, with reported remission rates ranging from the high 60s to high 90s[18,27–33] following transsphenoidal surgery. Surgical options include microscopic approaches via either sublabial[34] or endonasal[35] exposure, as well as the endoscopic approach.[36] While some centers continue to use the sublabial approach,[37] the endonasal is the more common of the microscopic approaches because of the decreased incisional morbidity. Recurrences may be treated with repeat transsphenoidal surgery, as well as radiosurgery or radiation therapy with interim medical therapy until radiation therapy takes effect.[38] Refractory cases may be considered for bilateral adrenalectomy.

Microscopic Endonasal Approach

The microscopic approach offers the advantage of a binocular stereoscopic view with superior optics. After induction of general anesthesia, the patient is positioned supine with the head on a gel headrest or in 3-point fixation. Navigation is provided by either fluoroscopy or frameless stereotaxy.

The posterior septal mucosa is infiltrated with local anesthetic containing epinephrine, and incised opposite the middle turbinate. The mucosa is lifted with a periosteal elevator, and the posterior septum fractured. A piece of the bony septum may be retained for later use. A self-retaining nasal speculum provides retraction as the anterior wall of the sphenoid sinus is drilled to provide enough room for later insertion and manipulation of appropriately sized curettes.

The sella is identified, paying attention to remain midline, using the location of bony septations and the carotid impressions in the superolateral walls of the sphenoid sinus as guides. A laser Doppler probe may be used to help identify the position of the cavernous carotid arteries, especially in cases of medially located cavernous sinuses.[39–41] The central region of entry into the sella is chosen, and the shell of bone over the face of the sella is thinned with a drill and removed with microcurettes and Kerrison punches. The dura is bipolarly coagulated and sharply opened in a cruciate fashion.

Tumor fragments are dissected free and delivered from the sella using an assortment of ring curettes. Because approximately 90% of tumors in CD are microadenomas,[42] care should be taken to obtain sufficient specimen for histopathological analysis. The surface of the pituitary gland is closely inspected for residual fragments of adenoma. If no

---

Box 3
Tumors most frequently associated with ectopic ACTH syndrome

Foregut carcinoid (bronchopulmonary, thymic)

Small cell lung carcinoma

Pancreatic or appendiceal carcinoid

Medullary thyroid carcinoma

Islet cell tumor

Undifferentiated neuroendocrine tumor

Pheochromocytoma

Olfactory esthesioneuroblastoma

obvious tumor is visualized, serial frozen-section biopsies are performed. If these remain negative, some advocate for hemi-hypophysectomy on the side predicted by the preoperative BIPSS.[43]

Following resection, hemostasis is obtained with oxidized cellulose or other hemostatic agents. Fat harvested from a separate abdominal incision is used to pack the sella, which is then covered with a piece of previously harvested septal bone, titanium mesh, or other synthetic plug. If cerebrospinal fluid (CSF) leak is suspected, a layer of fibrin glue or other sealant may be applied. The mucosal flap is reapproximated, and the nasal passage inspected before completion of the procedure.

Endoscopic Approach

The endoscopic approach offers the advantage of a wider field of view and the capacity to inspect regions of the sella with angled fiber bundles. Access into the sphenoid sinus is similar to that described above, although a nasal speculum is not required. The majority of situations favor a 0° degree 4-mm endoscope, which can be affixed to the operating table with an articulating arm or held by the assistant, allowing the surgeon to use conventional bimanual techniques.

Recent improvements in endoscope technology have provided much clearer high-definition visualization compared with the early monocular endoscopes. Three-dimensional videoscopes are also being developed. Several centers have reported remission rates similar to those of microscopic approaches.[36,44–50]

OUTCOMES
Initial Remission

One challenge in identifying success rates of transsphenoidal surgery for CD is that no standardized remission criteria exist. Varying stringencies of criteria used may contribute to observed variations in remission rates (**Table 1**). Proposed biochemical criteria for remission include low or undetectable serum cortisol, low plasma ACTH, low 24-hour UFC, low or normal cortisol following dexamethasone suppression, and combinations of these variables.[5,28,29,51–53]

Timing of postoperative laboratory investigation also varies, with some studies defining remission by hormone levels as much as 6 months postoperatively, whereas others characterize remission by values obtained early after the operation. In general, remission rates of 67% to 97% are reported.[5,28,29,42,52–66] Although pediatric CD is rare, similar remission rates have been documented in pediatric populations.[60,67,68]

A strategy of early repeat operation in patients with initial treatment failure has been investigated and shown to result in remission in 67% to 71% of patients with treatment failure after initial operation.[69,70] In such cases, positive BIPSS may be important to confirm the presence of pituitary adenoma. Because CD has serious associated morbidity and mortality and postponing a repeat operation may increase technical difficulty owing to scar tissue and altered anatomy,[71] early reoperation may offer substantial benefits. Conversely, complications such as hypopituitarism and CSF leak may be higher with repeat operation,[69,70] and occasional patients may achieve delayed remission in the weeks after the initial procedure, suggesting that reexploration should not be considered until the postoperative cortisol levels have plateaued in a persistently elevated range.[33]

Factors Predicting Initial Remission

Several factors have been linked to likelihood of successful outcome. A body of evidence points to higher remission rates in surgical patients with microadenomas than in those with macroadenomas,[5,42,53,59,62,72] although other studies have failed to find such a difference.[55,58] Overall, larger tumors may have worse outcomes,[28,60,73] even within the macroadenoma category alone,[74] perhaps because larger adenomas are more likely to be invasive. Patients with invasive tumors are less likely to achieve remission after transsphenoidal surgery.[61,75] Invasion of the cavernous sinus or suprasellar tumor extension results consistently in a higher incidence of persistent disease.[28,74]

Intraoperative identification of an adenoma is an important positive prognostic factor,[42,57,76,77] and allows selective adenomectomy to be performed rather than a potentially more morbid procedure such as partial or total hypophysectomy. Intraoperative ultrasonography has been successfully used to increase intraoperative adenoma localization and results in higher remission rates in some reports.[78] Identification of adenoma on preoperative MRI,[58] histopathology,[42,54,55,57,63] both MRI and intraoperatively,[53] or MRI and histology together[57] have also been linked to improved chance of remission. Failure to identify an adenoma may signal unusual pathology or misdiagnosis of a condition such as pseudo-CS that is unlikely to be cured by pituitary surgery, but in the presence of strict diagnostic criteria is more likely related to an incomplete exploration, or an undetected and invasive tumor.

Initial transsphenoidal surgery is often reported to have a higher chance of success than repeat surgery performed for treatment failure or

Table 1
Published surgical series for CD with remission and recurrence rates

Authors,[Ref.] Year	N	Follow-Up (mo)	Remission Rate (%)	Definition of Remission[a]	Recurrence Rate (%)	Time to Recurrence (mo)
Ciric et al,[94] 2012	136	69.9	83.4	Cortisol <5.3 Steroid requirement	9.4	80.3
Honegger et al,[59] 2012	83	38.2	84.3	Normal or decreased UFC Cortisol <2 with LDDST	6.7	37
Sun et al,[95] 2012	119	36.8	86.6	Cortisol ≤5 60mo cortisol ≤normal Normal UFC Suppression with LDDST	4.9	38.9
Yamada et al,[96] 2012	124	60	90.3	Cortisol ≤5 or Cortisol ≤2 with LDDST	3.6	45
Lindsay et al,[84] 2011	331	126	98.2	Cortisol <5	12	50.4
Ammini et al,[55] 2011	97	18–132	66.7	Cortisol <5	18.5	25.2
Storr et al,[68] 2011	183	N/S	72.2	Cortisol ≤normal	22.9	N/S
Alwani et al,[97] 2011	45	56.5	67	Suppression with LDDST Normal UFC Steroid requirement	6.7	13.5
Valassi et al,[33] 2010	620	45	76.1	UFC <80 Cortisol normal Cortisol <5 with LDDST	13	N/S
Jagannathan et al,[66] 2009	261	84	97	UFC or cortisol ≤normal	2.3	56
Fomekong et al,[58] 2009	40	86	80	Normal UFC Steroid requirement	9.4	54
Patil et al,[82] 2008	215	45	85.6%	Normal UFC Steroid requirement	17.4	39
Prevedello et al,[77] 2008	167	39	80	Cortisol and UFC ≤normal	13	50
Atkinson et al,[98] 2008	42	30	86	Hypocortisolism	11.1	57.6
Hofmann et al,[42] 2008	426	72.3	68.5	Cortisol ≤2 LDDST	15	73.2
Rollin et al,[62] 2007	108	72	83.3	Steroid dependence Cortisol <3 with LDDST Clinical remission	6.8	44
Acebes et al,[54] 2007	44	49	89	Clinical remission Cortisol and UFC ≤normal	7.7	54.6
Esposito et al,[53] 2006	40	33	80	Cortisol ≤5	3.1	21

Study			Remission criteria		
Atkinson et al,[56] 2005	63	115.2	71.4	UFC ≤127 Cortisol suppressed after LDDST	22.2	62.4
Salenave et al,[99] 2004	54	19.9	82.7	Cortisol ≤3.5 11-desoxycortisol <10 µg/dL in metyrapone test Negative insulin tolerance test Peak cortisol <20 after CRH stimulation Normal UFC Cortisol <2.7 with LDDST	19.5	19.9
Hammer et al,[28] 2004	289	133.2	82	Cortisol ≤5 basally or with LDDST UFC ≤normal	9	58.8
Pereira et al,[80] 2003	78	86	72	Steroid dependence or clinical remission Cortisol <3.6 with LDDST 2 consecutive normal UFC	9	84
Flitsch et al,[100] 2003	147	61	93	Cortisol ≤normal	5.5	44
Chen et al,[72] 2003	174	>60	80	Cortisol ≤3	6.3	27
Yap et al,[65] 2002	97	92	68.5	Cortisol undetectable (<2)	11.5	36.3
Shimon et al,[63] 2002	82	50.4	78	Clinical remission UFC normal Cortisol <5 with LDDST	5	44
Rees et al,[61] 2002	53	72	77	Cortisol <2	5	24.5
Chee et al,[57] 2001	61	88	78.7	Cortisol normal Clinical remission Cortisol <3.6 with LDDST	14.6	76.1
Barbetta et al,[52] 2001	68	57.5	90	Cortisol and UFC ≤normal Normal LDDST Steroid requirement	21	36
Swearingen et al,[5] 1999	161	96	85	Cortisol <5 UFC <20	7	68.4
Semple and Laws,[87] 1999	105	N/S	75.2	Cortisol <normal Steroid requirement	N/S	N/S
Invitti et al,[29] 1999	236	28	69	Cortisol and UFC ≤normal	17	115

Abbreviations: LDDST, low-dose dexamethasone suppression test; N/S, not specified.
[a] Units for cortisol are µg/dL, units for UFC are µg/24 h.

recurrence.[5,29,42,53,62] Repeat surgery may also be associated with a higher rate of complications such as CSF leak.[53] However, some studies specifically addressing the issue of repeat surgery have found a substantial remission rate of 62% to 87.5%,[63,76,79] thus surgical intervention should not be excluded in patients with treatment failure or recurrence.

Several biochemical parameters have been proposed to predict remission. Early postoperative cortisol[75] and ACTH levels may have prognostic value. In one study, ACTH greater than 34 pg/mL on postoperative day 1 had sensitivity of 80% and specificity of 97.4% for not achieving remission within 6 months, whereas cortisol greater than 20 μg/dL had sensitivity of 100% and specificity of 90%.[54] Another study found that patients who had less than 3 μg/dL cortisol on postoperative day 3 following low-dose dexamethasone suppression retained 93% remission at 5 years, whereas those who merely normalized cortisol had all experienced recurrence by that time.[72] Pereira and colleagues[80] suggested that a cortisol level below 5 μg/dL measured at 3 months after surgery is the optimal cutoff for predicting remission at 6 months with sensitivity of 94% and specificity of 79%. Preoperative ACTH has been reported to be higher in patients with postoperative hypercortisolemia.[74]

Several technical factors may contribute to operative success. One group reported using the pseudocapsule formed by compressed normal anterior pituitary cells as a surgical capsule in encapsulated adenomas confined to the anterior pituitary. This technique gave excellent results, with initial remission of 96.6% and 100% following early repeat surgery for initial treatment failures,[66] with a recurrence of only 2.3% at a mean of 7 years. A technique using preoperative MRI and BIPSS for localization and intraoperative frozen sections achieved 100% remission in 18 patients.[81] The contribution of surgical experience to surgical success is somewhat controversial, with several studies showing no changes in outcome over a surgeon's career,[42,57] and several others reporting improvement with experience.[61,65]

Recurrence

Despite initial surgical success, several patients develop recurrent disease. Because patients can develop recurrent disease many years after initial surgery, the rate of recurrence depends on the length of follow-up. Recurrent disease appears in 3% to 22% of patients at a mean of 1.75 to 9.6 years.[5,28,29,52–58,61–63,65,77,80]

As in the case for initial remission, the criteria for determining recurrence are also variable.

Recurrence continues to increase over time with long-term follow-up.[28,29,56,77,80,82] For example, one study showed recurrence of 0.5%, 6.7%, 20.8%, and 25.5% at 1, 2, 3, and 5 years, respectively, and ultimate recurrence of 46% in patients followed for at least 5 to 13 years. Recurrence may be higher in repeat operations. A study of early repeat surgery for failed initial transsphenoidal adenoma resection reported a 30% recurrence rate, perhaps reflecting a more treatment refractory characteristic of this subset of patients.[70] The recurrence rate may also be spuriously elevated if initial remission criteria were too lax, such as inclusion of patients with normal cortisol, because such patients may never have actually achieved initial remission.

Factors Predicting Recurrence

The vast majority of recurrent tumors are located at the same or adjacent location to the original tumor, suggesting that microscopic tumor remnants are the cause of many recurrences.[76,83] Histologic evidence of dural invasion has been reported in 45.4% of surgeries for pituitary adenomas; therefore, undetected dural invasion may contribute to unnoticed and unresected tumor tissue.[73,83] Dural invasion increases with adenoma size, patient age, and male gender.[73] Microadenomas may recur at a lower rate than macroadenomas,[5] perhaps because they are less likely to be invasive. However, conflicting evidence exists on this point, with one small study showing excellent long-term remission rates in patients with macroadenomas,[51] and several studies showing no difference in recurrence rates between microadenomas and macroadenomas.[65]

Postoperative cortisol and ACTH levels have been studied as predictors of long-term remission. Some investigators have found that patients with hypocortisolism in the postoperative period have lower rates of recurrence than subjects with normalized cortisol,[52,74,82] and that patients with long-term remission have lower cortisol levels on postoperative days 3 to 5.[84] One study found 97% sustained remission in patients with serum cortisol less than 5 μg/dL within the first 2 postoperative days, albeit with a relatively brief follow-up of 33 months.[54] Another study reported no recurrence during a median follow-up period of 40 months in patients who had undetectable postoperative serum cortisol.[85] However, undetectable postoperative cortisol does not exclude the chance of recurrence at a later date,[56,65] and in one study where postoperative cortisol predicted remission at 6 months, it was not related to long-term remission.[80] Some studies have suggested subnormal ACTH as a predictor of sustained remission, whereas others have not found this measure to be particularly useful.[53] High postoperative ACTH as well as cortisol and ACTH levels following CRH stimulation have been related to recurrence.[29,84]

COMPLICATIONS

Overall, transsphenoidal surgery for CD has a rate of serious morbidity of 1.8% to 15% and mortality of 0% to 1.9%.[5,28,61,62,65,80,86,87] A nationwide study of inpatient data found in-hospital mortality of 0.7%, 2.9% adverse outcomes (death or discharge other than to home), and morbidity of 42.1% following transsphenoidal surgery for CD.[88] However, untreated CD also results in significant morbidity and mortality, making appropriate treatment essential. Patients who are successfully surgically treated have long-term mortality similar to the general population,[5] whereas those with persistent disease have increased mortality.[28] Patients with CD who undergo transsphenoidal surgery may have higher immediate and delayed complication rates than patients with other pituitary tumors who undergo this operation,[89] perhaps because of the higher incidence of medical comorbidities in the CD population and the effects of cortisol withdrawal.

Endocrine

Hypothalamic-pituitary-adrenal axis dysfunction (adrenal insufficiency) is anticipated after successful transsphenoidal surgery for CD, and is generally reversible within 6 to 18 months postoperatively. Deficiency of at least one pituitary hormone is reported in 8.6% to 53% of patients.[5,28,61,62] Hypopituitarism likely depends on the procedure performed, with much lower rates in selective adenomectomy and increasing rates with extensive exploration.[59] In some series the rate approaches 100% for subtotal or total hypophysectomy.[79] The rate of hypopituitarism may also be increased in repeat surgeries.[62]

Normal corticotroph function is inhibited by adenoma hypersecretion and thus patients will require glucocorticoid replacement following successful surgery, although normal cortisol function is usually regained within 6 to 18 months.[90] The timing of initiation of glucocorticoid replacement varies between centers. Some physicians prefer to observe patients for biochemical or clinical hypocortisolism before initiating glucocorticoid replacement therapy, whereas others begin patients on a low-dose glucocorticoid immediately following surgery, allowing earlier discharge with outpatient follow-up to determine pituitary function and remission status.[51]

Diabetes insipidus (DI) is one of the most common postoperative endocrine disturbances. Transient DI occurs in 6% to 75% while permanent DI is less common and generally occurs in 1% to 15%, requiring long-term use of desmopressin.[5,28,29,53,56–59,61–65,75,77,86,87] Secretion from the syndrome of inappropriate antidiuretic hormone also occurs fairly frequently, so patients should be monitored for hyponatremia. Deficiency of new gonadotropin, thyroid, and growth hormone can also occur.

Neurologic

Neurologic symptoms occur in 5.6% of patients.[88] Vision loss may occur because of damage to the optic apparatus or its vasculature as well as vasospasm,[91] and occurs in 0.7% to 4% of patients.[58,61,86,87] Cranial nerve injury most commonly occurs from exploration of the cavernous sinus, with damage most frequently occurring to the sixth cranial nerve.[87] A 0.7% rate of cranial nerve injury has been reported nationally.[88] Cranial nerve palsies may be transient or permanent. A risk of carotid artery injury exists and has been reported at 0% to 2.5%.[53,75,86]

Infectious

Chronic sinusitis may occur in as many as 1.5% to 8.5% of patients.[66,86] Antibiotics are the first line of treatment, but up to half of patients may require surgical intervention to achieve cure.[92] Meningitis is a serious complication that is uncommonly observed postoperatively but is an associated risk of CSF leak. Incidence is reported at 0.4% to 7.9%.[28,56,64–66,86] Patients who have packing of the surgical cavity with a fat graft have a risk for infection or wound breakdown at the graft donor site.

CSF Rhinorrhea

CSF rhinorrhea may be apparent intraoperatively or postoperatively. It is treated by CSF drainage with a lumbar drain, and packing with a fat graft if noted intraoperatively or in persistent cases. If conservative measures fail, reexploaration is required. This complication occurs in 0% to 13% of patients.[5,28,56,57,61,63,64,66,77,86–88]

Nasal Complications

Patients may develop postoperative epistaxis. Occasionally the bleeding is severe enough to require nasal packing or vessel cauterization. Severe epistaxis occurs in 0.4% to 3.4% of patients.[5,53,57,66,86,87] Perforation of the nasal septum can occur with certain surgical approaches. Incidence has been reported at 1.6% to 9.3%.[57,75,86,87]

Thromboembolic

Thromboembolic disease may occur at a higher rate in CD than in other surgical patients, because of a hypercoagulable state that occurs with hypercortisolism as well as the greater rate of obesity associated with CD. Thus it is important that patients undergoing transsphenoidal surgery for CD receive appropriate deep vein thrombosis (DVT) prophylaxis, such as sequential compression devices and/or subcutaneous low molecular weight heparin. DVT or pulmonary embolism has been reported in 1% to 6% of cases.[56,58,61,65,75,87,93] Before treatment, patients with CD have an incidence of thromboembolic disease of 14.1 per 1000 person years.[93] CD patients have a higher postoperative rate of thromboembolic events than patients undergoing pituitary surgery for nonfunctioning adenomas.[93]

SUMMARY

Given the significant morbidity of untreated CS, it is imperative to determine its cause and begin therapy in a timely fashion. CD, or overproduction of ACTH by a pituitary adenoma, remains for the most part a surgical disease, with high remission rates and low complication rates following either microscopic or endoscopic transsphenoidal surgery. Reoperation, radiosurgery, and radiation therapy with interim medical therapy are options for recurrences, with bilateral adrenalectomy reserved for failures of other treatments. New medical treatments may hold promise as well (see the article by Fleseriu elsewhere in this issue on Medical management of persistent and recurrent CD).

REFERENCES

1. Clayton RN, Raskauskiene D, Reulen RC, et al. Mortality and morbidity in Cushing's disease over 50 years in Stoke-on-Trent, UK: audit and meta-analysis of literature. J Clin Endocrinol Metab 2011;96(3):632–42.

2. Etxabe J, Vazquez JA. Morbidity and mortality in Cushing's disease: an epidemiological approach. Clin Endocrinol (Oxf) 1994;40(4):479–84.

3. Lindholm J, Juul S, Jorgensen JO, et al. Incidence and late prognosis of Cushing's syndrome: a population-based study. J Clin Endocrinol Metab 2001; 86(1):117–23.

4. Mancini T, Kola B, Mantero F, et al. High cardiovascular risk in patients with Cushing's syndrome according to 1999 WHO/ISH guidelines. Clin Endocrinol (Oxf) 2004;61(6):768–77.

5. Swearingen B, Biller BM, Barker FG 2nd, et al. Long-term mortality after transsphenoidal surgery for Cushing disease. Ann Intern Med 1999;130(10):821–4.

6. Arnaldi G, Angeli A, Atkinson AB, et al. Diagnosis and complications of Cushing's syndrome: a consensus statement. J Clin Endocrinol Metab 2003; 88(12):5593–602.

7. Newell-Price J, Bertagna X, Grossman AB, et al. Cushing's syndrome. Lancet 2006;367(9522):1605–17.

8. Nieman LK, Biller BM, Findling JW, et al. The diagnosis of Cushing's syndrome: an Endocrine Society Clinical Practice Guideline. J Clin Endocrinol Metab 2008;93(5):1526–40.

9. Raff H, Findling JW. A physiologic approach to diagnosis of the Cushing syndrome. Ann Intern Med 2003;138(12):980–91.

10. Nieman LK, Ilias I. Evaluation and treatment of Cushing's syndrome. Am J Med 2005;118(12):1340–6.

11. Mericq MV, Cutler GB Jr. High fluid intake increases urine free cortisol excretion in normal subjects. J Clin Endocrinol Metab 1998;83(2):682–4.

12. Findling JW, Raff H. Screening and diagnosis of Cushing's syndrome. Endocrinol Metab Clin North Am 2005;34(2):385–402 ix-x.

13. Findling JW, Raff H. Cushing's Syndrome: important issues in diagnosis and management. J Clin Endocrinol Metab 2006;91(10):3746–53.

14. Nunes ML, Vattaut S, Corcuff JB, et al. Late-night salivary cortisol for diagnosis of overt and subclinical Cushing's syndrome in hospitalized and ambulatory patients. J Clin Endocrinol Metab 2009;94(2): 456–62.

15. Yanovski JA, Cutler GB Jr, Chrousos GP, et al. Corticotropin-releasing hormone stimulation following low-dose dexamethasone administration. A new test to distinguish Cushing's syndrome from pseudo-Cushing's states. JAMA 1993;269(17): 2232–8.

16. Valassi E, Swearingen B, Lee H, et al. Concomitant medication use can confound interpretation of the combined dexamethasone-corticotropin releasing hormone test in Cushing's syndrome. J Clin Endocrinol Metab 2009;94(12):4851–9.

17. Ilias I, Torpy DJ, Pacak K, et al. Cushing's syndrome due to ectopic corticotropin secretion: twenty years' experience at the National Institutes of Health. J Clin Endocrinol Metab 2005;90(8):4955–62.

18. Biller BM, Grossman AB, Stewart PM, et al. Treatment of adrenocorticotropin-dependent Cushing's syndrome: a consensus statement. J Clin Endocrinol Metab 2008;93(7):2454–62.

19. Hall WA, Luciano MG, Doppman JL, et al. Pituitary magnetic resonance imaging in normal human volunteers: occult adenomas in the general population. Ann Intern Med 1994;120(10):817–20.

20. Nieman LK, Oldfield EH, Wesley R, et al. A simplified morning ovine corticotropin-releasing hormone stimulation test for the differential diagnosis of adrenocorticotropin-dependent Cushing's syndrome. J Clin Endocrinol Metab 1993;77(5):1308–12.

21. Nieman LK, Chrousos GP, Oldfield EH, et al. The ovine corticotropin-releasing hormone stimulation test and the dexamethasone suppression test in the differential diagnosis of Cushing's syndrome. Ann Intern Med 1986;105(6):862–7.

22. Oldfield EH, Doppman JL, Nieman LK, et al. Petrosal sinus sampling with and without corticotropin-releasing hormone for the differential diagnosis of Cushing's syndrome. N Engl J Med 1991;325(13): 897–905.

23. Findling JW, Kehoe ME, Shaker JL, et al. Routine inferior petrosal sinus sampling in the differential diagnosis of adrenocorticotropin (ACTH)-dependent Cushing's syndrome: early recognition of the occult ectopic ACTH syndrome. J Clin Endocrinol Metab 1991;73(2):408–13.

24. Grant P, Dworakowska D, Carroll P. Maximising the accuracy of inferior petrosal sinus sampling: validation of the use of prolactin as a marker of pituitary venous effluent in the diagnosis of Cushing's disease. Clin Endocrinol (Oxf) 2012;76(4):555–9.

25. Mulligan GB, Eray E, Faiman C, et al. Reduction of false-negative results in inferior petrosal sinus sampling with simultaneous prolactin and corticotropin measurement. Endocr Pract 2011;17(1):33–40.

26. Sharma ST, Raff H, Nieman LK. Prolactin as a marker of successful catheterization during IPSS in patients with ACTH-dependent Cushing's syndrome. J Clin Endocrinol Metab 2011;96(12):3687–94.

27. Buchfelder M, Schlaffer S. Pituitary surgery for Cushing's disease. Neuroendocrinology 2010; 92(Suppl 1):102–6.

28. Hammer GD, Tyrrell JB, Lamborn KR, et al. Transsphenoidal microsurgery for Cushing's disease: initial outcome and long-term results. J Clin Endocrinol Metab 2004;89(12):6348–57.

29. Invitti C, Pecori Giraldi F, de Martin M, et al. Diagnosis and management of Cushing's syndrome: results of an Italian multicentre study. Study Group of the Italian Society of Endocrinology on the Pathophysiology of the Hypothalamic-Pituitary-Adrenal Axis. J Clin Endocrinol Metab 1999;84(2):440–8.

30. Liubinas SV, Porto LD, Kaye AH. Management of recurrent Cushing's disease. J Clin Neurosci 2011;18(1):7–12.

31. Patil CG, Veeravagu A, Prevedello DM, et al. Outcomes after repeat transsphenoidal surgery for recurrent Cushing's disease. Neurosurgery 2008;63(2):266–70 [discussion: 270–1].

32. Pouratian N, Prevedello DM, Jagannathan J, et al. Outcomes and management of patients with Cushing's disease without pathological confirmation of tumor resection after transsphenoidal surgery. J Clin Endocrinol Metab 2007;92(9):3383–8.

33. Valassi E, Biller BM, Swearingen B, et al. Delayed remission after transsphenoidal surgery in patients with Cushing's disease. J Clin Endocrinol Metab 2010;95(2):601–10.

34. Hardy J. Transphenoidal microsurgery of the normal and pathological pituitary. Clin Neurosurg 1969;16:185–217.

35. Griffith HB, Veerapen R. A direct transnasal approach to the sphenoid sinus. Technical note. J Neurosurg 1987;66(1):140–2.

36. Jho HD. Endoscopic transsphenoidal surgery. J Neurooncol 2001;54(2):187–95.

37. Kerr PB, Oldfield EH. Sublabial-endonasal approach to the sella turcica. J Neurosurg 2008; 109(1):153–5.

38. Starke RM, Williams BJ, Vance ML, et al. Radiation therapy and stereotactic radiosurgery for the treatment of Cushing's disease: an evidence-based review. Curr Opin Endocrinol Diabetes Obes 2010;17(4):356–64.

39. Dusick JR, Esposito F, Malkasian D, et al. Avoidance of carotid artery injuries in transsphenoidal surgery with the Doppler probe and micro-hook blades. Neurosurgery 2007;60(4 Suppl 2):322–8 [discussion: 328–9].

40. Yamasaki T, Moritake K, Hatta J, et al. Intraoperative monitoring with pulse Doppler ultrasonography in transsphenoidal surgery: technique application. Neurosurgery 1996;38(1):95–7 [discussion: 97–8].

41. Yamasaki T, Moritake K, Nagai H, et al. Integration of ultrasonography and endoscopy into transsphenoidal surgery with a "picture-in-picture" viewing system—technical note. Neurol Med Chir (Tokyo) 2002;42(6):275–7 [discussion: 278].

42. Hofmann BM, Hlavac M, Martinez R, et al. Long-term results after microsurgery for Cushing disease: experience with 426 primary operations over 35 years. J Neurosurg 2008;108(1):9–18.

43. Utz AL, Swearingen B, Biller BM. Pituitary surgery and postoperative management in Cushing's disease. Endocrinol Metab Clin North Am 2005; 34(2):459–78, xi.

44. Kabil MS, Eby JB, Shahinian HK. Fully endoscopic endonasal vs. transseptal transsphenoidal pituitary surgery. Minim Invasive Neurosurg 2005;48(6): 348–54.

45. Netea-Maier RT, van Lindert EJ, den Heijer M, et al. Transsphenoidal pituitary surgery via the endoscopic technique: results in 35 consecutive patients with Cushing's disease. Eur J Endocrinol 2006;154(5):675–84.

46. Rudnik A, Kos-Kudla B, Larysz D, et al. Endoscopic transsphenoidal treatment of hormonally active pituitary adenomas. Neuro Endocrinol Lett 2007;28(4):438–44.

47. Dehdashti AR, Gentili F. Current state of the art in the diagnosis and surgical treatment of Cushing disease: early experience with a purely endoscopic endonasal technique. Neurosurg Focus 2007;23(3):E9.

48. Dehdashti AR, Ganna A, Karabatsou K, et al. Pure endoscopic endonasal approach for pituitary adenomas: early surgical results in 200 patients and comparison with previous microsurgical series. Neurosurgery 2008;62(5):1006–15 discussion: 1015–7].

49. Gondim JA, Schops M, de Almeida JP, et al. Endoscopic endonasal transsphenoidal surgery: surgical results of 228 pituitary adenomas treated in a pituitary center. Pituitary 2010;13(1):68–77.

50. Wagenmakers MA, Netea-Maier RT, van Lindert EJ, et al. Repeated transsphenoidal pituitary surgery (TS) via the endoscopic technique: a good therapeutic option for recurrent or persistent Cushing's disease (CD). Clin Endocrinol (Oxf) 2009;70(2): 274–80.

51. Tritos NA, Biller BM, Swearingen B. Management of Cushing disease. Nat Rev Endocrinol 2011;7(5): 279–89.

52. Barbetta L, Dall'Asta C, Tomei G, et al. Assessment of cure and recurrence after pituitary surgery for Cushing's disease. Acta Neurochir (Wien) 2001; 143(5):477–81 [discussion: 481–2].

53. Esposito F, Dusick JR, Cohan P, et al. Clinical review: early morning cortisol levels as a predictor of remission after transsphenoidal surgery for Cushing's disease. J Clin Endocrinol Metab 2006; 91(1):7–13.

54. Acebes JJ, Martino J, Masuet C, et al. Early postoperative ACTH and cortisol as predictors of remission in Cushing's disease. Acta Neurochir (Wien) 2007;149(5):471–7 [discussion: 477–9].

55. Ammini AC, Bhattacharya S, Sahoo JP, et al. Cushing's disease: results of treatment and factors affecting outcome. Hormones (Athens) 2011;10(3):222–9.

56. Atkinson AB, Kennedy A, Wiggam MI, et al. Long-term remission rates after pituitary surgery for Cushing's disease: the need for long-term surveillance. Clin Endocrinol (Oxf) 2005;63(5):549–59.

57. Chee GH, Mathias DB, James RA, et al. Transsphenoidal pituitary surgery in Cushing's disease: can we predict outcome? Clin Endocrinol (Oxf) 2001; 54(5):617–26.

58. Fomekong E, Maiter D, Grandin C, et al. Outcome of transsphenoidal surgery for Cushing's disease: a high remission rate in ACTH-secreting macroadenomas. Clin Neurol Neurosurg 2009;111(5):442–9.

59. Honegger J, Schmalisch K, Beuschlein F, et al. Contemporary microsurgical concept for the treatment of Cushing's disease: endocrine outcome in 83 consecutive patients. Clin Endocrinol (Oxf) 2012;76(4):560–7.

60. Kanter AS, Diallo AO, Jane JA Jr, et al. Single-center experience with pediatric Cushing's disease. J Neurosurg 2005;103(Suppl 5):413–20.

61. Rees DA, Hanna FW, Davies JS, et al. Long-term follow-up results of transsphenoidal surgery for Cushing's disease in a single centre using strict criteria for remission. Clin Endocrinol (Oxf) 2002;56(4):541–51.

62. Rollin G, Ferreira NP, Czepielewski MA. Prospective evaluation of transsphenoidal pituitary surgery in 108 patients with Cushing's disease. Arq Bras Endocrinol Metabol 2007;51(8):1355–61.

63. Shimon I, Ram Z, Cohen ZR, et al. Transsphenoidal surgery for Cushing's disease: endocrinological follow-up monitoring of 82 patients. Neurosurgery 2002;51(1):57–61 [discussion: 61–2].

64. Trainer PJ, Lawrie HS, Verhelst J, et al. Transsphenoidal resection in Cushing's disease: undetectable serum cortisol as the definition of successful treatment. Clin Endocrinol (Oxf) 1993;38(1):73–8.

65. Yap LB, Turner HE, Adams CB, et al. Undetectable postoperative cortisol does not always predict long-term remission in Cushing's disease: a single centre audit. Clin Endocrinol (Oxf) 2002;56(1):25–31.

66. Jagannathan J, Smith R, DeVroom HL, et al. Outcome of using the histological pseudocapsule as a surgical capsule in Cushing disease. J Neurosurg 2009;111(3):531–9.

67. Joshi SM, Hewitt RJ, Storr HL, et al. Cushing's disease in children and adolescents: 20 years of experience in a single neurosurgical center. Neurosurgery 2005;57(2):281–5 [discussion: 281–5].

68. Storr HL, Alexandraki KI, Martin L, et al. Comparisons in the epidemiology, diagnostic features and cure rate by transsphenoidal surgery between paediatric and adult-onset Cushing's disease. Eur J Endocrinol 2011;164(5):667–74.

69. Locatelli M, Vance ML, Laws ER. Clinical review: the strategy of immediate reoperation for transsphenoidal surgery for Cushing's disease. J Clin Endocrinol Metab 2005;90(9):5478–82.

70. Ram Z, Nieman LK, Cutler GB Jr, et al. Early repeat surgery for persistent Cushing's disease. J Neurosurg 1994;80(1):37–45.

71. Hofmann BM, Hlavac M, Kreutzer J, et al. Surgical treatment of recurrent Cushing's disease. Neurosurgery 2006;58(6):1108–18 [discussion: 1108–18].

72. Chen JC, Amar AP, Choi S, et al. Transsphenoidal microsurgical treatment of Cushing disease: postoperative assessment of surgical efficacy by application of an overnight low-dose dexamethasone suppression test. J Neurosurg 2003;98(5): 967–73.

73. Meij BP, Lopes MB, Ellegala DB, et al. The long-term significance of microscopic dural invasion in 354 patients with pituitary adenomas treated with transsphenoidal surgery. J Neurosurg 2002;96(2): 195–208.

74. Cannavo S, Almoto B, Dall'Asta C, et al. Long-term results of treatment in patients with ACTH-secreting pituitary macroadenomas. Eur J Endocrinol 2003; 149(3):195–200.

75. De Tommasi C, Vance ML, Okonkwo DO, et al. Surgical management of adrenocorticotropic hormone-secreting macroadenomas: outcome and challenges in patients with Cushing's disease or Nelson's syndrome. J Neurosurg 2005;103(5): 825–30.

76. Nakane T, Kuwayama A, Watanabe M, et al. Long term results of transsphenoidal adenomectomy in patients with Cushing's disease. Neurosurgery 1987;21(2):218–22.

77. Prevedello DM, Pouratian N, Sherman J, et al. Management of Cushing's disease: outcome in patients with microadenoma detected on pituitary magnetic resonance imaging. J Neurosurg 2008; 109(4):751–9.

78. Watson JC, Shawker TH, Nieman LK, et al. Localization of pituitary adenomas by using intraoperative ultrasound in patients with Cushing's disease and no demonstrable pituitary tumor on magnetic resonance imaging. J Neurosurg 1998;89(6):927–32.

79. Friedman RB, Oldfield EH, Nieman LK, et al. Repeat transsphenoidal surgery for Cushing's disease. J Neurosurg 1989;71(4):520–7.

80. Pereira AM, van Aken MO, van Dulken H, et al. Long-term predictive value of postsurgical cortisol concentrations for cure and risk of recurrence in Cushing's disease. J Clin Endocrinol Metab 2003; 88(12):5858–64.

81. Lim JS, Lee SK, Kim SH, et al. Intraoperative multiple-staged resection and tumor tissue identification using frozen sections provide the best result for the accurate localization and complete resection of tumors in Cushing's disease. Endocrine 2011;40(3):452–61.

82. Patil CG, Prevedello DM, Lad SP, et al. Late recurrences of Cushing's disease after initial successful transsphenoidal surgery. J Clin Endocrinol Metab 2008;93(2):358–62.

83. Dickerman RD, Oldfield EH. Basis of persistent and recurrent Cushing disease: an analysis of findings at repeated pituitary surgery. J Neurosurg 2002; 97(6):1343–9.

84. Lindsay JR, Oldfield EH, Stratakis CA, et al. The postoperative basal cortisol and CRH tests for prediction of long-term remission from Cushing's disease after transsphenoidal surgery. J Clin Endocrinol Metab 2011;96(7):2057–64.

85. Trainer PJ, Besser GM. Differential diagnosis in Cushing's syndrome: the role of inferior petrosal sinus sampling. Eur J Med 1993;2(5):261–3.

86. Ciric I, Ragin A, Baumgartner C, et al. Complications of transsphenoidal surgery: results of a national survey, review of the literature, and personal experience. Neurosurgery 1997;40(2):225–36 [discussion: 236–7].

87. Semple PL, Laws ER Jr. Complications in a contemporary series of patients who underwent transsphenoidal surgery for Cushing's disease. J Neurosurg 1999;91(2):175–9.

88. Patil CG, Lad SP, Harsh GR, et al. National trends, complications, and outcomes following transsphenoidal surgery for Cushing's disease from 1993 to 2002. Neurosurg Focus 2007;23(3):E7.

89. Aulinas A, Colom C, Ybarra J, et al. Immediate and delayed postoperative morbidity in functional and non-functioning pituitary adenomas. Pituitary 2011. [Epub ahead of print].

90. Fitzgerald PA, Aron DC, Findling JW, et al. Cushing's disease: transient secondary adrenal insufficiency after selective removal of pituitary microadenomas; evidence for a pituitary origin. J Clin Endocrinol Metab 1982;54(2):413–22.

91. Barrow DL, Tindall GT. Loss of vision after transsphenoidal surgery. Neurosurgery 1990;27(1):60–8.

92. Batra PS, Citardi MJ, Lanza DC. Isolated sphenoid sinusitis after transsphenoidal hypophysectomy. Am J Rhinol 2005;19(2):185–9.

93. Stuijver DJ, van Zaane B, Feelders RA, et al. Incidence of venous thromboembolism in patients with Cushing's syndrome: a multicenter cohort study. J Clin Endocrinol Metab 2011;96(11):3525–32.

94. Ciric I, Zhao JC, Du H, et al. Transsphenoidal surgery for Cushing disease: experience with 136 patients. Neurosurgery 2012;70(1):70–81.

95. Sun Y, Sun Q, Fan C, et al. Diagnosis and therapy for Cushing's disease with negative dynamic MRI finding: a single-centre experience. Clin Endocrinol (Oxf) 2012;76(6):868–76.

96. Yamada S, Fukuhara N, Nishioka H, et al. Surgical management and outcomes in patients with Cushing disease with negative pituitary magnetic resonance imaging. World Neurosurg 2012;77(3–4): 525–32.

97. Alwani RA, de Herder WW, de Jong FH, et al. Rapid decrease in adrenal responsiveness to ACTH stimulation after successful pituitary surgery in patients with Cushing's disease. Clin Endocrinol (Oxf) 2011; 75(5):602–7.

98. Atkinson JL, Young WF Jr, Meyer FB, et al. Sublabial transseptal vs transnasal combined endoscopic microsurgery in patients with Cushing disease and MRI-depicted microadenomas. Mayo Clin Proc 2008;83(5):550–3.

99. Salenave S, Gatta B, Pecheur S, et al. Pituitary magnetic resonance imaging findings do not influence surgical outcome in adrenocorticotropin-secreting microadenomas. J Clin Endocrinol Metab 2004;89(7):3371–6.

100. Flitsch J, Knappe UJ, Ludecke DK. The use of postoperative ACTH levels as a marker for successful transsphenoidal microsurgery in Cushing's disease. Zentralbl Neurochir 2003;64(1):6–11.

Medical Management of Persistent and Recurrent Cushing Disease

Maria Fleseriu, MD[a,b],*

KEYWORDS

- Cushing disease • Failed transphenoidal surgery • Recurrent Cushing disease
- Somatostatin receptor ligands • Pasireotide • Glucocorticoid receptor antagonist • Mifepristone
- Adrenal steroidogenesis inhibitors

KEY POINTS

- The prevalence of Cushing disease seems to be higher than previously thought.
- Morbidity and mortality are significantly increased in untreated hypercortisolemia.
- Transphenoidal surgery, in the hands of experienced neurosurgeons, is currently considered the first-line treatment of choice.
- A significant number of patients with Cushing disease could require additional medical treatment at some point in their disease course (either after failed pituitary surgery or after disease recurrence, which can be seen as late as 20 years after initial treatment).
- New therapeutic agents, such as pasireotide (a multiligand somatostatin receptor ligand that targets the corticotroph adenoma itself) and mifepristone (a glucocorticoid receptor antagonist), have recently been approved in Europe (pasireotide for treatment of Cushing disease) and the United States (mifepristone for treatment of hyperglycemia associated with Cushing syndrome).
- Individualized, multidisciplinary management to normalize devastating disease effects of hypercortisolemia is required.

INTRODUCTION

Cushing syndrome (CS) is a severe clinical state produced by prolonged and inappropriate exposure to endogenous or exogenous cortisol. The exogenous cause is usually identifiable; in contrast, diagnosis of excessive pituitary adrenocorticotropic hormone (ACTH) secretion sometimes is more complicated, especially in the early disease phase. The true incidence and prevalence of CS is difficult to estimate because of the rarity of the disorder, its insidious onset. Diagnosis is also complicated by nonspecificity and high prevalence of clinical symptoms in the general population. Furthermore, the diagnostic work-up of suspected CS requires a variety of combined biochemical tests, which often have inadequate sensitivity and specificity. Early data suggested a prevalence of 0.7 to 2.4 per million.[1] However, several recent studies have suggested

Disclosure: MF serves as investigator on research grants to OHSU from Corcept Therapeutics, Inc and Novartis. She also serves as an ad hoc consultant to Novartis.
[a] Department of Medicine, Oregon Health & Science University, 3181 Southwest Sam Jackson Park Road (BTE 472), Portland, OR 97239, USA; [b] Department of Neurological Surgery, Oregon Health & Science University, 3181 Southwest Sam Jackson Park Road (BTE 472), Portland, OR 97239, USA
* Northwest Pituitary Center, Oregon Health & Science University, 3181 Southwest Sam Jackson Park Road (BTE 472), Portland, OR 97239.
E-mail address: fleseriu@ohsu.edu

a much higher prevalence for Cushing disease (CD) and CS.[2,3]

Moreover, epidemiologic studies in Belgium and England have revealed that the prevalence of clinically relevant pituitary tumors is 3.5- to 5-fold higher than previously estimated with an incidence rate of approximately 76 to 100 per million.[4,5] ACTH-secreting adenomas represent approximately 10% to 15% of all pituitary tumors; therefore, CD rates could be substantially higher than previously estimated.[1,6] Additionally, screening for CS in certain patient populations has revealed a prevalence of up to 3% to 11% in patients with diabetes, obesity, and osteoporosis.[7–9]

The most common etiology (70%–80%) of CS is CD, caused by an ACTH-secreting pituitary adenoma. Women are affected more than men (5:1), with peak incidence at 25 to 40 years of age.

MORBIDITY AND MORTALITY

CS is associated with increased cardiovascular morbidity and mortality. Chronic hypercortisolemia is responsible for a higher incidence of hypertension, glucose intolerance, diabetes mellitus, central obesity, hyperlipidemia, and hypercoagulability.[10] Recent evidence also suggests that increased cardiovascular risk may persist even after long-term CS remission.[11–16]

In a 2011 study, Clayton and colleagues[17] calculated standardized mortality ratio for a group of their own patients; persistent CD (adjusted for age and gender) versus CD in remission was 10.7 versus 3.3, respectively. Standardized mortality ratio data for six other studies they reviewed were 5.5 versus 1.2 in persistent CD versus CD in remission. Hypertension and diabetes mellitus were risk factors for worse outcome, as well as disease persistence and older age at diagnosis.[17] In another review of three larger studies,[18] patients with persistent CD experienced a marked increase in mortality rate compared with those experiencing initial cure (mortality rate of 3.25).

These results suggest that in patients with persistent CD early and aggressive intervention to prevent excessive mortality is required.

TREATMENT
Successful Management

For as long as CS has been described, the syndrome has presented a challenge to physicians and patients alike. Treatment goals for CD include the reversal of clinical features, the normalization of cortisol levels with minimal morbidity while preserving pituitary function, and long-term disease control without recurrence.[19] In a small number of patients with macroadenomas, removal of the tumor mass represents an additional treatment goal.

First-line therapy in most cases is transphenoidal surgery (TSS), but even in the hands of the most experienced neurosurgeon, cure rates can range from 65% to 90% for microadenomas (with even lower percentage cure rates for macroadenomas). Unfortunately, cure rates have been noted to drop further with longer follow-up.[20,21] The outcomes of TSS for CD have recently been reviewed in detail.[22,23] An accurate measurement of real outcome data is hampered by different definitions of cure or interval assessments in various studies.[24] For example, postoperative patients could be considered as in complete remission or cured, remission with relapse, or not cured with persistent hypercortisolism.[25,26]

Furthermore, even for patients who are "cured," the risk of relapse over time is relatively high with long-term follow-up.[14,27,28] Thus, a diagnosis of remission rather than "cured" is preferable. Unfortunately, there is no ideal predictor of what could be considered permanent remission. Postoperative adrenal insufficiency has been shown to be less reliable than initially thought.[6] Conversely, a normal or slightly high postoperative cortisol level is not an absolute indicator of not being in remission. A recent multicenter study showed that 5.6% of patients, who had an initial normal or slightly high urine free cortisol (UFC) level, developed a delayed and persistent cortisol decrease after an average of 1 month postoperatively.[14] An immediate postoperative cortisol level, especially if high, could be important for a decision regarding early repeat surgery.[6,14,29]

If first-line surgery is unsuccessful, the next treatment step is presently somewhat dependent on the patient or treatment center preference. In all cases of persistent or recurrent CD, successful treatment requires close collaboration between endocrinologists, neurosurgeons, radiation oncologists, and general surgeons (**Fig. 1**).

Screening tests and localization tests are fraught with false-positives and negative results. If a patient fails surgery (unless pathology is positive for ACTH-secreting adenoma), a diagnosis reconfirmation is recommended[6] before any further treatment decision can be made.

Medical Treatment

Recently, medical treatment has played a more important role in controlling cortisol excess and its devastating physiologic effects.[21,30] Results of two large phase III prospective trials conducted over the last few years have been published that

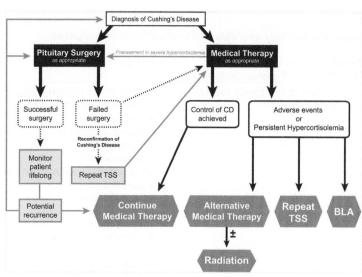

Fig. 1. Treatment of Cushing disease. BLA, bilateral adrenalectomy; CD, Cushing disease; TSS, transphenoidal surgery.

could have an impact on treatment perspective (reviewed in detail next).

Pasireotide (Signifor) has been approved in Europe for treatment of CD and mifepristone (Korlym) has been approved by the US Food and Drug Administration for hyperglycemia associated with endogenous CS. Currently, uses of medication include preparation for surgery (to control the metabolic effects of hypercortisolemia) or as adjunctive treatment after surgery.[31] Medications are also of use in patients who are unwilling or have contraindications to surgery and are awaiting effects of radiation.[6] Mirroring the treatment approach to acromegaly (to a different extent), primary medical therapy (that is replacing surgery) has also been used in patients with CD in clinical practice or research clinical trials.[32–36] It is essential that patients be counseled about the need for lifelong medical therapy in such cases because hypercortisolemia recurs on treatment discontinuation.

A brief review of treatment options after failed first-line TSS for CD is detailed next. The remainder of the discussion focuses on medical therapy.

Repeat TSS is a good option in selected cases, achieving remission in 43% to 70% of patients.[23,37,38] The risk of hypopituitarism is higher after repeat surgery compared with the first TSS, and ranges from 41% to 50%.[39,40]

Radiation (conventional and stereotactic) plays a role in patients with large tumors that invade the cavernous sinus or in patients who experience relapse after an initial cure with no observed tumor on magnetic resonance imaging.[6] Radiation therapy outcome studies in patients with CD have been summarized by Tritos and colleagues.[23] Up

to 86% of patients experienced hypercortisolemia remission and tumor growth was controlled in most cases. Unfortunately, similar to the surgical series, different criteria and assessment timelines were used to measure remission. Effects of radiation are usually observed at 2 to 5 years and patients require interim medical treatment to control hypercortisolemia.[25] Besides the general risks related to radiation, hypopituitarism was observed in almost half of the patients at 5 years.[41]

Bilateral adrenalectomy (BLA), the first reported treatment for CS, offers quick control of hypercortisolemia. Currently, laparoscopic BLA has a role in patients who have failed all other options, or in women who wish to become pregnant.[42] Despite being a definite treatment for CS, patients experience permanent adrenal insufficiency with a need for lifelong glucocorticoid and mineralocorticoid replacement. In addition, corticotroph tumor progression is observed in up to 30% of cases.[43]

MEDICAL THERAPY

Mechanism of action and a summary of drugs commercially available and under clinical investigation are provided in **Table 1** and **Fig. 2**.

Modulation of ACTH Release

ACTH hypersecretion is still under hypothalamic control in CD, thus the potential therapeutic role for neuromodulatory agents. Bromocriptine, cyproheptadine, octreotide, and valproate have yielded variable efficacy and only marginal results.[44,45] Spontaneous remission of CD could explain discrepant results in small studies.

Table 1
A summary of drugs, commercially available and under clinical investigation

A	Glucocorticoid receptor blocker (act to block effects of hypercortisolemia)	Mifepristone
B	Modulate ACTH (act at the tumor level to modulate ACTH release)	Somatostatin receptor ligands: • Pasireotide–SOM 230 • Octreotide Dopamine agonists • Cabergoline • Bromocriptine Other agents tried but not uniformly effective • GABA agonists • Valproic acid • Serotonin antagonists • PPAR gamma In vitro/animal models • Alpha 1 adrenergic receptor antagonist • Retinoic acid • EGFR inhibitors
C	Inhibitors of steroidogenesis (blockage of adrenal enzymes implicated in cortisol synthesis)	• Ketoconazole • Mitotane (approved in Europe) • Etomidate • Metyrapone • Ketoconazole + Metyrapone + Etomidate • Aminoglutethimide (no longer available) • Trilostane (no longer available) In clinical trials • LCI (www.clinicaltrials.gov)
D	Combination therapy using drugs from different groups	• Pasireotide + Cabergoline + Ketoconazole

Recently, studies have shown that the dopamine D_2 receptor is expressed in 75% of corticotroph adenomas[46] and somatostatin receptor SSTR5 is predominantly expressed in cultured human corticotroph adenoma cells.[47,48] These data have renewed interest in dopamine agonists and somatostatin receptor ligands (SRLs) as potential CD therapeutic agents (see later).

Cyproheptadine is a histamine and serotonin (5-HT) antagonist previously used in patients with Nelson syndrome. It has been postulated that ACTH secretion is under a degree of serotoninergic central nervous control or that cyproheptadine has a direct inhibitory effect on corticotropin-releasing hormone (CRH) and vasopressin secretion from the hypothalamus (in vitro studies).[49]

One patient with CD was remarkably controlled for a period of 11 years,[50] but other patients have experienced disappointing results.[19,44] Doses have varied between 12 and 24 mg/d. The most commonly encountered side effects are sleepiness and weight gain, which represent the main cause for treatment discontinuation.

Valproic acid is an antiepileptic agent that inhibits γ-aminobutyric acid aminotransferase. Earlier studies showed a significant reduction in ACTH levels,[51] but chronic administration was not associated with similar results.[45] As is the case with other neuromodulatory agents, the exact mechanism of action is not well understood, but most likely acts at the hypothalamic level or on CRH secretion.

Peroxisome proliferator-activated receptor (PPAR)-γ is a member of the nuclear receptor superfamily, and functions as a transcription factor. ACTH-secreting adenomas highly express PPAR-γ.[52] Despite initial reports that PPAR-γ ligands could play a role in treating CD,[53,54] current results do not sufficiently support routine clinical use.[19,55]

Dopamine agonists: bromocriptine and cabergoline

Bromocriptine and cabergoline have shown in vitro inhibition of ACTH secretion in corticotroph tumor cells.[46] Bromocriptine is a potent dopamine receptor agonist and cortisol levels are reduced after just one dose; however, long-term cortisol

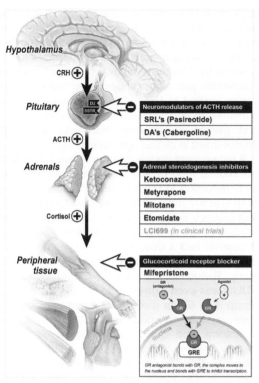

Fig. 2. Mechanism of action and targets for therapy in Cushing disease. ACTH, adrenocorticotropic hormone; DA, dopamine agonist; GR, glucocorticoid receptor; GRE, glucocorticoid response elements; SRL, somatostatin receptor ligand.

reduction results are at best 30% to 50%.[44,56] Bromocriptine effectiveness was initially reported for Nelson syndrome[57] and in CD with associated tumor shrinkage, but long-term response was limited.[58] In 12 patients with CD after BLA (no evidence of a pituitary adenoma), plasma ACTH showed a small but significant overall reduction after bromocriptine therapy.[59] Addition of cyproheptadine did not offer additional benefits.

Dopamine agonist use is associated with adverse effects, such as nasal congestion, nausea, and postural hypotension, although a gradual increase in dose could minimize these effects.

Cabergoline has recently been added to the treatment armamentarium in patients with CD who have failed surgery. It has a much longer half-life and a very high affinity and specificity for D_2 receptors. Short-term results have been encouraging in monotherapy and in combination therapy (reviewed elsewhere in this article).

As with bromocriptine, cabergoline efficacy (0.5 mg twice a week) was initially reported for Nelson syndrome.[60] In this particular case, bromocriptine treatment had failed and 12 mg/d cyproheptadine for 18 months significantly decreased ACTH levels

and partially improved pigmentation, but was ultimately stopped because of adverse effects.

In multiple CD case reports, treatment with cabergoline resulted in a short-term response in up to 75%[61,62] of patients. In long-term studies cabergoline has been found to induce a complete response in selected patients (25%–40%) in studies lasting 6 to 24 months.[62,63]

Retrospectively, Godbout and colleagues[35] studied 30 patients with CD (first-line treatment for three patients) treated with cabergoline over the long term. Initial dosing was 0.5 to 1 mg/wk, which was increased up to 6 mg/wk in 80% of patients, a much higher dose than previously reported. Complete response to treatment (normal serial UFC) was initially observed in 36.6% of patients; however, after a mean of 37.7 months, just 9 (30%) of 30 patients were considered controlled (mean dose was 2.1 mg/wk) (**Fig. 3**). It was also noted that the patients with a partial initial response were not controlled at follow-up and that two patients presented an escape phenomenon at 2 and 5 years, respectively. Severity of disease was not shown to influence outcome. Cabergoline was well tolerated overall. Interestingly, despite theoretical concerns, no significant cardiac valvulopathy was seen in this study or in Pivonello's study[63]; longer-term studies are needed to elucidate the potential cardiac involvement.

Somatostatin-receptor ligands
Native somatostatin (binds to all five somatostatin receptors subtypes with high affinity) has been

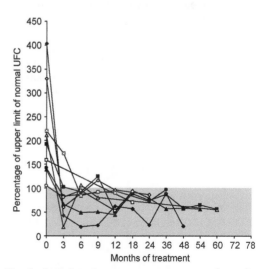

Fig. 3. Complete long-term response to cabergoline monotherapy in nine patients with Cushing disease. (*From* Godbout A, Manavela M, Danilowicz K, et al. Cabergoline monotherapy in the long-term treatment of Cushing's disease. Eur J Endocrinol 2010;163(5):709–16; with permission.)

shown to inhibit CRH-stimulated ACTH release in normal rat pituitary cells, when incubated in serum-deprived conditions or after pretreatment with a glucocorticoid-receptor blocking agent.[64]

Octreotide, an SRL that predominantly targets SSTR2 and has been extensively used with other neuroendocrine tumors, was also studied in a variety of CS cases. In vitro, octreotide-inhibited CRH stimulated ACTH secretion but in vivo did not have any effects on basal or CRH-stimulated ACTH. This discrepancy could be related to down-regulation of SSTR2 by hypercortisolemia[65] and could explain some of the positive results observed in Nelson syndrome versus CD.[66]

Predominant expression of SSTR5 mRNA in cultured human corticotroph adenoma cells[47] prompted an alternative approach using an SST5 ligand.[67]

Pasireotide (SOM 230) is a novel multireceptor-targeted SRL that has shown efficacy in patients with acromegaly and CD when administered by subcutaneous injection.[68,69] Pasireotide (Fig. 4) demonstrates high binding affinity for SST1, SST2, SST3, and SST5, and has a 40-fold higher affinity for SST5 than octreotide.[70]

Pasireotide has been found to exhibit enhanced potency in murine corticotroph cells as evidenced by cyclic adenosine monophosphate accumulation and calcium oscillations (important markers of ACTH secretion).[71,72] Pasireotide action seems to be determined primarily by SST5, whereas the ligand effect on SST2 is negligible. Cell proliferation and ACTH secretion were also suppressed by pasireotide in primary cultures of human corticotroph tumors.[67] In a phase II, proof-of-concept, open-label, single-arm, multicenter study, the in vivo efficacy of pasireotide was evaluated in 39 subjects with either de novo or with persistent or recurrent CD.[68] Pasireotide, 600 µg, was given subcutaneously twice daily for 15

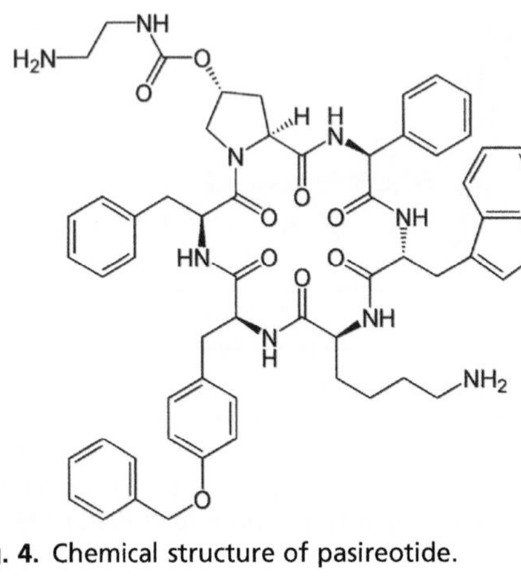

Fig. 4. Chemical structure of pasireotide.

days: mean UFC level decreased in 76% of subjects and normalized in 17%. Responders seemed to have higher pasireotide exposure than nonresponders. The authors noted a trend toward lower baseline UFC levels as predictive of a response to pasireotide with significantly greater reductions in serum cortisol in UFC responders versus nonresponders. In addition, reductions in serum cortisol and plasma ACTH were seen with significant improvement in clinical symptomatology.

A subsequent double-blinded phase III trial with pasireotide (600 or 900 µg twice daily) revealed UFC reduction in most patients.[34] Normalization of UFC at 6 months without the need for dose titration (primary endpoint) was achieved in 14.6% of the 600-µg group and 16.3% of the 900-µg group. If patients had a dose increase at Month 3, this percentage increased to 16% and 29%, respectively. Response rate in mild CD (UFC >1.5–2 XULN) was even higher, up to 50% in the 900-µg group (Fig. 5). As mean UFC decreased, clinical signs (systolic and diastolic blood pressure) and symptoms and quality of life improved. Low-density lipoprotein cholesterol and weight decreased significantly ($P<.001$). Serum and salivary cortisol and plasma ACTH were also reduced. Of utmost significance, if present, response was rapid and sustained; responders (based on UFC levels) were identified early in most cases, within 2 months of treatment. Tumor volume also decreased, by up to 43.8% (95% confidence interval, decrease range 68.4%–19.2%). Adverse effects were similar to that of other SRLs (mostly transient gastrointestinal discomfort), except for hyperglycemia; 73% of subjects had a hyperglycemia-related adverse effect and 6% discontinued the study because of such events. In these patients, close monitoring of glucose levels and prompt treatment for hyperglycemia is essential. Thirteen (8%) subjects had an adverse effect of hypocortisolism that was responsive to a dose reduction. Based on these study results, pasireotide (Signifor) has recently been recommended by the Committee for Medicinal Products for Human Use of the European Medicines Agency for approval to treat CD in Europe.[73] Clinical studies using monthly pasireotide long-acting-release in CD are ongoing (www.clinicaltrials.gov). This drug represents an important advance in treating CD with a pituitary-directed therapy that decreases ACTH, cortisol values, and corticotroph tumor volume.

Potential new receptor targets: in vitro and animal models
Retinoic acid receptors are important drug targets for cancer therapy and prevention.[74,75] Retinoic acid

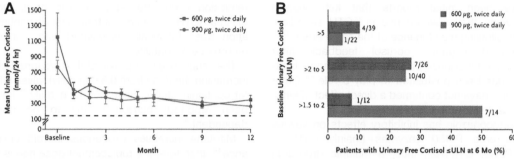

Fig. 5. Mean change in urinary free cortisol levels from baseline to Month 12 and proportion of patients with normalized levels at Month 6. ULN, upper limit of normal. (*From* Colao A, Petersenn S, Newell-Price J, et al. A 12-month phase 3 study of pasireotide in Cushing's disease. N Engl J Med 2012;366:914–24; with permission.)

has been shown in vitro and in animal studies to have a potent inhibitory effect on corticotroph tumor growth, plasma ACTH, and corticosterone secretion.[75,76] α_1-Adrenergic receptor antagonists have also been shown to decrease plasma ACTH and decrease tumor growth in murine pituitary cells.[77]

The epidermal growth factor receptor (EGFR) family has recently been studied as a therapeutic target for CD. Melmed's group[78] showed in surgically resected human and canine corticotroph cultured tumors that blocking EGFR activity with gefitinib (an EGFR tyrosine kinase inhibitor) attenuated pro-opiomelanocortin expression, inhibited corticotroph tumor cell proliferation, and induced apoptosis. In mice, gefitinib treatment decreased tumor size and corticosterone levels and reversed signs of hypercortisolemia, including elevated glucose levels and excess omental fat. These results indicate that inhibiting EGFR signaling may be a novel strategy for treating CD.[78] Efficacy in patients with CD has not yet been tested in clinical trials.

Drugs that Inhibit Steroidogenesis

These drugs decrease cortisol production by complete or partial direct inhibition of adrenal steroidogenesis: ketoconazole, mitotane, etomidate, metyrapone, trilostane, and aminoglutethimide. However, metyrapone, aminoglutethimide, and trilostane are no longer available in the United States. Combinations of these drugs may have additive or synergistic effects, achieving similar results with lower doses and less adverse effects.

Ketoconazole is an imidazole derivative that impairs steroid hormone synthesis by blocking mitochondrial P-450–dependent enzyme systems (inhibition of 17,20-lyase, adrenal 11β-hydroxylase, 17-hydroxylase and side chain cleavage).

Excluding those studies with less than five patients, there are now more than 150 patients

with CD who have been treated with ketoconazole.[33,79] Remission rates vary from 30% to 90%.[33] However, some study results may have been biased by previous pituitary radiation treatment.[80]

The first large retrospective study of patients with CD treated with ketoconazole included 28 patients with CD. Twelve patients were treated for more than 6 months with good results overall; all patients had undergone pituitary irradiation.[80] Ketoconazole has also been used in three patients older than 75 years of age with good results and no adverse effects.[81]

In most of the initial studies, dose ranged from 200 to 1200 mg/d.[82] Liver toxicity was also variable and ranged from 12% to 50%.[83–86] In addition to liver problems (hepatic dyscrazia and elevated transaminases), gastrointestinal disturbances, gynecomastia, and sexual side effects were also observed. Ketoconazole is contraindicated in pregnant women.

In the largest study to date,[33] 38 patients with CD treated long-term (range, 6–72 months; mean, 23 months) with ketoconazole were reviewed, most as primary therapy (21 patients); the other 17 patients had previously undergone TSS. Ketoconazole dose was 200 to 1200 mg daily with 45% of patients considered responders based on the intention-to-treat analysis. Five patients stopped taking the drug within 1 week because of intolerance. Interestingly, 5 of 15 patients who did not have a pituitary adenoma initially had a visible tumor after 20 to 30 months of treatment. There was no adrenal insufficiency with the titration used in the study. Responders were identified early in the treatment course (all controlled patients responded within 3 months of the treatment start). Unfortunately, none of the initial biochemical parameters were good predictors of response.

An ACTH increase is expected with most adrenal steroidogenesis inhibitor drugs but there have been initial reports that ketoconazole prevents the expected rise in ACTH secretion, thus allowing maintenance of the same dose.[26,87] Reduced negative cortisol feedback after enhanced response of ACTH to CRH administration has been postulated to play a role.[88] Other studies have not confirmed a direct effect of ketoconazole on ACTH.[89]

Ketoconazole has inhibitory effects on several cytocrome P-450 enzymes (mainly CYP3A4, CYP2C9, CYP1A2); thus, a multiple drug-drug interaction is possible. The most frequently used medications, which require dose adjustments, are most benzodiazepines; calcium channel blockers; statins (excluding pravastatin and fluvastatin); warfarin; phenytoin; and fluoxetine.[90]

Ketoconazole absorption requires an acidic environment, precluding the use of proton pump inhibitors or H_2 receptor blockers. Because of over-the-counter availability of both of these drug classes, it is important that this is discussed with patients before starting treatment (**Box 1**).

Mitotane (o'p'-DDD) is an adrenocorticolytic drug that also inhibits the same enzymes as etomidate. It is mainly used to treat adrenocortical carcinoma, but it seems to have some suppressive ACTH effects. Eighty percent of patients treated with mitotane and pituitary radiation have been reported as in remission.[91]

In a recent retrospective large cohort of 76 patients with CD treated with mitotane at a single center, 24-hour UFC normalization was observed in 48 (72%) patients, with a median follow-up of 6.7 months. Adverse events led to discontinuation in 29% of patients. A pituitary adenoma became visible during treatment in 12 patients (25%) with initial negative pituitary imaging allowing subsequent TSS. Fortunately, 29% of patients were in

---

Box 1
Clinical practice

- Ketoconazole at a dose of 200 mg two or three times daily, and check liver function and 24-hour UFC within 1 week.

- If clinical signs of adrenal insufficiency, measure morning cortisol as soon as possible, stop drug for 1 day. Start replacement glucocorticoids if needed.

- If UFC still high, increase to 400 mg twice daily.

- If not well tolerated or no effect in 2 to 3 months, switch to a different drug.

- Consider possible combination therapy.

Data from references.[6,25,33,44]

---

remission even after stopping the drug; high plasma ACTH at the time of treatment discontinuation was statistically associated with a lower recurrence probability.[32]

The usual dose is approximately 4 g/d (gradually increasing the dose from 0.5–1 g daily), given with fat-containing food. Doses of 12 g daily[92] have been reported; nausea seems to be dose dependent.[44]

Mitotane increases exogenous steroid clearance[44]; therefore, the replacement dose needs to be adjusted. There are also induced changes in corticosteroid-binding globulin, potentially making plasma cortisol measurements less reliable. Adverse effects are represented by gastrointestinal symptoms, rash, confusion, gynecomastia, and hepatotoxicity.

Mitotane is completely contraindicated in women who are planning pregnancy over several years because the drug has been detected in adipose tissue long after discontinuation.[93] Sometimes mitotane spares aldosterone secretion, a potential advantage over surgical adrenalectomy.

Metyrapone (not commercially available compassionate use) inhibits 11β-hydroxylase when used in single or combination therapy[94,95] with good results overall, in up to 75% of patients.[19] Doses range from 500 to 6000 mg daily. Adverse effects are mainly hirsutism and acne in women, dizziness, gastrointestinal upset, and hypokalemia. Although contraindicated in pregnancy, it is the agent most frequently used in CS associated with pregnancy.[96] Compensatory increases in ACTH are seen, mostly at the beginning of the treatment.[95]

Trilostane, a 3β-hydroxysteroid dehydrogenase selective inhibitor, is probably not a potent inhibitor.[97] Trilostane is no longer available in the United States.

Aminoglutethimide, an anticonvulsant, inhibits the side chain cleavage of cortisol biosynthesis (cholesterol to pregnenolone). Dosage varies between 250 mg twice to three times daily. Initial falls in cortisol levels are usually overcome by an increase in ACTH. An early study in 39 patients showed a remission rate of 46%. Adverse effects are gastrointestinal symptoms, headache, dizziness, depression, and blurred vision. Aminoglutethimide is no longer available in the United States.

The hypnotic drug etomidate has a strong inhibitory effect that inhibits cholesterol chain cleavage and 11-deoxycortisol β-hydroxylase and it is the only parenteral and intravenous option for CS treatment.[98] Intravenously administered etomidate in a low nonhypnotic dose (0.03 mg/kg etomidate in a bolus injection, followed by constant infusion of 0.3 mg/kg/h for 24 hours) decreased serum cortisol concentrations in a dose-dependent manner in subjects who were hypercortisolemic and eucortisolemic.[99]

Etomidate also has α-adrenergic activities, which may contribute to the cardiovascular stability in these patients.[100] Etomidate as a single line of therapy has been reported in patients with CS of other origins and use in 11 CD cases has been reported.[99,101–103] Because of very rapid onset of action, etomidate is a good option in severe emergent cases.

Etomidate has also been successfully used in patients (especially children) who developed liver enzymes abnormalities on ketoconazole.[104] Cortisol decrease can be seen within 12 to 24 hours of treatment[99,102] and glucocorticoid replacement to prevent adrenal insufficiency is warranted after 24 hours of etomidate infusion.[98] Adverse effects are dominated by sedation, pain at the infusion site, anaphylactic reactions, coughing, hiccups, nausea, myoclonus, and vomiting (www.drugs.com).[98]

LCI699 is an inhibitor of aldosterone synthase and 11β-hydroxilase, currently under investigation in a proof of concept study in patients with CD (www.clinicaltrials.gov).

Combination of adrenal steroidogenesis inhibitors

Recently, a triple drug combination as an alternative to urgent adrenalectomy has been discussed.[79] Eleven patients with CD with severe disease were simultaneously started on mitotane (3–5 g per 24 hour), metyrapone (3–4.5 g per 24 hour), and ketoconazole (400–1200 mg per 24 hour). UFC was noted to decrease very rapidly (within days). Clinical improvement permitted five patients to undergo pituitary surgery. Side effects were tolerable and no more so than with each medication alone (despite high doses).

Monitoring patients being treated with an adrenal steroidogenesis inhibitor

The fine line between eucortisolemia and abnormal cortisol can be hard to maintain in some cases.[6,22,23,25,30,44,105] Although still debatable, most authors agree that a mean normal serum or 24-hour UFC should be the aim of therapy. An initial dose should be slowly increased for tolerability. Later in the course of treatment, for most steroid synthesis inhibitors, it is necessary to increase the dose because the set point for negative feedback is higher in corticotroph tumors than in the normal pituitary. Frequent cortisol monitoring is necessary to diagnose adrenal insufficiency and breakthrough hypercortisolism in patients previously controlled (drug escape vs disease progression).

Another approach widely used is total blockade of glucocorticoid synthesis (hypocortisolism/adrenal insufficiency) and replacement with glucocorticoids. A possible drug holiday to evaluate CS remission in patients previously radiated is also recommended.

Glucocorticoid Receptor Blocker: Mifepristone

Mifepristone is a steroid that binds competitively to glucocorticoid, androgen, and progestin receptors (**Fig. 6**).[44] It blocks the action of cortisol by binding to the glucocorticoid receptor.[106]

Mifepristone use with CD was previously limited to just five cases (53 isolated or small series cases of mifepristone use to treat CS reported).[107–109] However, the recent SEISMIC study of mifepristone use (reviewed later) included 43 subjects with CD.[110]

Most patients with CS in the case series had received previous treatments, such as surgery, chemotherapy, or other therapeutic interventions, including a variety of anticortisolic drugs, without success. A majority of patients in these reports showed resolution of or significant improvement in somatic features of CS (buffalo hump, central obesity, moon facies, peripheral edema, striae). Many showed improvements in blood glucose levels and diabetes, including reductions in the use of antidiabetic medications or changing from insulin use to oral antidiabetic drugs. Improvements in depression and rapid resolution of psychiatric symptoms were also frequently reported.

Although mifepristone was used previously to treat other forms of CS,[109] the first CD case was reported in 2001.[108] The patient noticed a significant improvement in symptoms with heart failure amelioration and resolution of severe depression. Furthermore, diabetes control improved (HbA_{1c} decreased from 10.4% to 6.9%). Castinetti and colleagues[107] reviewed four patients with CD treated with mifepristone: rapid improvement of clinical signs was observed in three patients and

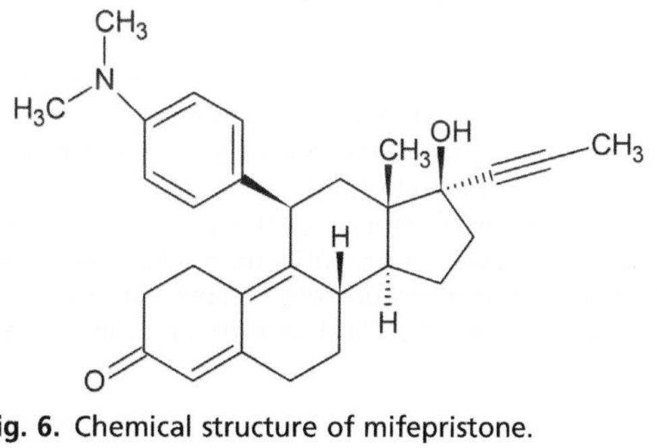

Fig. 6. Chemical structure of mifepristone.

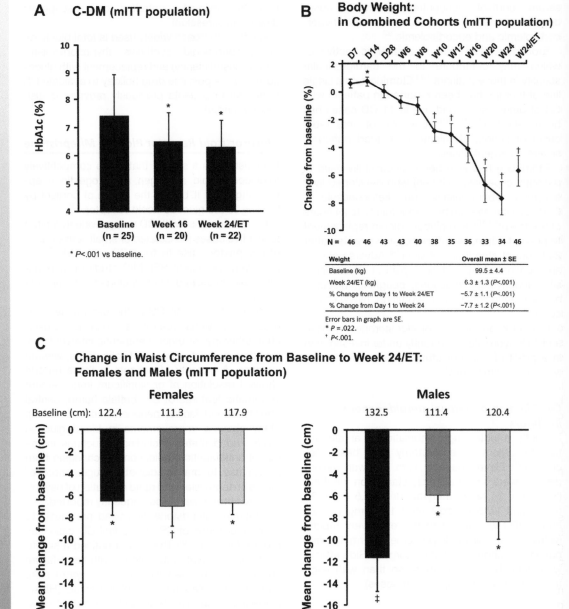

Fig. 7. (A) Changes in glucose-related outcomes. HbA$_{1c}$ significantly decreased from baseline to week 24/early termination (P<.001). Data shown as mean ± SD. (B, C) Changes in weight and body composition. Results demonstrated a significant reduction in body weight from baseline to week 24/early termination (P<.001). Data shown as mean ± SE. To multiply insulin values to pmol/L multiply by 6.945. C-DM, patients with CS and type 2 diabetes/impaired glucose tolerance; C-HT, patients with CS and a diagnosis of hypertension; ET, early termination; HbA$_{1c}$, glycated hemoglobin A$_{1c}$; MITT, modified intent to treat. (*Adapted from* Fleseriu M, Biller BM, Findling JW, et al. Mifepristone, a glucocorticoid receptor antagonist, produces clinical and metabolic benefits in patients with Cushing's syndrome. J Clin Endocrinol Metab 2012;97(6):2039–2049; with permission.)

psychosis improved in 1 week in one patient. Cortisol and ACTH increases were observed in all patients (as expected by physiologic mechanism). Mifepristone dose ranged from 400 to 2000 mg/d over 6 to 24 months.

A serious potential side effect of mifepristone treatment is adrenal insufficiency. Adrenal insufficiency (hypotension) and signs of adrenal insufficiency (nausea, vomiting, or lethargy without hypotension) were noted for some patients: these episodes responded to dexamethasone treatment. The most commonly reported adverse effect was new or worsening hypokalemia, which responded to large doses of supplemental potassium and spironolactone.

In a recent 24-week multicenter, open-label trial in 50 subjects with CS that included 43 subjects with CD who had failed multimodal standard therapy, mifepristone was studied at a dose of 300 to 1200 mg daily (SEISMIC study)[110,111]; at the final study visit, mean dose was 732 ± 366 mg/d. Twenty-two subjects received the maximum dose of 1200 mg/d. The study included two groups: subjects with glucose intolerant or diabetes and subjects who had a diagnosis of hypertension but had a normal glucose tolerance. Diabetes control improved significantly, from a mean ($\pm$ SD) baseline HbA_{1c} of $7.43 \pm 1.52\%$ to $6.29 \pm 0.99\%$ at the end of the study despite concomitant decreases in antidiabetes medications (Fig. 7A). Furthermore, mean ($\pm$ SE) body weight change from baseline (99.5 kg) to week 24/early termination was $-5.7 \pm 7.4\%$ (see Fig. 7B) (24 patients lost $\geq 5\%$, 12 of whom lost $\geq 10\%$, but 10 patients gained an average of $3.6 \pm 3.9\%$). Waist circumference also decreased significantly by 6.8 ± 5.8 cm in women and 8.4 ± 5.9 cm in men (see Fig. 7C). In the hypertensive group, 38% of subjects had a change of at least 5% in diastolic blood pressure over baseline. Overall, 87% of the subjects had significant improvement in clinical status. Insulin resistance, depression, cognition, and quality of life also improved. Common adverse events were fatigue, nausea, headache, low potassium, arthralgia, vomiting, edema, and endometrial thickening in women. Adrenal insufficiency was reported in only two subjects, but mifepristone was decreased or interrupted and glucocorticoids were administered in several cases.[111] Because of mifepristone's mechanism of action, blocking the glucocorticoid receptor, cortisol measurements would not be reliable for any assessments (either for efficacy or adrenal insufficiency). Hypokalemia and edema may develop because of excess mineralocorticoid effect, but seem to respond well to potassium and mineralocorticoid antagonist medications (ie, spironolactone, eplerenone).

Although not providing a cure, mifepristone treatment over 24 weeks diminishes the clinical impact of hypercortisolism and improves the associated cardiometabolic, psychiatric, and somatic abnormalities associated with the syndrome. Notably, the psychiatric and metabolic comorbidities may resolve rapidly and can dramatically improve patient's clinical status.[94,107] Longer-term studies are needed to assess benefit-risk ratio profile with prolonged treatment.

Combination Treatment Between Drugs with Different Mechanisms of Action

Several of the aforementioned drugs can be used as a single therapy; however, in general results are improved when drugs are used in combination. A combined treatment with ketoconazole and octreotide was reported to have additive effect in improving clinical features and reducing cortisol production in three out of four patients with severe ACTH-dependent hypercortisolism.[112]

Subsequently, combined treatment of SRLs and a dopamine agonist in a patient with no response to either agent also supports the hypothesis that somatostatin and dopamine receptor interact and that agonists may potentiate actions.[113] Some preliminary data also suggested a potential use of dopamine agonists alone or in combination with ketoconazole.[62,85] Feelders and colleagues[114] combined all of the aforementioned drugs in an 80-day trial in 17 patients with CD: pasireotide monotherapy induced UFC normalization in five patients with pasireotide. In nonresponsive patients, cabergoline was added and normalized in an additional four patients. The addition of low-dose ketoconazole increased the number of patients with a complete response to 88% after a further 2 months. Low doses of each therapy could allow also for fewer adverse events.

SUMMARY

The incidence of CD could be higher than previously thought. Severe complications (central adiposity, cardiovascular, diabetes, neuropsychiatric, bone disease) are a challenge if the disease is left untreated. Mortality is increased overall; however, results improve after treatment. This emphasizes the need for individualized, multidisciplinary management to normalize hypercortisolemia or manage devastating effects. Morbidity can persist even after remission.

Recently approved medications and ongoing research studies that involve innovative medical therapeutic agents, and strategies targeting the corticotroph adenoma itself, or that block the effects of cortisol in the periphery, provide hope for future treatment options.

ACKNOWLEDGMENTS

The author thanks Shirley McCartney, PhD, for professional assistance with the manuscript, and Andy Rekito, MS, for illustrative services.

REFERENCES

1. Lindholm J, Juul S, Jorgensen JO, et al. Incidence and late prognosis of Cushing's syndrome: a population-based study. J Clin Endocrinol Metab 2001; 86(1):117–23.
2. Arnardottir S, Sigurjonsdottir HA. The incidence and prevalence of Cushing's disease may be higher than previously thought: results from a retrospective study in Iceland 1955 through 2009. Clin Endocrinol (Oxf) 2011;74(6):792–3.
3. Bolland MJ, Holdaway IM, Berkeley JE, et al. Mortality and morbidity in Cushing's syndrome in New Zealand. Clin Endocrinol (Oxf) 2011;75(4): 436–42.
4. Daly AF, Rixhon M, Adam C, et al. High prevalence of pituitary adenomas: a cross-sectional study in the province of Liege. J Clin Endocrinol Metab 2006;91(12):4769–75.
5. Fernandez A, Karavitaki N, Wass JA. Prevalence of pituitary adenomas: a community-based, cross-sectional study in Banbury (Oxfordshire, UK). Clin Endocrinol (Oxf) 2010;72(3):377–82.
6. Blevins LS Jr, Sanai N, Kunwar S, et al. An approach to the management of patients with residual Cushing's disease. J Neurooncol 2009; 94(3):313–9.
7. Catargi B, Rigalleau V, Poussin A, et al. Occult Cushing's syndrome in type-2 diabetes. J Clin Endocrinol Metab 2003;88(12):5808–13.
8. Chiodini I, Mascia ML, Muscarella S, et al. Subclinical hypercortisolism among outpatients referred for osteoporosis. Ann Intern Med 2007;147(8): 541–8.
9. Leibowitz G, Tsur A, Chayen SD, et al. Pre-clinical Cushing's syndrome: an unexpected frequent cause of poor glycaemic control in obese diabetic patients. Clin Endocrinol (Oxf) 1996;44(6):717–22.
10. Arnaldi G, Angeli A, Atkinson AB, et al. Diagnosis and complications of Cushing's syndrome: a consensus statement. J Clin Endocrinol Metab 2003;88(12):5593–602.
11. Barahona MJ, Sucunza N, Resmini E, et al. Persistent body fat mass and inflammatory marker increases after long-term cure of Cushing's syndrome. J Clin Endocrinol Metab 2009;94(9): 3365–71.
12. De Leo M, Pivonello R, Auriemma RS, et al. Cardiovascular disease in Cushing's syndrome: heart versus vasculature. Neuroendocrinology 2010; 92(Suppl 1):50–4.
13. Toja PM, Branzi G, Ciambellotti F, et al. Clinical relevance of cardiac structure and function abnormalities in patients with Cushing's syndrome before and after cure. Clin Endocrinol (Oxf) 2011;76(3): 332–8.
14. Valassi E, Biller BM, Swearingen B, et al. Delayed remission after transsphenoidal surgery in patients with Cushing's disease. J Clin Endocrinol Metab 2010;95(2):601–10.
15. Pivonello R, De Martino MC, De Leo M, et al. Cushing's syndrome: aftermath of the cure. Arq Bras Endocrinol Metabol 2007;51(8):1381–91.
16. Valassi E, Biller BM, Klibanski A, et al. Adipokines and cardiovascular risk in Cushing's syndrome. Neuroendocrinology 2011;95(3):187–206.
17. Clayton RN, Raskauskiene D, Reulen RC, et al. Mortality and morbidity in Cushing's disease over 50 years in Stoke-on-Trent, UK: audit and meta-analysis of literature. J Clin Endocrinol Metab 2011;96(3):632–42.
18. Sughrue ME, Chang EF, Gabriel RA, et al. Excess mortality for patients with residual disease following resection of pituitary adenomas. Pituitary 2011; 14(3):276–83.
19. Biller BM, Grossman AB, Stewart PM, et al. Treatment of adrenocorticotropin-dependent Cushing's syndrome: a consensus statement. J Clin Endocrinol Metab 2008;93(7):2454–62.
20. Chandler WF, Schteingart DE. Controversies in the management of Cushing's disease. Clin Neurosurg 1986;33:553–62.
21. Chee GH, Mathias DB, James RA, et al. Transsphenoidal pituitary surgery in Cushing's disease: can we predict outcome? Clin Endocrinol (Oxf) 2001; 54(5):617–26.
22. Aghi MK. Management of recurrent and refractory Cushing disease. Nat Clin Pract Endocrinol Metab 2008;4(10):560–8.
23. Tritos NA, Biller BM, Swearingen B. Management of Cushing disease. Nat Rev Endocrinol 2011;7(5): 279–89.
24. Czepielewski MA, Rollin GA, Casagrande A, et al. Criteria of cure and remission in Cushing's disease: an update. Arq Bras Endocrinol Metabol 2007; 51(8):1362–72.
25. Fleseriu M, Loriaux DL, Ludlam WH. Second-line treatment for Cushing's disease when initial pituitary surgery is unsuccessful. Curr Opin Endocrinol Diabetes Obes 2007;14(4):323–8.
26. Utz AL, Swearingen B, Biller BM. Pituitary surgery and postoperative management in Cushing's disease. Endocrinol Metab Clin North Am 2005; 34(2):459–78, xi.

27. Atkinson AB, Kennedy A, Wiggam MI, et al. Long-term remission rates after pituitary surgery for Cushing's disease: the need for long-term surveillance. Clin Endocrinol (Oxf) 2005;63(5):549–59.

28. Patil CG, Prevedello DM, Lad SP, et al. Late recurrences of Cushing's disease after initial successful transsphenoidal surgery. J Clin Endocrinol Metab 2008;93(2):358–62.

29. Hoybye C, Grenback E, Thoren M, et al. Transsphenoidal surgery in Cushing disease: 10 years of experience in 34 consecutive cases. J Neurosurg 2004;100(4):634–8.

30. Miller JW, Crapo L. The medical treatment of Cushing's syndrome. Endocr Rev 1993;14(4):443–58.

31. Pivonello R, De Martino MC, De Leo M, et al. Cushing's syndrome. Endocrinol Metab Clin North Am 2008;37(1):135–49, ix.

32. Baudry C, Coste J, Khalil RB, et al. Results of 1, Ortho-1, para′-Dichloro-Diphenyl-Dichloroethane (O, p′DDD) treatment in 76 patients with Cushing disease. Presented at ENDO 2011. Boston, June 4, 2011.

33. Castinetti F, Morange I, Jaquet P, et al. Ketoconazole revisited: a preoperative or postoperative treatment in Cushing's disease. Eur J Endocrinol 2008;158(1):91–9.

34. Colao A, Petersenn S, Newell-Price J, et al. Pasireotide (SOM230) demonstrates efficacy in patients with Cushing disease: results from a large, randomized-dose, double-blind, phase III study. Presented at ENDO 2011. Boston, June 4, 2011.

35. Godbout A, Manavela M, Danilowicz K, et al. Cabergoline monotherapy in the long-term treatment of Cushing's disease. Eur J Endocrinol 2010; 163(5):709–16.

36. Colao A, Petersenn S, Newell-Price J, et al. A 12-month phase 3 study of pasireotide in Cushing's disease. N Engl J Med 2012;366(10):914–24.

37. Invitti C, Pecori Giraldi F, de Martin M, et al. Diagnosis and management of Cushing's syndrome: results of an Italian multicentre study. Study group of the Italian Society of Endocrinology on the pathophysiology of the hypothalamic-pituitary-adrenal axis. J Clin Endocrinol Metab 1999;84(2):440–8.

38. Hofmann BM, Fahlbusch R. Treatment of Cushing's disease: a retrospective clinical study of the latest 100 cases. Front Horm Res 2006;34:158–84.

39. Ram Z, Nieman LK, Cutler GB Jr, et al. Early repeat surgery for persistent Cushing's disease. J Neurosurg 1994;80(1):37–45.

40. Friedman RB, Oldfield EH, Nieman LK, et al. Repeat transsphenoidal surgery for Cushing's disease. J Neurosurg 1989;71(4):520–7.

41. Losa M, Picozzi P, Redaelli MG, et al. Pituitary radiotherapy for Cushing's disease. Neuroendocrinology 2010;92(Suppl 1):107–10.

42. Young WF Jr, Thompson GB. Laparoscopic adrenalectomy for patients who have Cushing's syndrome. Endocrinol Metab Clin North Am 2005;34(2):489–99.

43. Assie G, Bahurel H, Coste J, et al. Corticotroph tumor progression after adrenalectomy in Cushing's disease: a reappraisal of Nelson's syndrome. J Clin Endocrinol Metab 2007;92(1):172–9.

44. Nieman LK. Medical therapy of Cushing's disease. Pituitary 2002;5(2):77–82.

45. Colao A, Pivonello R, Tripodi FS, et al. Failure of long-term therapy with sodium valproate in Cushing's disease. J Endocrinol Invest 1997;20(7):387–92.

46. Pivonello R, Ferone D, de Herder WW, et al. Dopamine receptor expression and function in corticotroph pituitary tumors. J Clin Endocrinol Metab 2004;89(5):2452–62.

47. Hofland LJ, van der Hoek J, Feelders R, et al. The multi-ligand somatostatin analogue SOM230 inhibits ACTH secretion by cultured human corticotroph adenomas via somatostatin receptor type 5. Eur J Endocrinol 2005;152(4):645–54.

48. Gatto F, Hofland LJ. The role of somatostatin and dopamine D2 receptors in endocrine tumors. Endocrine 2011;18(6):R233–51.

49. Suda T, Tozawa F, Mouri T, et al. Effects of cyproheptadine, reserpine, and synthetic corticotropin-releasing factor on pituitary glands from patients with Cushing's disease. J Clin Endocrinol Metab 1983;56(6):1094–9.

50. Tanakol R, Alagol F, Azizlerli H, et al. Cyproheptadine treatment in Cushing's disease. J Endocrinol Invest 1996;19(4):242–7.

51. Koppeschaar HP, Croughs RJ, Thijssen JH, et al. Response to neurotransmitter modulating drugs in patients with Cushing's disease. Clin Endocrinol (Oxf) 1986;25(6):661–7.

52. Heaney AP. PPAR-gamma in Cushing's disease. Pituitary 2004;7(4):265–9.

53. Ambrosi B, Dall'Asta C, Cannavo S, et al. Effects of chronic administration of PPAR-gamma ligand rosiglitazone in Cushing's disease. Eur J Endocrinol 2004;151(2):173–8.

54. Pecori Giraldi F, Scaroni C, Arvat E, et al. Effect of protracted treatment with rosiglitazone, a PPAR-gamma agonist, in patients with Cushing's disease. Clin Endocrinol (Oxf) 2006;64(2):219–24.

55. Mannelli M, Cantini G, Poli G, et al. Role of the PPAR-gamma system in normal and tumoral pituitary corticotropic cells and adrenal cells. Neuroendocrinology 2010;92(Suppl 1):23–7.

56. Mercado-Asis LB, Yasuda K, Murayama M, et al. Beneficial effects of high daily dose bromocriptine treatment in Cushing's disease. Endocrinol Jpn 1992;39(4):385–95.

57. Lamberts SW, Birkenhager JC. Bromocriptine in Nelson's syndrome and Cushing's disease. Lancet 1976;2(7989):811.

58. Bevan JS, Webster J, Burke CW, et al. Dopamine agonists and pituitary tumor shrinkage. Endocr Rev 1992;13(2):220–40.

59. Whitehead HM, Beacom R, Sheridan B, et al. The effect of cyproheptadine and/or bromocriptine on plasma ACTH levels in patients cured of Cushing's disease by bilateral adrenalectomy. Clin Endocrinol (Oxf) 1990;32(2):193–201.

60. Casulari LA, Naves LA, Mello PA, et al. Nelson's syndrome: complete remission with cabergoline but not with bromocriptine or cyproheptadine treatment. Horm Res 2004;62(6):300–5.

61. Godbout A, Manavela M, Danilowicz K, et al. Long-term therapy with cabergoline in Cushing's disease [abstract: P2–130]. Presented at the Endocrine Society's 90th meeting. San Francisco, 2008.

62. Vilar L, Naves LA, Azevedo MF, et al. Effectiveness of cabergoline in monotherapy and combined with ketoconazole in the management of Cushing's disease. Pituitary 2010;13(2):123–9.

63. Pivonello R, De Martino MC, Cappabianca P, et al. The medical treatment of Cushing's disease: effectiveness of chronic treatment with the dopamine agonist cabergoline in patients unsuccessfully treated by surgery. J Clin Endocrinol Metab 2009; 94(1):223–30.

64. Lamberts SW, Zuyderwijk J, den Holder F, et al. Studies on the conditions determining the inhibitory effect of somatostatin on adrenocorticotropin, prolactin and thyrotropin release by cultured rat pituitary cells. Neuroendocrinology 1989;50(1): 44–50.

65. Stalla GK, Brockmeier SJ, Renner U, et al. Octreotide exerts different effects in vivo and in vitro in Cushing's disease. Eur J Endocrinol 1994;130(2): 125–31.

66. van der Hoek J, Waaijers M, van Koetsveld PM, et al. Distinct functional properties of native somatostatin receptor subtype 5 compared with subtype 2 in the regulation of ACTH release by corticotroph tumor cells. Am J Physiol Endocrinol Metab 2005;289(2):E278–87.

67. Batista DL, Zhang X, Gejman R, et al. The effects of SOM230 on cell proliferation and adrenocorticotropin secretion in human corticotroph pituitary adenomas. J Clin Endocrinol Metab 2006;91(11): 4482–8.

68. Boscaro M, Ludlam WH, Atkinson B, et al. Treatment of pituitary-dependent Cushing's disease with the multireceptor ligand somatostatin analog pasireotide (SOM230): a multicenter, phase II trial. J Clin Endocrinol Metab 2009;94(1):115–22.

69. Petersenn S, Schopohl J, Barkan A, et al. Pasireotide (SOM230) demonstrates efficacy and safety in patients with acromegaly: a randomized, multicenter, phase II trial. J Clin Endocrinol Metab 2010;95(6):2781–9.

70. Murray RD, Kim K, Ren SG, et al. The novel somatostatin ligand (SOM230) regulates human and rat anterior pituitary hormone secretion. J Clin Endocrinol Metab 2004;89(6):3027–32.

71. Ben-Shlomo A, Schmid H, Wawrowsky K, et al. Differential ligand-mediated pituitary somatostatin receptor subtype signaling: implications for corticotroph tumor therapy. J Clin Endocrinol Metab 2009;94(11):4342–50.

72. Ben-Shlomo A, Wawrowsky KA, Proekt I, et al. Somatostatin receptor type 5 modulates somatostatin receptor type 2 regulation of adrenocorticotropin secretion. J Biol Chem 2005;280(25):24011–21.

73. The European Medicines Agency. Signifor. Available at: http://www.ema.europa.eu/ema/index.jsp?curl=pages/medicines/human/medicines/002052/smops/Positive/human_smop_000326.jsp&mid=WC0b01ac058001d127&jsenabled='''true. Accessed January 23, 2012.

74. Altucci L, Gronemeyer H. The promise of retinoids to fight against cancer. Nat Rev Cancer 2001;1(3): 181–93.

75. Labeur M, Paez-Pereda M, Arzt E, et al. Potential of retinoic acid derivatives for the treatment of corticotroph pituitary adenomas. Rev Endocr Metab Disord 2009;10(2):103–9.

76. Paez-Pereda M, Kovalovsky D, Hopfner U, et al. Retinoic acid prevents experimental Cushing syndrome. J Clin Invest 2001;108(8):1123–31.

77. Fernando MA, Heaney AP. Alpha1-adrenergic receptor antagonists: novel therapy for pituitary adenomas. Mol Endocrinol 2005;19(12):3085–96.

78. Fukuoka H, Cooper O, Ben-Shlomo A, et al. EGFR as a therapeutic target for human, canine, and mouse ACTH-secreting pituitary adenomas. J Clin Invest 2011;121(12):4712–21.

79. Kamenicky P, Droumaguet C, Salenave S, et al. Mitotane, metyrapone, and ketoconazole combination therapy as an alternative to rescue adrenalectomy for severe ACTH-dependent Cushing's syndrome. J Clin Endocrinol Metab 2011; 96(9):2796–804.

80. Sonino N, Boscaro M, Paoletta A, et al. Ketoconazole treatment in Cushing's syndrome: experience in 34 patients. Clin Endocrinol (Oxf) 1991;35(4): 347–52.

81. Berwaerts JJ, Verhelst JA, Verhaert GC, et al. Corticotropin-dependent Cushing's syndrome in older people: presentation of five cases and therapeutical use of ketoconazole. J Am Geriatr Soc 1998; 46(7):880–4.

82. Chou SC, Lin JD. Long-term effects of ketoconazole in the treatment of residual or recurrent Cushing's disease. Endocr J 2000;47(4):401–6.

83. Loli P, Berselli ME, Tagliaferri M. Use of ketoconazole in the treatment of Cushing's syndrome. J Clin Endocrinol Metab 1986;63(6):1365–71.

84. McCance DR, Hadden DR, Kennedy L, et al. Clinical experience with ketoconazole as a therapy for patients with Cushing's syndrome. Clin Endocrinol (Oxf) 1987;27(5):593–9.

85. Colao A, Di Sarno A, Marzullo P, et al. New medical approaches in pituitary adenomas. Horm Res 2000;53(Suppl 3):76–87.

86. Sonino N, Boscaro M, Merola G, et al. Prolonged treatment of Cushing's disease by ketoconazole. J Clin Endocrinol Metab 1985;61(4):718–22.

87. Tabarin A, Navarranne A, Guerin J, et al. Use of ketoconazole in the treatment of Cushing's disease and ectopic ACTH syndrome. Clin Endocrinol (Oxf) 1991;34(1):63–9.

88. Boscaro M, Sonino N, Rampazzo A, et al. Response of pituitary-adrenal axis to corticotrophin releasing hormone in patients with Cushing's disease before and after ketoconazole treatment. Clin Endocrinol (Oxf) 1987;27(4):461–7.

89. Feldman D. Ketoconazole and other imidazole derivatives as inhibitors of steroidogenesis. Endocr Rev 1986;7(4):409–20.

90. AHFS Consumer Medication Information. Ketoconazole. Available at: http://www.mhra.gov.uk/Publications/Safetyguidance/DrugSafetyUpdate/CON028267. Accessed January 23, 2012.

91. Schteingart DE, Tsao HS, Taylor CI, et al. Sustained remission of Cushing's disease with mitotane and pituitary irradiation. Ann Intern Med 1980;92(5):613–9.

92. Luton JP, Mahoudeau JA, Bouchard P, et al. Treatment of Cushing's disease by O, p'DDD. Survey of 62 cases. N Engl J Med 1979;300(9):459–64.

93. Leiba S, Weinstein R, Shindel B, et al. The protracted effect of o, p'-DDD in Cushing's disease and its impact on adrenal morphogenesis of young human embryo. Ann Endocrinol (Paris) 1989;50(1):49–53.

94. Schteingart DE. Drugs in the medical treatment of Cushing's syndrome. Expert Opin Emerg Drugs 2009;14(4):661–71.

95. Verhelst JA, Trainer PJ, Howlett TA, et al. Short and long-term responses to metyrapone in the medical management of 91 patients with Cushing's syndrome. Clin Endocrinol (Oxf) 1991; 35(2):169–78.

96. Karaca Z, Tanriverdi F, Unluhizarci K, et al. Pregnancy and pituitary disorders. Eur J Endocrinol 2010;162(3):453–75.

97. Engelhardt D, Weber MM. Therapy of Cushing's syndrome with steroid biosynthesis inhibitors. J Steroid Biochem Mol Biol 1994; 49(4–6):261–7.

98. Heyn J, Geiger C, Hinske CL, et al. Medical suppression of hypercortisolemia in Cushing's syndrome with particular consideration of etomidate. Pituitary 2012;15(2):117–25.

99. Schulte HM, Benker G, Reinwein D, et al. Infusion of low dose etomidate: correction of hypercortisolemia in patients with Cushing's syndrome and dose-response relationship in normal subjects. J Clin Endocrinol Metab 1990; 70(5):1426–30.

100. Paris A, Philipp M, Tonner PH, et al. Activation of alpha 2B-adrenoceptors mediates the cardiovascular effects of etomidate. Anesthesiology 2003; 99(4):889–95.

101. Herrmann BL, Mitchell A, Saller B, et al. Transsphenoidale hypophysektomie bei einer patientin mit einem ACTH-produzierenden hypophysenadenom und einer "empty Sella" nach vorbehandlung mit etomidat. Dtsch Med Wochenschr 2001;126(9): 232–4 [in German].

102. Mettauer N, Brierley J. A novel use of etomidate for intentional adrenal suppression to control severe hypercortisolemia in childhood. Pediatr Crit Care Med 2009;10(3):e37–40.

103. Allolio B, Schulte HM, Kaulen D, et al. Nonhypnotic low-dose etomidate for rapid correction of hypercortisolaemia in Cushing's syndrome. Klin Wochenschr 1988;66(8):361–4.

104. Dabbagh A, Sa'adat N, Heidari Z. Etomidate infusion in the critical care setting for suppressing the acute phase of Cushing's syndrome. Anesth Analg 2009;108(1):238–9.

105. Trainer PJ, Eastment C, Grossman AB, et al. The relationship between cortisol production rate and serial serum cortisol estimation in patients on medical therapy for Cushing's syndrome. Clin Endocrinol (Oxf) 1993;39(4):441–3.

106. Johanssen S, Allolio B. Mifepristone (RU 486) in Cushing's syndrome. Eur J Endocrinol 2007; 157(5):561–9.

107. Castinetti F, Fassnacht M, Johanssen S, et al. Merits and pitfalls of mifepristone in Cushing's syndrome. Eur J Endocrinol 2009;160(6):1003–10.

108. Chu JW, Matthias DF, Belanoff J, et al. Successful long-term treatment of refractory Cushing's disease with high-dose mifepristone (RU 486). J Clin Endocrinol Metab 2001;86(8):3568–73.

109. Nieman LK, Chrousos GP, Kellner C, et al. Successful treatment of Cushing's syndrome with the glucocorticoid antagonist RU 486. J Clin Endocrinol Metab 1985;61(3):536–40.

110. Fleseriu M, Biller B, Findling J, et al. Mifepristone, a glucocorticoid receptor antagonist, produces clinical and metabolic benefits in patients with refractory Cushing syndrome: results from the study of the efficacy and Safety of Mifepristone in the Treatment of Endogenous Cushing Syndrome (SEISMIC). Presented at ENDO 2011. Boston, June 4, 2011.

111. Fleseriu M, Biller BM, Findling JW, et al. Mifepristone, a glucocorticoid receptor antagonist, produces

clinical and metabolic benefits in patients with Cushing's syndrome. J Clin Endocrinol Metab 2012;97(6): 2039–49.

112. Vignati F, Loli P. Additive effect of ketoconazole and octreotide in the treatment of severe adrenocorticotropin-dependent hypercortisolism. J Clin Endocrinol Metab 1996;81(8):2885–90.

113. Rocheville M, Lange DC, Kumar U, et al. Receptors for dopamine and somatostatin: formation of hetero-oligomers with enhanced functional activity. Science 2000;288(5463):154–7.

114. Feelders RA, de Bruin C, Pereira AM, et al. Pasireotide alone or with cabergoline and ketoconazole in Cushing's disease. N Engl J Med 2010;362(19):1846–8.

Medical Versus Surgical Management of Prolactinomas

Michael C. Oh, MD, PhD, Sandeep Kunwar, MD,
Lewis Blevins, MD, Manish K. Aghi, MD, PhD*

KEYWORDS

- Prolactinomas • Pituitary adenoma • Dopamine agonist • Bromocriptine • Cabergoline
- Transsphenoidal surgery

KEY POINTS

- Prolactinomas are the most common endocrine active adenomas, comprising 40% of pituitary tumors.
- Prolactinomas present a unique challenge for clinicians given the relatively comparable efficacy of medical management versus transsphenoidal surgery.
- A full endocrine laboratory panel should be obtained, especially for macroprolactinomas, as stalk compression can cause hypopituitarism.
- Small, asymptomatic prolactinomas may be observed with close hormonal and radiographic monitoring, whereas symptomatic prolactinomas require treatment.
- Dopamine agonists have become the standard treatment for symptomatic prolactinomas, including macroprolactinomas causing mass-effect symptoms such as visual loss.
- Although most patients with prolactinomas respond to medical therapy, 10% to 20% do not respond to dopamine agonist therapy in terms of prolactin normalization, and may require surgery.
- Transsphenoidal surgery is recommended if (1) the tumor is cystic, (2) inadequate prolactin reduction or tumor growth occurs despite high doses of dopamine agonists, (3) a female patient is planning pregnancy, (4) there is intratumoral hemorrhage with mass effect or apoplexy, (5) the patient presents with rapid visual loss or rapid visual loss occurs on dopamine agonist therapy, or (6) the patient opts for surgical resection rather than medical management.

INTRODUCTION

Pituitary tumors represent 10% to 15% of primary intracranial neoplasms,[1] of which more than 90% are benign pituitary adenomas with World Health Organization grade I.[1–3] Among endocrine active adenomas (EAAs), prolactinomas are the most common, comprising 40% of pituitary tumors.[4,5] One study, for example, determined that among 46 pituitary macroadenomas found incidentally, 15% were prolactinomas based on laboratory evaluation.[6] Given that autopsy and imaging studies suggest that pituitary tumors are up to 700 times more prevalent (16.7%, or 1 out of 6 people in the general population) than suggested by registry studies,[7,8] prolactinomas can be a large component of practice for pituitary neurosurgeons and neuroendocrinologists.

Prolactinomas present a unique challenge for clinicians given the relatively comparable efficacy of medical management versus transsphenoidal surgery.[9,10] In fact, currently prolactinomas are the only brain tumors for which remission, defined as biochemical and radiographic remission in an endocrine active tumor, can be achieved by medical

Department of Neurological Surgery, California Center for Pituitary Disorders, University of California, 400 Parnassus Avenue, A-808, San Francisco, CA, 94143, USA
* Corresponding author. Department of Neurological Surgery, University of California, San Francisco, 505 Parnassus Avenue, M770, Box 0112, San Francisco, CA 94143.
E-mail address: AghiM@neurosurg.ucsf.edu

Neurosurg Clin N Am 23 (2012) 669–678
http://dx.doi.org/10.1016/j.nec.2012.06.010

therapy alone. After initial studies proving the efficacy of dopamine agonists as medical therapy for prolactinomas,[11] these medications came to be viewed by many as the first-line therapy for prolactinomas. Over the years, however, several indications have arisen for surgery to treat prolactinomas. The surgical approach to prolactinomas is typically via a transseptal transsphenoidal corridor achieved through microscopic or endoscopic exposure. This article reviews the recent advancements in medical and surgical management of prolactinomas.

CLINICAL FINDINGS OF PROLACTINOMAS
Symptoms Associated with Prolactinomas

Prolactinomas are the most common EAAs, comprising 40% of pituitary tumors.[4,5] Symptoms associated with prolactinomas are due to 2 factors: (1) the endocrine effects of prolactin oversecretion and (2) the mass effect on the surrounding structures. Endocrine symptoms include decreased libido, galactorrhea, gynecomastia, amenorrhea in females, and infertility. Because amenorrhea is readily detected in women and decreased libido is often not reported by men, women more often present with microprolactinomas whereas men often present with macroprolactinomas. The prevalence of prolactinomas is generally higher is women as well,[12,13] possibly because endocrine symptoms are more easily detected in women than in men. Asymptomatic microprolactinomas grow slowly in general and may not require treatment, as only 9 of 139 (7%) women in 6 studies with microprolactinomas had tumor growth during untreated follow-up averaging 8 years.[4]

Patients with large macroprolactinomas, however, may present with symptoms of mass effect, including bitemporal hemianopsia caused by suprasellar extension with compression of the optic chiasm (**Fig. 1**), headache potentially attributable to stretching of the nearby dura or diaphragm sella, hypopituitarism caused by compression of portal vessels, the pituitary stalk, or the pituitary gland, and cranial neuropathies resulting from parasellar extension with cavernous sinus invasion. Hypopituitarism, most often manifesting as hypogonadism, may be present in 43% of patients with macroadenomas.[14] Though acutely reversible, prolonged compression of the optic chiasm can lead to optic-nerve atrophy, permanent visual-field deficits, and decreased visual acuity. Cranial neuropathies may include ptosis, ophthalmoplegia, and diplopia from compression of the cranial nerves III, VI, and IV, in the order of frequency.[15]

Radiological Findings

The radiographic features of prolactinomas are identical to those of other pituitary adenomas, and are best detected on gadolinium-enhanced magnetic resonance imaging (MRI). Prolactinomas may be isointense or slightly hypointense compared with the pituitary gland on T1-weighted images. While pituitary adenomas such as prolactinomas enhance with gadolinium on T1-weighted images, their enhancement is typically less than that of the pituitary gland or the stalk (**Fig. 2**). A convex outline along the pituitary gland or deviation of the pituitary stalk away from the adenoma may or may not be present.

Diagnostic Investigations

A full endocrine laboratory panel should be obtained, especially for macroprolactinomas, as stalk compression can cause hypopituitarism. For example, large nonfunctioning pituitary adenomas (NFPAs) may mimic the clinical picture of macroprolactinomas by the stalk effect, whereby compressing the portal vessels can inhibit delivery of dopamine from the hypothalamus to pituitary lactotrophs.[12] Dopamine inhibits prolactin release from the pituitary gland and, thus, the stalk effect can lead to excessive release of prolactin, causing large NFPAs to sometimes present with laboratory hyperprolactinemia that is sometimes clinically symptomatic.

In general, the degree of prolactin elevation correlates with tumor size. Most patients with prolactin greater than 150 mg/L have prolactinomas, whereas macroprolactinomas can have levels well above 250 mg/L. In some giant prolactinomas, prolactin levels may be extremely high, saturating the immunoradiometric assays and leading to falsely low levels. Performing assays with diluted serum samples can prevent this "hook effect."

Differential Diagnosis

The differential diagnosis in a patient with elevated serum prolactin and a pituitary tumor on MRI is prolactinoma versus NFPA with stalk effect. Although serum prolactin may improve or normalize in stalk-effect patients treated medically, the associated NFPA will usually not regress and the associated mass effect will not improve in the way it would with a prolactinoma treated medically. There is a linear correlation between adenoma size and a serum prolactin below which the stalk effect should be suspected and above which prolactinoma should be suspected,[16] but this correlation is not perfect, particularly with cystic adenomas

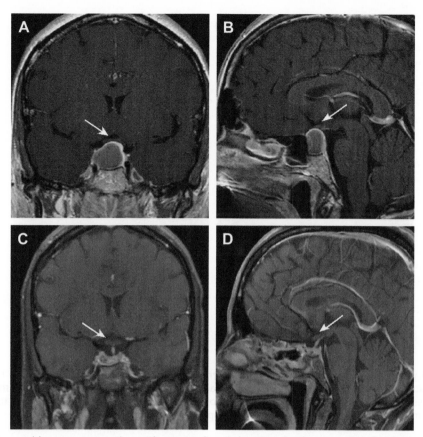

Fig. 1. A 38-year-old woman presenting with amenorrhea. Laboratory workup revealed elevated prolactin at 85 ng/mL, suggesting that the tumor was a cystic microprolactinoma rather than a cystic nonfunctioning pituitary adenoma with stalk effect. Gadolinium-enhanced T1-weighted images (*A, B*) confirmed a cystic lesion with suprasellar extension and compression of the optic chiasm (*arrows*). Although with bromocriptine her prolactin level normalized to 14.1 ng/mL, the tumor size did not respond to medical treatment. Normalization of serum prolactin to medical treatment suggested that this lesion is indeed a prolactinoma. She underwent transsphenoidal resection of the tumor with decompression of the cystic component (*C, D*), which resulted in decompression of the optic chiasm (*arrows*). Surgical pathology confirmed the lesion as prolactinoma.

(see **Fig. 1**). Other different diagnoses include other EAAs (adenomas releasing adrenocorticotropin or growth hormones and, rarely, gonadotropins or thyroid-stimulating hormones), hypophysitis, Rathke cleft cyst, craniopharyngioma, meningioma, and metastases.

MANAGEMENT OF PROLACTINOMAS

With increasing prevalence of pituitary incidentalomas from more frequent imaging for other reasons, such as headaches, trauma, and vertigo, studies delineating the natural progression history of microprolactinomas will become more important for management stratification. The evidence to date suggests that asymptomatic microprolactinomas grow slowly and may not warrant treatment. Only 9 of 139 (7%) women in 6 studies with

microprolactinomas had tumor growth during untreated follow-up averaging 8 years.[4] In another study observing 30 women with hyperprolactinemia for an average of 5.2 years, one-third (10 of 30) of patients had a decrease in prolactin levels during the observation period.[17] Thus, small, asymptomatic prolactinomas may be observed with close hormonal and radiographic monitoring, whereas symptomatic prolactinomas require treatment.

Dopamine Agonist Therapy

Prolactinomas are tumors of lactotrophs, whose production of prolactin is normally inhibited by dopamine from the hypothalamus and enhanced by estrogen. Understanding the regulation of lactotrophs by dopamine has led to the development of drugs to treat prolactinomas. Prolactinoma cells

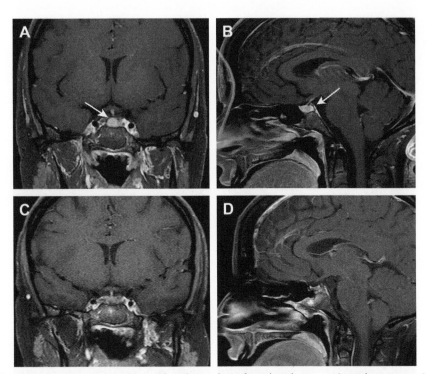

Fig. 2. A 29 year-old woman presenting with galactorrhea, found to have a microadenoma on MRI. Despite medical treatment, the tumor size increased. (*A, B*) Gadolinium-enhanced T1-weighted images show a 7-mm enhancing lesion (*arrows*). She underwent transsphenoidal resection with complete removal of the lesion (*C, D*), with normalization of prolactin levels by way of dopamine agonists.

express dopamine D2 receptors which, when activated, cause cell death, decrease cellular metabolism, and decrease prolactin gene synthesis, thereby inhibiting prolactin production and secretion. Furthermore, prolactinoma cell size decreases as well as a result of decreased cytoplasmic, nuclear, and nucleolar areas, with involution of endoplasmic reticulum and Golgi complex,[18,19] which may be responsible for reduction in tumor size in response to dopamine agonists. Thus, dopamine agonists have been used to treat prolactinomas with great success over the last 4 decades.

Indeed, over the last 25 years dopamine agonists have become the standard treatment for symptomatic prolactinomas, including macroprolactinomas causing mass-effect symptoms such as visual loss. In 1985, a prospective multicenter trial showed that the dopamine agonist bromocriptine, an ergoline derivative that activates dopamine D1 and D2 receptors, normalized prolactin levels in 18 of 27 patients.[11] Tumors decreased in size as early as 6 weeks after administration. Tumor size decreased by more than 50% in 13 patients (46%), 50% in 5 patients (18%), and 10% to 25% in 9 patients (36%).[11] Of note, visual fields improved in 9 of 10 patients who had deficits, confirming that medical

treatment can treat tumor mass effect as well. These results with medical therapy resemble those achieved with surgery,[9,10] and a meta-analysis of 34 series showed that 73.7% of microadenomas and 32.4% of macroadenomas had normal prolactin levels 1 to 12 weeks following surgery.[20] Although a randomized trial directly comparing medical with surgical treatment has not been performed, based on the results of these studies demonstrating comparable efficacy of surgery versus medical therapy, dopamine agonist therapy has replaced surgery as the first-line therapy for prolactinomas, including macroprolactinomas with symptomatic mass effect (**Fig. 3**).

Another dopamine agonist that has recently supplanted bromocriptine is cabergoline, a more potent and longer-acting dopamine D2 receptor agonist than bromocriptine. Cabergoline only requires once- or twice-weekly oral administration, and has a very low side-effect profile. A direct comparison of cabergoline with bromocriptine in a randomized multicenter trial involving 459 women showed that cabergoline is more effective and better tolerated than bromocriptine.[21] Normal prolactin levels were achieved in 59% of women treated with bromocriptine, whereas cabergoline restored normal prolactin in 83%.[21] Amenorrhea

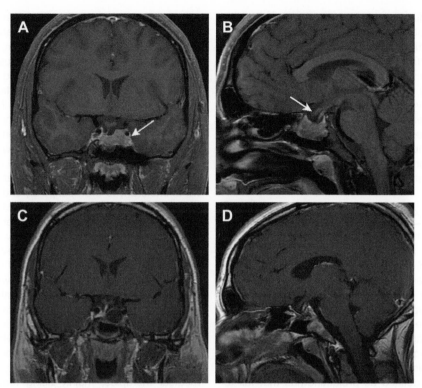

Fig. 3. A 30-year-old man presenting with left ocular headaches and decreased libido. Further workup revealed elevated prolactin well above 1000 ng/mL with a 3-cm macroprolactinoma on MRI. He was started on cabergoline with a consequent 50% reduction in tumor size. Gadolinium-enhanced T1-weighted images showed invasion into the left cavernous sinus (*A, arrow*), and a partially empty sella with slight downward herniation of the optic chiasm (*B, arrow*). He remained stable on medical treatment until he presented with spontaneous cerebrospinal fluid rhinorrhea. He underwent transsphenoidal tumor resection with septal repair for the rhinorrhea (*C, D*). He improved symptomatically but his prolactin level remained elevated, at 130 ng/mL.

persisted in 7% of women taking cabergoline versus 16% for bromocriptine, and 3% stopped cabergoline because of drug intolerance versus 12% for bromocriptine.[21] These findings were confirmed by another multicenter, randomized double-blind study involving 120 women, in which prolactin normalization occurred in 93% of patients taking cabergoline and 48% of patients taking bromocriptine.[22] As a consequence of these 2 randomized trials, cabergoline has replaced bromocriptine as the dopamine agonist of choice for prolactinomas, with surgery reserved for prolactinomas resistant to medical therapy.

Furthermore, a recent prospective study showed that higher cabergoline doses can restore prolactin to normal levels irrespective of previous treatment with other dopamine agonists.[23] Even patients previously resistant to other dopamine agonists responded to cabergoline, with 35% of patients in remission within a year.[23] Cabergoline is also more effective than bromocriptine in its ability to be withdrawn without prolactin elevation after prolactin has normalized, the ultimate goal

with medically managed prolactinomas. Although no randomized comparison has been done, numerous series have reported 0% to 44% rates of maintaining normal prolactin 2 to 48 months after bromocriptine withdrawal, compared with 10% to 69% rates of maintaining normal prolactin 3 to 60 months after cabergoline withdrawal.[24]

Other dopamine agonists with clinical benefit exist, such as pergolide mesylate and quinagolide (CV 205-502). Neither of these drugs is available in the United States, however, and pergolide was voluntarily removed from the US market in 2007 because of concerns over increased incidence of serious restrictive cardiac valvular disease with high doses of pergolide used in patients with Parkinson disease.[25]

Prognosis

Overall, approximately 80% to 90% of patients with microprolactinomas and 70% of patients with macroprolactinomas can achieve normalized prolactin level, reduced tumor size, and restoration of gonadal function with bromocriptine.[26] Results are even better with cabergoline, with 95% and 80% of patients normalizing prolactin levels in microprolactinomas and macroprolactinomas, respectively.[26] Tumor volume can decrease dramatically, even in macroprolactinomas, with rapid improvements in headache and visual field, with complete tumor shrinkage with cabergoline in about one-third of patients with macroprolactinomas.[24] Thus the short-term and long-term prognosis for prolactinoma patients is good when managed with medial therapy alone.

Dopamine Agonist–Resistant Prolactinomas

Although most patients with prolactinomas respond to medical therapy, data suggest that 10% to 20% do not respond to dopamine agonist therapy in terms of prolactin normalization, or are intolerant of the medication owing to nausea and postural hypotension.[27–29] Moreover, an even higher percentage of patients do not respond to dopamine agonists through reduction in tumor size. Although no clear consensus exists, dopamine agonist–resistant prolactinomas (DARPs) have been defined as prolactinomas that fail to normalize prolactin levels despite greater than 15 mg of daily bromocriptine for at least a 3-month period,[30–32] while cabergoline resistance is present when prolactin levels fail to normalize despite greater than 1.5 to 2.0 mg of weekly cabergoline.[33,34] The exact definition for dopamine agonist resistance has been difficult to establish, as it is unclear which criteria, such as prolactin level normalization, tumor volume reduction, or reestablishment of hormonal function without complete normalization of prolactin level (ie, reestablishment of menses or pregnancy in women), should be used. Nonetheless, DARPs make up a considerable portion of prolactinomas, with different clinical behavior and management.

Although they are more commonly macroprolactinomas,[33] DARPs can be microprolactinomas as well. DARPs also do not metastasize and are not associated with pituitary carcinomas. Thus DARPs are benign pituitary tumors with distinct biochemical and cellular makeup that favor a larger, more invasive, and more proliferative tumor in comparison with dopamine-responsive prolactinomas.[29]

The main therapy for DARPs after failing initial dopamine agonist therapy consists of more intense medical therapies. First, the dose of current dopamine agonist being used may be increased, as long as there is a response shown in prolactin level to higher doses of dopamine agonist. Moreover, patients currently unresponsive to bromocriptine may respond to cabergoline. Prolactin normalized in 95% of patients previously untreated or intolerant to bromocriptine with cabergoline at 6 months, while 58% of patients previously resistant to cabergoline at a lower dose responded at higher doses of cabergoline.[23] More importantly, by 12 months of treatment nearly all of the patients (99.3%) in the group resistant to bromocriptine responded to high doses of cabergoline, although a much higher dose of cabergoline was required compared with other groups (mean cabergoline dose of 2 mg/wk in previously untreated; 0.9 mg/ wk in intolerant to bromocriptine; and 5.2 mg/wk in bromocriptine-resistant groups).[23] Most patients (83%), however, are managed sufficiently with low doses of cabergoline (0.5–1.5 mg/wk).[33] About 11% of remaining patients achieved normal prolactin levels with higher doses of cabergoline (up to 7 mg/wk, but most by 3.5 mg/wk) while the remaining 6% remained resistant to cabergoline.[33] Thus, overall most patients (94%) can be controlled with cabergoline doses of less than 3.5 mg per week. For the remaining 6% who are resistant to high doses of dopamine agonists, surgery and radiation therapy are available. Alternative medical therapies, mainly using temozolomide, an alkylating agent used in glioblastoma multiforme, have been reported in a small number of case studies.[35–37]

SURGICAL TREATMENT OF PROLACTINOMAS

Transsphenoidal surgery is recommended for prolactinomas if (1) the tumor is cystic, as cysts will not shrink with dopamine agonist therapy (see **Fig. 1**); (2) inadequate prolactin reduction or tumor growth occurs despite high doses of dopamine agonist (DARPs); (3) a female patient is planning pregnancy, which may be difficult to achieve on dopamine agonists; (4) there is intratumoral hemorrhage with mass effect or apoplexy,[38] which will not resolve with dopamine agonist therapy; (5) the patient presents with rapid visual loss or rapid visual loss occurs on dopamine agonist therapy; or (6) the patient opts for surgical resection rather than medical management after discussion of risks, benefits, and alternatives to both treatments with a neurosurgeon and endocrinologist. Even in the absence of these conditions, a patient with a newly diagnosed prolactinoma should be made aware that surgery and medicine are two treatment alternatives, and should understand the risks and benefits of each before committing to an initial treatment choice. The goal of surgical resection of prolactinomas is to completely remove all surgically accessible portions of the tumor.

A retrospective study evaluated surgical outcomes of patients who required surgery because of intolerance to dopamine agonist therapy or because patients had DARPs.[39] Among patients who were intolerant to dopamine agonist therapy, 67% had normalization of prolactin levels following surgery, whereas only 36% of patients with DARPs achieved prolactin normalization after surgery. This result is likely due to the fact that more macroprolactinomas were present in the groups with DARPs (74%). In fact, patients with microprolactinomas had good outcomes following surgery, as 84% of patients with microprolactinomas achieved normal prolactin levels following surgery. This finding is corroborated by other studies that achieved 73% to 90% remission rates following transsphenoidal surgery for microprolactinomas.[40–42]

Another debate concerns whether prolactinomas causing intractable headaches should be considered for surgical resection. Headache is present in 33% to 72% of patients with pituitary tumor[14,43,44] and 48% of patients with primary and metastatic brain tumor,[45] similar to the 47% prevalence of headache in the general population.[46] A retrospective study reviewed 41 patients with pituitary microadenomas to determine whether headache improved following transsphenoidal surgery.[47] This study showed that 85% of patients had headache improvement while 58% had complete resolution. EAA patients had similar improvement in headache. Given the relatively low morbidity of transsphenoidal surgery and the potential to improve headache, surgery may be appropriate for microprolactinoma patients with intractable headaches.

Microscopic Versus Endoscopic Approaches

For the past few decades, surgery for pituitary tumors involved using a microscope with an endonasal speculum via a transseptal transsphenoidal approach with fluoroscopy or neuronavigation used for intraoperative localization, although transcranial approaches were used in 10% of cases for large pituitary tumors with significant extrasellar components.[48] Over the last decade endoscopic pituitary surgery has gained popularity, based on proposed advantages over microscope-based surgery, including angled scopes improving visualization and resection of tumor in the suprasellar, infrasellar, and parasellar (lateral to the sella) spaces.[49] For example, a 36-patient series reported a 72% gross total resection rate of pituitary tumors invading the cavernous sinus using the endoscopic approach.[49] The endoscopic approach has also been reported to offer better preservation of sinonasal function, reduced length of stay

in hospital, decreased pain postoperatively, less blood loss, and less lumbar drain usage.[50] The microscope, however, allows a 3-dimensional view of the surgical field, whereas an endoscope with a monitor may provide inferior resolution. Furthermore, postoperative pain, complications, blood loss, and length of hospital stay are already quite low with the microscopic-based surgery.[50]

Arguments for or against the endoscopic versus microscope-based approaches have not been tested by randomized studies. A meta-analysis of 9 studies showed that pituitary tumors can be removed endoscopically, with good short-term outcomes and low complication rates.[51] Complete tumor removal was achieved in 78%, with 81% to 84% remission rates for EAAs. Visual-field deficits improved in 62% to 100% of patients with deficits. A retrospective cohort study found that endoscopic and microscopic pituitary tumor resection produced similar operative results and complication rates.[50] Thus, endoscopy may allow an experienced neurosurgeon to completely resect tumors invading the cavernous sinus that were previously incompletely resectable, but for noninvasive adenomas. For now the choice between endoscopic and microscope-based surgery falls on surgeon preference, institutional experience, and available resources. It is hoped that long-term studies in the future with a large sample size will compare endoscopic with microscope-based pituitary surgery, and will allow an informed choice between the two methods while accounting for patient-specific and tumor-specific factors.

RADIATION TREATMENT OF PROLACTINOMAS

Radiation, in the form of either fractionated radiation therapy delivered in multiple treatments or stereotactic radiosurgery given in single or few treatments, is rarely used for prolactinomas, given the efficacies of medical and surgical treatments. Moreover, given the high incidence of significant side effects, including hypopituitarism from damage to the stalk, increased risk of strokes and secondary brain tumors, and damage to the optic nerve,[12] radiation therapy or radiosurgery are usually reserved for recurrences following surgery or medical treatment, or if a patient is a poor surgical candidate because of other medical comorbidities. Radiation therapy or radiosurgery may be an option for malignant pituitary carcinomas[12] or DARPs that have failed to respond to higher doses of multiple dopamine agonists.

Previous studies have shown that fractionated stereotactic radiotherapy (FSRT) and Gamma Knife stereotactic radiosurgery (SRS) are both effective means to control recurrent pituitary adenomas, including prolactinomas, after surgery or medical treatment.[52] Tumor control rates with FSRT for pituitary adenomas can be as high as 95%, but with 1% to 3% risk of damage to the optic nerve and 50% to 100% risk of hypopituitarism.[52–54] In comparison, the risk of hypopituitarism seems to be lower with SRS than with FSRT, ranging from 0% to 36%,[55] whereas the risk of visual deficits may be slightly higher with SRS.[56] With SRS, radiographic prolactinoma control rate, in one study, was 100%, whereas biochemical remission defined by a prolactin level of less than 13 ng/mL in men and less than 27 ng/mL in women was 64%.[57] Although the definition of biochemical remission varies, previous studies have reported 13% to 83% remission rates for patients with prolactinomas who were intolerant or unresponsive to dopamine agonist therapy following SRS.[38,57] Thus, SRS is considered the first-line radiotherapy for pituitary adenomas when both surgery and medical therapies fail. FSRT is considered for large tumors (>3.5 cm) or for tumors less than 5 mm from the optic chiasm.[52]

SUMMARY

Prolactinomas are unique, being the only brain tumor for which remission can typically be achieved through medical management. However, surgery has a clear role in the management of prolactinomas, and patients are ultimately best served when neurosurgeons and neuroendocrinologists work together to inform patients of risks and benefits, allowing patients to make personalized choices in their health care. Further research is also needed to improve current management for the rare subset of prolactinomas resistant to dopamine agonists.

REFERENCES

1. Monson JP. The epidemiology of endocrine tumours. Endocr Relat Cancer 2000;7(1):29–36.
2. CBTRUS. 2009-2010 CBTRUS Statistical report: primary brain and central nervous system tumors diagnosed in the United States in 2004-2006. 2010. Available at: http://www.cbtrus.org. Accessed April 4, 2010.
3. DeLellis RA, Lloyd RV, Heitz PU, et al. World Health Organization classification of tumours: tumours of endocrine organs. Lyon (France): IARC; 2004.
4. Colao A. Pituitary tumours: the prolactinoma. Best Pract Res Clin Endocrinol Metab 2009;23(5):575–96.
5. Gillam MP, Molitch ME, Lombardi G, et al. Advances in the treatment of prolactinomas. Endocr Rev 2006;27(5):485–534.
6. Fainstein Day P, Guitelman M, Artese R, et al. Retrospective multicentric study of pituitary incidentalomas. Pituitary 2004;7(3):145–8.
7. Daly AF, Burlacu MC, Livadariu E, et al. The epidemiology and management of pituitary incidentalomas. Horm Res 2007;68(Suppl 5):195–8.
8. Ezzat S, Asa SL, Couldwell WT, et al. The prevalence of pituitary adenomas: a systematic review. Cancer 2004;101(3):613–9.
9. Losa M, Mortini P, Barzaghi R, et al. Surgical treatment of prolactin-secreting pituitary adenomas: early results and long-term outcome. J Clin Endocrinol Metab 2002;87(7):3180–6.
10. Tyrrell JB, Lamborn KR, Hannegan LT, et al. Transsphenoidal microsurgical therapy of prolactinomas: initial outcomes and long-term results. Neurosurgery 1999;44(2):254–61 [discussion: 261–3].
11. Molitch ME, Elton RL, Blackwell RE, et al. Bromocriptine as primary therapy for prolactin-secreting macroadenomas: results of a prospective multicenter study. J Clin Endocrinol Metab 1985;60(4):698–705.
12. Casanueva FF, Molitch ME, Schlechte JA, et al. Guidelines of the Pituitary Society for the diagnosis and management of prolactinomas. Clin Endocrinol (Oxf) 2006;65(2):265–73.
13. Daly AF, Rixhon M, Adam C, et al. High prevalence of pituitary adenomas: a cross-sectional study in the province of Liege, Belgium. J Clin Endocrinol Metab 2006;91(12):4769–75.
14. Ferrante E, Ferraroni M, Castrignanò T, et al. Nonfunctioning pituitary adenoma database: a useful resource to improve the clinical management of pituitary tumors. Eur J Endocrinol 2006;155(6):823–9.
15. Kim SH, Lee KC. Cranial nerve palsies accompanying pituitary tumour. J Clin Neurosci 2007;14(12):1158–62.
16. Klijn JG, Lamberts SW, de Jong FH, et al. The importance of pituitary tumour size in patients with hyperprolactinaemia in relation to hormonal variables and extrasellar extension of tumour. Clin Endocrinol (Oxf) 1980;12(4):341–55.
17. Schlechte J, Dolan K, Sherman B, et al. The natural history of untreated hyperprolactinemia: a prospective analysis. J Clin Endocrinol Metab 1989;68(2):412–8.
18. Bassetti M, Spada A, Pezzo G, et al. Bromocriptine treatment reduces the cell size in human macroprolactinomas: a morphometric study. J Clin Endocrinol Metab 1984;58(2):268–73.
19. Tindall GT, Kovacs K, Horvath E, et al. Human prolactin-producing adenomas and bromocriptine: a histological, immunocytochemical, ultrastructural, and morphometric study. J Clin Endocrinol Metab 1982;55(6):1178–83.
20. Molitch ME. Medical management of prolactin-secreting pituitary adenomas. Pituitary 2002;5(2):55–65.

21. Webster J, Piscitelli G, Polli A, et al. A comparison of cabergoline and bromocriptine in the treatment of hyperprolactinemic amenorrhea. Cabergoline Comparative Study Group. N Engl J Med 1994;331(14):904–9.

22. Pascal-Vigneron V, Weryha G, Bosc M, et al. Hyperprolactinemic amenorrhea: treatment with cabergoline versus bromocriptine. Results of a national multicenter randomized double-blind study. Presse Med 1995;24(16):753–7 [in French].

23. Ono M, Miki N, Kawamata T, et al. Prospective study of high-dose cabergoline treatment of prolactinomas in 150 patients. J Clin Endocrinol Metab 2008;93(12):4721–7.

24. Colao A, Pivonello R, Di Somma C, et al. Medical therapy of pituitary adenomas: effects on tumor shrinkage. Rev Endocr Metab Disord 2009;10(2):111–23.

25. Van Camp G, Flamez A, Cosyns B, et al. Treatment of Parkinson's disease with pergolide and relation to restrictive valvular heart disease. Lancet 2004; 363(9416):1179–83.

26. Colao A, di Sarno A, Pivonello R, et al. Dopamine receptor agonists for treating prolactinomas. Expert Opin Investig Drugs 2002;11(6):787–800.

27. Molitch ME. Dopamine resistance of prolactinomas. Pituitary 2003;6(1):19–27.

28. Molitch ME. Pharmacologic resistance in prolactinoma patients. Pituitary 2005;8(1):43–52.

29. Oh MC, Aghi MK. Dopamine agonist-resistant prolactinomas. J Neurosurg 2011;114(5):1369–79.

30. Brue T, Pellegrini I, et al. Prolactinomas and resistance to dopamine agonists. Horm Res 1992;38(1–2):84–9.

31. Morange I, Barlier A, Pellegrini I, et al. Prolactinomas resistant to bromocriptine: long-term efficacy of quinagolide and outcome of pregnancy. Eur J Endocrinol 1996;135(4):413–20.

32. Pellegrini I, Rasolonjanahary R, Gunz G, et al. Resistance to bromocriptine in prolactinomas. J Clin Endocrinol Metab 1989;69(3):500–9.

33. Delgrange E, Daems T, Verhelst J, et al. Characterization of resistance to the prolactin-lowering effects of cabergoline in macroprolactinomas: a study in 122 patients. Eur J Endocrinol 2009;160(5):747–52.

34. Di Sarno A, Landi ML, Cappabianca P, et al. Resistance to cabergoline as compared with bromocriptine in hyperprolactinemia: prevalence, clinical definition, and therapeutic strategy. J Clin Endocrinol Metab 2001;86(11):5256–61.

35. Hagen C, Schroeder HD, Hansen S, et al. Temozolomide treatment of a pituitary carcinoma and two pituitary macroadenomas resistant to conventional therapy. Eur J Endocrinol 2009;161(4):631–7.

36. Neff LM, Weil M, Cole A, et al. Temozolomide in the treatment of an invasive prolactinoma resistant to dopamine agonists. Pituitary 2007;10(1):81–6.

37. Sheehan J, Rainey J, Nguyen J, et al. Temozolomide-induced inhibition of pituitary adenoma cells. J Neurosurg 2011;114(2):354–8.

38. Castinetti F, Regis J, Dufour H, et al. Role of stereotactic radiosurgery in the management of pituitary adenomas. Nat Rev Endocrinol 2009;6(4):214–23.

39. Hamilton DK, Vance ML, Boulos PT, et al. Surgical outcomes in hyporesponsive prolactinomas: analysis of patients with resistance or intolerance to dopamine agonists. Pituitary 2005;8(1):53–60.

40. Faria MA Jr, Tindall GT. Transsphenoidal microsurgery for prolactin-secreting pituitary adenomas. J Neurosurg 1982;56(1):33–43.

41. Hardy J, Beauregard H, Robert F, et al. Prolactin-secreting pituitary adenomas: transsphenoidal microsurgical treatment. Clin Neurosurg 1980;27:38–47.

42. Thomson JA, Davies DL, McLaren EH, et al. Ten year follow up of microprolactinoma treated by transsphenoidal surgery. BMJ 1994;309(6966):1409–10.

43. Abe T, Matsumoto K, Kuwazawa J, et al. Headache associated with pituitary adenomas. Headache 1998;38(10):782–6.

44. Scheithauer BW, Jaap AJ, Horvath E, et al. Clinically silent corticotroph tumors of the pituitary gland. Neurosurgery 2000;47(3):723–9 [discussion: 729–30].

45. Forsyth PA, Posner JB. Headaches in patients with brain tumors: a study of 111 patients. Neurology 1993;43(9):1678–83.

46. Jensen R, Stovner LJ. Epidemiology and comorbidity of headache. Lancet Neurol 2008;7(4):354–61.

47. Fleseriu M, Yedinak C, Campbell C, et al. Significant headache improvement after transsphenoidal surgery in patients with small sellar lesions. J Neurosurg 2009; 110(2):354–8.

48. Buchfelder M, Schlaffer S. Surgical treatment of pituitary tumours. Best Pract Res Clin Endocrinol Metab 2009;23(5):677–92.

49. Kitano M, Taneda M, Shimono T, et al. Extended transsphenoidal approach for surgical management of pituitary adenomas invading the cavernous sinus. J Neurosurg 2008;108(1):26–36.

50. Higgins TS, Courtemanche C, Karakla D, et al. Analysis of transnasal endoscopic versus transseptal microscopic approach for excision of pituitary tumors. Am J Rhinol 2008;22(6):649–52.

51. Tabaee A, Anand VK, Barrón Y, et al. Endoscopic pituitary surgery: a systematic review and meta-analysis. J Neurosurg 2009;111(3):545–54.

52. Sun DQ, Cheng JJ, Frazier JL, et al. Treatment of pituitary adenomas using radiosurgery and radiotherapy: a single center experience and review of literature. Neurosurg Rev 2011;34:181–9.

53. Kokubo M, Sasai K, Shibamoto Y, et al. Long-term results of radiation therapy for pituitary adenoma. J Neurooncol 2000;47(1):79–84.

54. Zierhut D, Flentje M, Adolph J, et al. External radiotherapy of pituitary adenomas. Int J Radiat Oncol Biol Phys 1995;33(2):307–14.

55. Sheehan JP, Jagannathan J, Pouratian N, et al. Stereotactic radiosurgery for pituitary adenomas: a review of

the literature and our experience. Front Horm Res 2006;34:185–205.

56. Sheehan JP, Niranjan A, Sheehan JM, et al. Stereotactic radiosurgery for pituitary adenomas: an intermediate review of its safety, efficacy, and role in the neurosurgical treatment armamentarium. J Neurosurg 2005;102(4):678–91.

57. Tanaka S, Link MJ, Brown PD, et al. Gamma knife radiosurgery for patients with prolactin-secreting pituitary adenomas. World Neurosurg 2010;74(1):147–52.

Hypopituitarism and Central Diabetes Insipidus
Perioperative Diagnosis and Management

Jessica K. Devin, MD

KEYWORDS

- Pituitary tumor • Adrenal insufficiency • Diabetes insipidus • Hyponatremia • Hypopituitarism

KEY POINTS

- Pituitary tumors have the capacity to result in hormone deficiencies and disorders of water metabolism secondary to their unique location.
- The evaluation of pituitary function before surgery is essential both to identify and treat life-threatening pituitary deficiencies and to rule out the presence of a hormone-secreting tumor.
- Patients who have recently received surgery in the pituitary region must be closely monitored for both diabetes insipidus and hyponatremia, so that these disorders may be promptly addressed.
- All patients who have undergone pituitary surgery require a thorough assessment of pituitary function at least 4 to 6 weeks after surgery to identify new deficits and recognize those that may have resolved.

INTRODUCTION

Pituitary tumors represent a unique class of intracranial neoplasms uniquely located to cause mass effect on vital nearby structures including, but not limited to, the pituitary gland and the hypothalamus, which may result in hormone deficiencies as well as disorders of water metabolism. Patients with pituitary lesions may present with hormone deficiencies before surgery, during surgery, or during the weeks following surgery. Disorders of water metabolism most commonly do not present until the postoperative period and usually are transient. The neurosurgeon's challenge is to safely remove the lesion, decompress nearby vital structures, and preserve or restore pituitary function. Close collaboration between neurosurgical, endocrine, and anesthetic teams is vital during the perioperative time period. This article reviews the perioperative evaluation and management of hormone deficiencies and disorders of water metabolism in patients with lesions of the pituitary region.

PREOPERATIVE ENDOCRINE EVALUATION OF PATIENTS UNDERGOING PITUITARY SURGERY

Pituitary tumors comprise approximately 15% of all intracranial neoplasms, and are clinically apparent in 18 per 100,000 persons.[1] The evaluation of pituitary function before surgery is essential both to identify and treat life-threatening pituitary deficiencies and to rule out the presence of a hormone-secreting tumor. Approximately 70% to 90% of patients with nonfunctioning pituitary macroadenomas have deficiencies in 1 or more pituitary hormones before surgery.[2] The evaluation requires assessment of the following anterior pituitary hormones: luteinizing hormone (LH), follicle-stimulating hormone (FSH), growth hormone (GH), prolactin, adrenocorticotropic hormone (ACTH), and thyroid-stimulating hormone (TSH).

Disclosures: The author does not have any financial disclosures.
Division of Diabetes, Endocrinology and Metabolism, Vanderbilt University Medical Center, 8017 Medical Center East, North Tower, 1215 21st Avenue South, Nashville, TN 37232, USA
E-mail address: jessica.devin@vanderbilt.edu

Neurosurg Clin N Am 23 (2012) 679–689
http://dx.doi.org/10.1016/j.nec.2012.06.001
1042-3680/12/$ – see front matter © 2012 Elsevier Inc. All rights reserved

Each of these hormones and their downstream mediators must be evaluated as discussed later. The most common deficiencies involve GH and the gonadotropins (LH and FSH). ACTH and TSH deficiencies are less common, but must be addressed before surgery when they occur. Central diabetes insipidus (DI) is present in only about 2% of patients on presentation and ideally is recognized before surgery. Although most nonfunctioning tumors of the sellar region represent nonfunctioning pituitary adenomas, the differential diagnosis of nonfunctioning lesions of the sellar region must be considered (**Box 1**).

HYPOPITUITARISM

The signs and symptoms of hormone deficiencies are often nonspecific and vague. In the interest of both time and resources, laboratory tests to screen for hormone deficiencies are used before surgery with dynamic testing reserved for the postoperative period. **Table 1.** addresses the signs and symptoms of hypopituitarism, along with the diagnosis and treatment pertinent to each hormone deficiency. Current recommendations state that all patients with a pituitary lesion, including asymptomatic patients with an incidentaloma, undergo clinical and laboratory evaluation for hypopituitarism.[3] A typical preoperative panel therefore includes TSH, free T4, LH, and

---

Box 1
Nonfunctioning lesions of the sellar region

- Gonadotropin-secreting pituitary tumor
- Null-cell adenoma
- Clinically silent hormone-producing adenoma
- Benign neoplasms
  - Craniopharyngioma
  - Meningioma
  - Chordoma
  - Germ cell tumor
  - Rathke cleft cyst
- Malignant neoplasms
  - Lymphoma
  - Metastatic disease (breast and lung)
  - Pituitary carcinoma
- Infiltrative diseases
  - Sarcoidosis
  - Lymphocytic hypophysitis
  - Granulomatous hypophysitis

---

testosterone in men versus FSH and estradiol in women, insulin-like growth factor (IGF)-1, prolactin, and an early morning ACTH and cortisol. Chen and colleagues[4] prospectively evaluated 385 patients with nonfunctioning pituitary adenomas undergoing surgery. Hypothyroidism, hypogonadism, and hypoprolactinemia were found in 36%, 41%, and 18% of patients respectively. GH deficiency (GHD) was suspected in 61%. One-third of the patients with hypothyroidism had hypocortisolism.

Central Adrenal Insufficiency

A random serum cortisol should be drawn between 8 and 9 AM to assess for insufficiency because the hypothalamic-pituitary-adrenal (HPA) axis activity is maximal during this time period. A careful history must be taken to rule out recently administered exogeneous glucocorticoids, because this interferes with the assay and renders the results uninterpretable. A serum cortisol level of less than 6 µg/dL in the morning should prompt the initiation before surgery of glucocorticoid replacement to ameliorate patients symptoms. A value greater than 18 µg/dL makes a diagnosis of adrenal insufficiency highly unlikely.[5] Intermediary values must be interpreted in the clinical context, with consideration of patient's symptoms, size and location of the lesion, and the presence of other hormone deficiencies. An intermediary level in the presence of additional hormone deficiencies should prompt initiation of glucocorticoid replacement before surgery with appropriate education regarding steroid adjustment in times of illness or additional dynamic testing. Additional testing must still be performed in the postoperative period in all cases.

Central Hypothyroidism

Central hypothyroidism is suspected by a less than normal or low normal free T4 with a low, normal, or slightly increased TSH. Dynamic testing with thyrotropin-releasing hormone (TRH) does not provide any advantage in the diagnosis of central hypothyroidism and may precipitate pituitary apoplexy in patients with macroadenomas.[6] Treatment of suspected central hypothyroidism should be initiated before surgery to minimize perioperative morbidity. Perioperative problems encountered in untreated hypothyroid patients include delayed clearance of anesthesia, electrolyte abnormalities, ileus, a decreased ability to increase respiratory drive, and neuropsychiatric disturbances. Thyroid hormone replacement can be initiated with once-daily oral L-thyroxine. If indicated, it is important to start glucocorticoid replacement before the start of thyroid hormone

Table 1
Diagnosis and treatment of hypopituitarism

Deficiency	Signs and Symptoms	Diagnosis	Treatment
GH	Fatigue, weight gain, decreased exercise endurance, poor sense of well-being, osteoporosis, hyperlipidemia	Serum IGF-1 less than the normal range Hypoglycemia-induced GH <5.1 ng/mL Arginine-stimulated GH<1.4 ng/mL Glucagon-stimulated GH <3 ng/mL	Daily subcutaneous injections starting at 0.4 mg/d (lower in the elderly) Titrate at intervals of 4–8 wk to IGF-1 within midnormal range Not replaced before surgery and contraindicated in presence of residual or enlarging tumor
ACTH	Nausea, anorexia, weight loss, fatigue and malaise, hyponatremia, and hypoglycemia	Preoperative morning serum cortisol <6 µg/dL ACTH-stimulated cortisol <18 µg/dL Hypoglycemia-induced cortisol <20 µg/dL	Oral hydrocortisone 15–20 mg/d, in divided doses with two-thirds given in the morning Dexamethasone 0.125–0.375 mg qhs Prednisone 3–5 mg/d
TSH	Weight gain, fatigue, constipation, menorrhagia, cold intolerance, dry skin, bradycardia	Serum free T4 in lower quartile of normal range or less than the lower limit of normal	Initiate at 1.6 µg/kg and titrate dose to serum free T4 upper half of the normal range
LH, FSH	Mood swings, impotence, vaginal dryness, hot flashes, decreased libido, osteoporosis	LH, FSH Serum free testosterone in men Serum estradiol in women	Cyclic estrogen and progesterone in premenopausal women Testosterone injections, gel, or patches in men Not replaced before surgery

Abbreviations: IGF, insulin-like growth factor; qhs, at bedtime.

replacement to avoid the risk of precipitating an adrenal crisis caused by the resulting increased metabolism of cortisol.

Central Hypogonadism

Hypogonadism is easily detected in premenopausal women by a history of oligomenorrhea or amenorrhea. An inappropriately normal or less than normal FSH in a postmenopausal woman additionally suggests the diagnosis. Treatment should not be initiated before surgery, and may increase the risk of perioperative venous thrombosis. Men with hypogonadism are usually diagnosed by a combination of less than normal testosterone and inappropriately normal or less than normal LH. If symptomatic, treatment may be initiated before surgery following a discussion of risks and benefits, but is generally held in the perioperative period. Continued need for replacement should then be assessed after surgery.

Growth Hormone Deficiency

GH secretion is pulsatile with a short half-life. Its level is undetectable in adults for nearly two-thirds of the day. A single less than normal GH level in an adult therefore does not suggest GHD. Hepatic IGF-1 is regulated primarily by GH and therefore as a single level may be used as a marker of endogenous GH secretion. A less than normal level suggests the presence of adult GHD, although this level may be influenced by nutritional status and age in normal subjects. Although it is helpful to use IGF-1 as a marker of pituitary function together with other laboratories in the preoperative period, reassessment after surgery, potentially with dynamic testing, is necessary before treatment with GH replacement is considered.[6] We therefore advocate assessment of IGF-1 before surgery, together with a single GH level, only if there is clinical concern for a GH–secreting pituitary adenoma.

Prolactin

Exclusion of pregnancy, prolactin-increasing medications, primary hypothyroidism, and polycystic ovarian syndrome is necessary to accurately interpret a preoperative prolactin level. A preoperative prolactin level greater than 200 μg/L in the setting of a tumor greater than 1 cm is diagnostic of a macroprolactinoma. A prolactin level less than this in the setting of a greater than 1 cm lesion is more likely to indicate stalk compression by a nonfunctioning tumor leading to a decrease in prolactin-inhibiting factors. An intermediary level, or an increase in the setting of a microadenoma (tumor<1 cm) may be worthy of a trial of dopamine agonist therapy, which can be both diagnostic and therapeutic. Prolactin deficiency (prolactin less than the lower limit of the normal range) is associated with severe hypopituitarism.[6]

DIABETES INSIPIDUS

The presence of DI is rare in the preoperative patient and should prompt consideration of a diagnosis of craniopharyngioma, Rathke cleft cyst, or an infiltrative process.[7] The synthesis of arginine vasopressin (AVP) occurs in the supraoptic and paraventricular nuclei of the hypothalamus, not within the posterior pituitary gland. Therefore destruction of the posterior pituitary destroys the nerve terminals of the AVP neurons; as this occurs, the site of AVP release shifts more superiorly on the stalk. Thus, slow-growing noninfiltrative lesions such as adenomas are unlikely to result in this complication.[8] The diagnosis is typically made before surgery by the presence of classic symptoms of polyuria and polydipsia with a high normal serum sodium and urine specific gravity less than 1.005, and a positive response to vasopressin treatment. The symptoms of DI may also be unmasked following initiation of glucocorticoid replacement; glucocorticoids inhibit the synthesis and secretion of AVP, thus adrenal insufficiency can result in increased levels of AVP, which are then lowered following initiation of glucocorticoid replacement.

PERIOPERATIVE MANAGEMENT OF PATIENTS WITH HYPOPITUITARISM

All patients who undergo pituitary surgery, whether or not they have a history of central adrenal insufficiency, should be treated during surgery as if their HPA function has been, or will remain, compromised. This condition may occur secondary to disruption of the anterior pituitary, the pituitary stalk, or the hypothalamus at the time of surgery.[9] Confirmation of residual pituitary tissue left in the sella by the neurosurgeon does not ensure preservation of normal pituitary function, because this tissue itself may be damaged.[2]

Most centers use a standardized protocol for perioperative administration of glucocorticoid as well as an early postoperative assessment of continued need for steroid coverage following discharge.[9] These protocols differ from center to center. A typical approach is to administer intravenous hydrocortisone (Solu-Cortef) 50 to 100 mg on the morning of surgery at the induction of anesthesia. This dose is then repeated at the conclusion of the procedure. Hydrocortisone 50 mg intravenously (IV) every 8 hours is then administered for the first 24 hours following surgery. Provided that the patient is making satisfactory postoperative recovery, the dose can then be decreased to 25 mg IV every 8 hours on the second postoperative day. Once patients are able to take oral medications, they may be transitioned to 20 mg of hydrocortisone by mouth in the morning and 10 mg in the afternoon. This dose, or a comparable replacement, is then taken until patients return for their postoperative visit and definitive assessment of the HPA axis with dynamic testing.

Several centers prefer to assess cortisol levels on the second or third postoperative days at least 24 hours after the last day of IV hydrocortisone to determine the need for continued glucocorticoid use after discharge. Although patients with an early morning cortisol level greater than 18 μg/dL rarely require ongoing steroid replacement, levels between 10 and 17 μg/dL are considered indeterminate and recommendations differ between institutions. One approach is to discharge patients with postoperative cortisol greater than 10 μg/dL on no steroid replacement, but provide them with prescriptions for hydrocortisone and educate them on symptoms of adrenal insufficiency. If these occur, patients are instructed to contact their physicians and obtain both a serum cortisol and serum sodium, because the symptoms of postoperative hyponatremia mimic those of adrenal insufficiency. If serum sodium returns less than normal, patients are appropriately treated with fluid restriction, with hospitalization if appropriate. If serum cortisol is less than 10 μg/dL, then hydrocortisone replacement is initiated.[3]

Khan and colleagues[10] advocate that a postoperative day cortisol value greater than 10 μg/dL accurately predicts integrity of the HPA axis and that these patients, within the appropriate clinical context, may be discharged without any glucocorticoid replacement. Each decision must be personalized and the presence of multiple anterior pituitary hormone deficiencies, including disorders of water metabolism, in the postoperative period should prompt discharge on glucocorticoid replacement regardless of the postoperative cortisol level. The type of pituitary lesion also predicts the likelihood of pituitary dysfunction; for example, patients with craniopharyngioma are more likely to experience hypopituitarism and DI. A morning cortisol level less than 10 μg/dL necessitates discharge on glucocorticoid replacement with instructions on management of the dose during times of illness.[7,11]

Marko and colleagues[12] uniquely prospectively assessed immediate day-of-surgery cortisol levels to assist in determination of the need for steroid replacement on discharge. Results were correlated with Cortrosyn stimulation testing performed 4 to 6 weeks after surgery. An immediate cortisol level of greater than 15 μg/dL was a predictor of adequate postoperative HPA axis function following transsphenoidal surgery, with a sensitivity of 98%, accuracy of 97%, and positive predictive value of 99%. This information may prove to be increasingly valuable as earlier discharges become more the norm.

A Cortrosyn stimulation test in the early postoperative period is not able to detect recent-onset central adrenal insufficiency because it relies on failure of the adrenal glands to respond appropriately to ACTH, which requires the presence of adrenocortical atrophy to develop secondary to ACTH deficiency and takes time. Klose and colleagues[13] showed that, out of 62 patients with a normal 250 μg Cortrosyn stimulation testing 1 week following surgery, 23 patients developed an abnormal response in the next 1 to 3 months. In the early postoperative period, the 1-μg Cortrosyn stimulation test has the same limitations. Changes in HPA function are therefore dynamic and reassessment of HPA function in the first 3 months after surgery is mandatory regardless of the protocol for glucocorticoid replacement used.[9]

The assessment of other anterior pituitary hormone deficiencies is generally reserved for the first postoperative visit. Those patients taking thyroid hormone replacement for preoperative central hypothyroidism should be continued on their thyroid hormone replacement after surgery. In those patients in whom new-onset hypopituitarism may be suspected (for example, a serum cortisol <10 μg/dL in the postoperative period and/or continued postoperative DI at the time of discharge), an assessment with a serum free T4 may be necessary 1 to 2 weeks following discharge, with replacement indicated following a significant decline in the free T4.

POSTOPERATIVE DIABETES INSIPIDUS

Polyuria is common following pituitary surgery; the primary differential diagnosis consists of central DI, hyperglycemia, diuresis characteristic of patients with acromegaly, and diuresis of intraoperative and postoperative fluids. The last 3 of these can adequately be ruled out by patient history and review of the intraoperative and nursing records. A postoperative hypotonic diuresis occurs in nearly one-third of patients immediately following surgery but is accompanied by neither hypernatremia nor excessive thirst.[9,14]

The cardinal clinical features of DI include polyuria, defined as the passage of more than 30 mL of urine per kilogram of body weight in a 24-hour period; dehydration or plasma hyperosmolarity; and intense thirst with resultant polydipsia. Laboratories reflect an increase in the serum sodium toward 145 mEq/L and always a decline in the urine specific gravity to less than 1.005. An increase in the urine specific gravity in the setting of a normal serum sodium should prompt consideration of hyperglycemia and glucosuria; alternatively, a stable or low normal serum sodium in the setting of a urine specific gravity more than 1.005 without accompanying thirst should prompt consideration of postoperative diuresis.

The incidence of DI following pituitary surgery at our institution is 18.5% and typically presents within 24 hours of surgery; this finding is comparable with that reported by other high-volume pituitary centers.[15] Postoperative DI can exhibit 1 of 3 patterns: transient, permanent, or triphasic. Transient DI accounts for most DI following surgery and is characterized by an abrupt onset of polyuria and polydipsia within the first postoperative day and typically resolves within several days to weeks. Minor injury to the posterior pituitary gland with resultant temporary inhibition of AVP release is thought to be the cause. Permanent DI presents similarly but does not resolve within 6 months of surgery and requires lifelong treatment. This condition occurs in approximately 3% of cases.[7] This form of DI results from extensive damage to the neurohypophyseal stalk and/or the hypothalamus and is most often seen in those patients with infiltrative lesions, suprasellar tumors, or in the setting of extensive resections.[14,15] Other predictors of DI include surgery for microadenomas secondary possibly to increased exploration, intraoperative cerebrospinal fluid leak, younger age, male sex, and intrasellar expansion of the tumor.[9]

The triphasic pattern of DI is characterized by an initial phase consisting of polyuria and polydipsia, followed by an interphase consisting of a period of antidiuresis and often hyponatremia, and a third phase of permanent or prolonged DI. The interphase of antidiuresis is thought to result from leakage of AVP from the injured hypothalamic neurons and occurs approximately 1 week after surgery, lasting 5 to 7 days. Severe hyponatremia may result during this time period, with symptoms including nausea, headache, and anorexia. Patients may experience transient DI followed by this interphase without the development of permanent DI. A full triphasic response is seen in 1.1% of patients and the biphasic response in 3.4% of patients.[14]

The treatment of postoperative DI most commonly involves the subcutaneous administration of aqueous vasopressin (Pitressin). This treatment is often preferred initially rather than desmopressin (1-desamino-8-D-arginine vasopressin; DDAVP) because of its short-acting nature. Most patients require 5 units of Pitressin every 6 to 8 hours. It is best initially to administer the medication on an as-needed basis because of the often transient nature of the DI. A single dose of vasopressin is often sufficient. If the patient continues to require repeated doses of Pitressin, DDAVP at 1 μg administered subcutaneously can then be used instead. This dose can last as long as 8 to 16 hours and should be provided on an as-needed basis. Lower doses are generally used in the elderly. Patients with DI and an intact thirst mechanism should be allowed free access to water (without administration of IV fluids) to allow their thirst to guide adequate replacement.

If DI persists at the time of discharge, a transition to DDAVP tablets or DDAVP nasal spray (provided that nasal packs have been removed) can be made. The nasal spray delivers a dose of 10 μg per spray; most patients start with 1 spray at bedtime, with a second spray added in the morning if necessary to control symptoms. For both the parenteral and intranasal preparations, increasing the dose increases the duration of effect rather than the magnitude.

DDAVP tablets are most effective in the setting of mild symptoms of polyuria and polydipsia, because they have more erratic bioavailability and patients often need larger doses. A typical dosage regimen starts with 0.1 mg twice daily and may be titrated as high as 0.3 mg twice daily. Potential side effects of DDAVP therapy include nausea, diarrhea, and abdominal cramps.

Patients should be appropriately educated on how to dose DDAVP. The purpose of the medication is mainly to keep patients comfortable and to avoid thirst and frequent urination. They should be told to allow their thirst mechanism to guide their fluid intake and to drink only when thirsty. We generally advise patients that DDAVP is meant to be used on an as-needed basis when the following 3 criteria are satisfied: (1) the patient is using the restroom often (every hour); (2) the patient's urine is clear, resembling water; and (3) the patient is experiencing thirst. The treatment of central DI is summarized in **Table 2**.

POSTOPERATIVE HYPONATREMIA

The differential diagnosis of hyponatremia following pituitary surgery may include the interphase of the previously mentioned triphasic response; syndrome of inappropriate antidiuretic hormone (SIADH) as a result of infection, stress, pain, or trauma to the central nervous system; overzealous

Table 2
Treatment of central DI

Formulation	Dosage	Use	Advantages	Disadvantages
Vasopressin (Pitressin)	5 units subcutaneous q6–8 h prn	Postoperative transient DI	Immediate bioavailability Short duration of action	Reaction at injection site Anti-AVP antibodies reported
DDAVP, SQ	1 μg SQ prn	Postoperative DI	Immediate bioavailability	Reaction at injection site
DDAVP, spray	1 spray qhs to 1 BID (10 μg/spray)	Maintenance medication	Allows for variable dosing	Generic formulation requires refrigeration Delivers fixed dose
DDAVP, oral tablets	0.1–0.3 mg PO BID–TID	Maintenance medication	Ease of Administration Alternative when nasal route not feasible	Erratic bioavailability May require large doses to achieve effect

Abbreviations: BID, twice a day; PO, by mouth; prn, as needed; q, every; SQ, subcutaneous; TID, 3 times a day.

administration of hypotonic fluids and/or DDAVP; and cerebral salt wasting. For reasons that are not understood, patients with Cushing disease have nearly a 3-fold higher risk of postoperative hyponatremia.[14] It is additionally important to rule out pseudohyponatremia secondary to hyperglycemia, hypothyroidism, and untreated central adrenal insufficiency. Cerebral salt wasting is characterized by a natriuresis and hypovolemia and is most commonly associated with subarachnoid disease.[15] Thus, these patients typically have high levels of urinary sodium and clinical signs and symptoms of dehydration.

Postoperative hyponatremia occurs in 9% to 24% of patients following pituitary surgery and peaks on the seventh postoperative day.[9,11,15] Most cases of postoperative hyponatremia secondary to inappropriate AVP release (ie, over-administration of DDAVP, SIADH, or the interphase) respond to fluid restriction. The combined oral and IV intake of fluids is typically restricted to less than 500 mL of the 24-hours urine outpatient. We prefer fluid restriction as the sole approach to the management of hyponatremia when the serum sodium exceeds 125 mEq/L. The fluid restriction is discontinued when the serum sodium exceeds 132 mEq/L or if there is clinical evidence of the development of DI. The sudden occurrence of DI indicates the third phase of the triphasic response and may lead to large increases in serum sodium; therapy is often required to control the rate of increase of the serum sodium even in patients who may still be hyponatremic.

A more severe and symptomatic hyponatremia associated with a rapid decline in serum sodium requires more aggressive treatment. Hypertonic saline may be administered to raise the serum sodium 0.5 mEq/L/h, although it may be reasonable to increase this rate to 1 to 2 mEq/L/h (not exceeding a total of 12 mEq/L in 24 hours) in patients with more acute hyponatremia and significant symptoms including change in level of consciousness or seizures. Once serum sodium exceeds 125 mEq/L, the patient may be treated with fluid restriction.

There is a new class of medications available that specifically targets AVP receptors and may be used in patients with hyponatremia attributable to SIADH. Two of these vaptans, conivaptan and tolvaptan, have been approved by the US Food and Drug Administration for treatment of both euvolemic and hypervolemic hyponatremia. There are currently limited retrospective data in the literature on the use of this class of therapeutics in postsurgical patients with sellar lesions. Potts and colleagues[16] published a series of 13

neurosurgical patients with SIADH who received conivaptan; 6 of these patients underwent endonasal transsphenoidal approach for resection of their lesions. Fluid restriction had previously been attempted in all patients and sodium chloride tablets with or without hypertonic saline in half without success. The mean pretreatment serum sodium in this subset was 124.7 ± 4.4 mEq/L and the mean time to achieve a 6-mEq/L increase in serum sodium was 10.2 ± 8.9 hours. Although conivaptan is approved as a 20-mg IV loading dose over 30 minutes followed by a 20-mg IV infusion over the next 24 hours, half of these patients responded sufficiently to the single 20-mg loading dose. Hyponatremia did not recur in any of these patients. Wright and colleagues[17] summarized their experience with treating euvolemic hyponatremia with conivaptan in the neurocritical care unit and found a sodium increase of greater than or equal to 6 mEq/L was reached in most patients within an average time of 13 hours. Vaptans should not be administered if there is any clinical suspicion for the presence of cerebral salt wasting because this represents a hypovolemic state. In addition, because of their mechanism of action, vaptans should not be administered to any patient with a history of DI. Side effects of vaptans include hypotension, infusion-site reaction with or without pyrexia, hyperkalemia, increased creatinine, and increased thirst. In neurosurgical patients, there is the additional risk of possible volume depletion that may compromise cerebral perfusion as well as the concern for rapid overcorrection of sodium leading to central pontine myelinosis. The cautious use of conivaptan in this population thus seems safe and effective but should only be used in the setting of careful monitoring of fluid status, blood pressure, and electrolytes.[16,17]

DISCHARGE INSTRUCTIONS FOR PATIENTS WHO HAVE UNDERGONE PITUITARY SURGERY

Patients who are discharged following pituitary surgery face several unique potential endocrine complications as outpatients. They must be made aware of the potential for these and how to appropriately manage each. These complications primarily involve disorders of water metabolism as well as the management of adrenal insufficiency.

Patients who are discharged on glucocorticoids should be advised of the necessary adjustments in times of illness. In general, patients should be asked to double the dose of glucocorticoid in the event of fever greater than 38.1°C. They should be advised to go to the nearest emergency room to receive stress dose steroids if they cannot take any medications by mouth because of nausea and vomiting. They should also be reminded, if indicated, to hold their glucocorticoid for 24 hours before their postoperative endocrinology assessment so that definitive testing of the HPA axis may be accurately performed.

All patients, regardless of their postoperative course, should be advised on the signs and symptoms of both hyponatremia and DI. However, the latter is unlikely to be apparent following discharge in the absence of other postoperative complications. Patients are advised that headache, nausea, vomiting, confusion, impaired concentration, and muscle aches may be caused by hyponatremia. Excessive urination and thirst may be related to the onset of DI. In each of these cases, patients are advised to contact their physicians immediately.

POSTOPERATIVE EVALUATION AND MANAGEMENT OF HYPOPITUITARISM AND DIABETES INSIPIDUS

All patients who have undergone pituitary surgery should have a thorough assessment of pituitary function following pituitary surgery both to identify new deficits that may have occurred and to identify those that may have resolved. Nearly one-third to one-half of preoperative pituitary deficits resolve after surgery, thus eliminating the need for lifelong hormone replacement therapy.[18,19] Factors associated with the recovery of pituitary function following surgery include the absence of residual tumor on postoperative imaging and no neurosurgical or pathologic evidence of invasive disorders.[18] Mild or recent onset, or clinically silent hormone deficiencies, as well as a complete resection, additionally predict a greater likelihood of regaining pituitary function.[9] The rate of deterioration of pituitary function following transsphenoidal surgery ranges from 15% to 30%.[18,19] Preoperative prolactin levels have been proposed to be a useful predictor of pituitary function after surgery. Patients with a mild preoperative increase in prolactin presumably secondary to stalk compression tend to be more likely to recover pituitary function. The mechanism underlying this finding is hypothesized to be that hypopituitarism in the setting of large adenomas is secondary to infundibular compression impairing the delivery of hypothalamic-stimulating hormones; this is subsequently relieved following surgery.[19]

Central Adrenal Insufficiency

Regardless of the approach taken with glucocorticoid replacement on discharge, all patients should receive a thorough assessment of the HPA axis with dynamic testing 4 to 6 weeks following surgery. Some patients require further testing 3 to 6 months later.

Several dynamic tests are available to assess the integrity of the HPA axis. The most commonly used tests include the standard and low-dose Cortrosyn stimulation test as well as the insulin-induced hypoglycemia test. Dynamic tests should not be performed until at least 4 weeks after surgery because the presence of pituitary edema in the early postoperative period may interfere with pituitary function. In addition, testing earlier may underdiagnose ACTH deficiency, given that adrenal atrophy may not yet have occurred. Patients should continue on any prescribed glucocorticoid until the time of dynamic testing, and are advised to hold steroid in the 24-hour period before testing.

A Cortrosyn-stimulated cortisol less than 18 μg/dL at 30 minutes (1-μg test) or at either the 30-minute or 60-minute time point (250-μg test) confirms central adrenal insufficiency. Although there has been some concern that the 250-μg Cortrosyn test represents a supraphysiologic stimulus and thus may not detect patients with partial insufficiency, there is equal concern that the 1-μg test has low specificity that may in part be explained by incomplete delivery of the dose of Cortrosyn.[20]

In the insulin-induced hypoglycemia test, regular human insulin is administered IV at 0.1 to 0.15 U/kg body weight; failure of the serum cortisol to increase to greater than 20 μg/dL in the following 90 minutes confirms the diagnosis of central adrenal insufficiency. This test is contraindicated in patients with known low baseline cortisol levels and in those patients with a history of ischemic heart disease or seizures. In addition, a physician must remain in attendance throughout the test. For these reasons, this test is increasingly seldom performed.

In the setting of a borderline test (peak serum cortisol 14–18 μg/dL) with the presence of other pituitary hormone deficiencies, daily treatment is continued for partial adrenal insufficiency. In the setting of no other pituitary hormone deficiencies, the patient may be provided with a prescription for glucocorticoids to take only in times of illness, and may be retested again at a later date.

Lifelong glucocorticoid replacement is recommended in patients with confirmed central adrenal insufficiency. Because the production of adrenal mineralocorticoids is regulated by the renin-angiotensin system, patients with central adrenal insufficiency do not require concomitant treatment with mineralocorticoids. As previously mentioned, lifelong therapy can be commenced with hydrocortisone in divided doses typically of 15 to

20 mg daily with two-thirds administered on rising, dexamethasone 0.125 to 0.375 mg at bedtime, or prednisone in doses of 3 to 5 mg/d. The recommended dose of glucocorticoid has trended downwards over the years. Patients receiving hydrocortisone-equivalent doses of less than 20 mg/d do not differ in metabolic endpoints from patients with intact HPA axes. A higher body mass index (BMI) and more unfavorable lipid profile are seen with increasing doses of hydrocortisone.[21]

Because there is no laboratory test to guide the choice and dose of replacement, the treating physician must rely entirely on these guidelines together with patient symptoms of over-replacement and under-replacement. It has been our experience that patients with persistent symptoms of hypocortisolism, particularly in the morning, on hydrocortisone or prednisone benefit from a change to the longer-acting dexamethasone. Patients with adrenal insufficiency are advised to obtain and wear a MedicAlert bracelet or similar form of jewelry stating that they have adrenal insufficiency and are steroid dependent. Patients are also educated regarding the appropriate adjustment of their steroid dose in the setting of injury, illness, and invasive medical procedures.

Central Hypothyroidism

The assessment of the pituitary-thyroid axis following pituitary surgery is straightforward and relies on the measurement of the serum free T4 at the 6-week postoperative visit. A serum TSH is of little value, because patients with central hypothyroidism have been shown to have biologically ineffective TSH that is either normal or greater than normal, as well as a less than normal TSH. Either a less than normal free T4 or a free T4 that has decreased to the lower quartile of the normal range in patients with clinical symptoms of hypothyroidism should prompt the initiation of replacement therapy. Therapy should be initiated following assessment of the HPA axis and after initiation of glucocorticoid replacement, if indicated, to avoid precipitation of an adrenal crisis. Patients taking oral estrogens may require a higher dose. A recent study recommended initiation of L-thyroxine at 1.6 μg/kg once daily with therapy titrated to a serum free T4 in the upper limit of the normal range because this results in a lower BMI and more favorable cholesterol profile.[22] TSH levels are not reliable indicators of adequate replacement in patients with a history of pituitary disease.[2,7]

In patients with preoperative central hypothyroidism, thyroid hormone replacement can be stopped at the postoperative visit and reassessed in 6 weeks in the presence of other indicators of postoperative pituitary function recovery.

Central Hypogonadism

The resumption of menses in women following pituitary surgery indicates a normal gonadal axis. Serum estradiol and FSH levels should be measured if menses does not resume within 3 months of surgery. Replacement therapy with cyclic estrogen and progesterone is indicated in premenopausal women to preserve bone mineral density, libido, sexual function, and to maintain an overall sense of well-being. A variety of options are available for women and should be guided based on their age, medical history, and patient preference. Although most premenopausal hypogonadal women take oral estrogen replacement therapy, evidence exists that this aggravates the waist/hip ratio and that oral estrogens reduce the action of GH on fat mass. In addition, women using oral contraceptives have lower IGF-1 levels and require twice the dose of GH replacement compared with patients receiving transdermal estradiol. Ethinyl estradiol seems to be a greater GH antagonist than other oral estrogens.[23] Postmenopausal women with laboratory evidence of central hypogonadism are the subject of debate regarding the pros and cons of hormone replacement therapy, similar to women with physiologic menopause.

Measurement of the serum total or free testosterone levels in conjunction with LH is required to confirm central hypogonadism in men. We generally prefer an assessment of at least 2 less than normal early morning testosterone levels, including a free testosterone in elderly or obese patients and patients with hyperinsulinemia. Testosterone replacement can be accomplished with regular intramuscular injections, or the application of transdermal patches and gels. Benefits of therapy include maintenance of muscle and bone mass, improvements in libido and sexual function, and improvements in overall sense of well-being. Therapy is not recommended in those patients with metastatic prostate cancer, breast cancer, an unevaluated prostate nodule, prostate-specific antigen greater than 4ng/mL (or greater than 3 ng/mL in men at high risk for prostate cancer), hematocrit greater than 50%, symptomatic benign prostatic hyperplasia, or poorly controlled heart failure. Therapy is selected based on patient preference, cost, and response to therapy. Therapy is titrated to a testosterone level within the midnormal range.[23]

Growth Hormone Deficiency

GHD can result in several nonspecific complaints in patients with a history of pituitary disease, including fatigue, weakness, decreased exercise tolerance, and weight gain. GH secretion is less likely to recover than gonadotropin, ACTH, or TSH secretion and may not present clinically until several years following pituitary surgery or radiation therapy.[24]

Serum IGF-1 levels are a useful screening test in the initial evaluation of patients with suspected GHD. IGF-1 results that are either low or in the lower quartile of the normal range in a patient with pituitary disease should prompt the performance of dynamic tests to confirm a suspected diagnosis of GHD. The arginine–GH-releasing hormone (GHRH) stimulation test used to be the most commonly used test to assess GH reserve. This test has since been replaced with other dynamic tests because of the increasing difficulty in obtaining GHRH (see **Table 1**). The likelihood of GHD increases in the setting of multiple pituitary hormone deficiencies; the presence of 3 or more other deficits with a low serum IGF-1 level is as specific for the diagnosis of GHD as dynamic testing. Dynamic testing is therefore not always necessary. In contrast, a normal IGF-1 level in patients with other pituitary hormone deficits does not effectively rule out GHD and these patients should always be further evaluated with dynamic testing.[25]

GH replacement is accomplished by the daily subcutaneous injection of recombinant human GH. In most patients, treatment may be initiated at 0.4 mg/d and titrated upwards every 4 to 8 weeks to achieve a serum IGF-1 level in the middle of the age-specific and gender-specific normal range. Women taking oral estrogens typically require higher doses, as do younger patients. Side effects may include fluid retention, arthralgias, and nerve entrapment syndromes and generally resolve with continued therapy. It is now recognized that important interactions occur between GH and other pituitary hormone replacements. Initiation of GH may unmask adrenal insufficiency or increase glucocorticoid requirements. GH may unmask central hypothyroidism or increase thyroxine requirements. Most premenopausal women with hypopituitarism take oral estrogens, which aggravates the metabolic abnormalities of GHD and induces a relative resistance to GH therapy. Alternatively, testosterone and GH replacement in men act synergistically and the combination of the 2 augments the IGF-1 increase. Other pituitary hormone deficiencies must therefore be monitored as well during the titration of GH replacement.[21]

GH replacement is contraindicated in the presence of an active malignancy and should not commence until therapy for the pituitary tumor is completed. Although it has long been a concern, there is still no compelling evidence that GH replacement therapy increases the risk of recurrent pituitary disease.[25]

Central Diabetes Insipidus

Patients with established DI should be evaluated in the weeks and months after surgery to determine whether their treatment is effective and to ensure that continued treatment is necessary. The previously mentioned recommendation that patients withhold their medication until symptoms recur both avoids the unwanted side effect of hyponatremia and provides continued reassurance that the medication is still necessary. Patients with DI are symptomatic when left untreated and report a resurgence of polyuria and polydipsia if their DDAVP is withheld for more than 12 hours.

The chronic pharmacologic management of the patient with DI is summarized in **Table 2**. Patients may note an increased vasopressin dose requirement in the setting of an upper respiratory infection, during a period of allergic rhinitis, and during pregnancy. Patients should be advised to avoid activities and habits that may lead to the ingestion of large amounts of fluids. Examples may include diet recommendations to ingest numerous glasses of water daily, drinking large amounts of beer at parties, and ingestion of hypotonic fluids during vigorous exercise. These scenarios carry a high risk of hyponatremia in patients treated with DDAVP.

REFERENCES

1. Blevins LS Jr, Shore D, Weinstein J, et al. Clinical presentation of pituitary tumors. In: Krisht AF, Tindall GT, editors. Pituitary disorders: comprehensive management. Baltimore (MD): Lippincott Williams & Wilkins; 1999. p. 145–61.
2. Singer PA, Sevilla LJ. Postoperative endocrine management of pituitary tumors. Neurosurg Clin North Am 2003;14(1):123–38.
3. Freda PU, Beckers AM, Katznelson L, et al. Pituitary incidentaloma: an Endocrine Society clinical practice guideline. J Clin Endocrinol Metab 2011;96(4): 894–904.
4. Chen L, White WL, Spetzler RF, et al. A prospective study of nonfunctioning pituitary adenomas: presentation, management, and clinical outcome. J Neurooncol 2011;102(1):129–38.
5. Karaca Z, Tanriverdi F, Atmaca H, et al. Can basal cortisol measurement be an alternative to the insulin tolerance test in the assessment of the hypothalamic-pituitary-adrenal axis before and after pituitary surgery? Eur J Endocrinol 2010;163(3): 377–82.

6. Pereira O, Bevan JS. Preoperative assessment for pituitary surgery. Pituitary 2008;11(4):347–51.

7. Vance ML. Perioperative management of patients undergoing pituitary surgery. Endocrinol Metab Clin North Am 2003;32(2):355–65.

8. Verbalis JG. Management of disorders of water metabolism in patients with pituitary tumors. Pituitary 2002;5(2):119–32.

9. Ausiello JC, Bruce JN, Freda PU. Postoperative assessment of the patient after transsphenoidal pituitary surgery. Pituitary 2008;11(4):391–401.

10. Khan MI, Habra MA, McCutcheon IE, et al. Random postoperative day 3 cortisol as a predictor of hypothalamic-pituitary-adrenal axis integrity after transsphenoidal surgery. Endocr Pract 2011; 17:1–25.

11. Nemergut EC, Dumont AS, Barry UT, et al. Perioperative management of patients undergoing trans-sphenoidal pituitary surgery. Anesth Analg 2005; 101(4):1170–81.

12. Marko NF, Hamrahian AH, Weil RJ. Immediate postoperative cortisol levels accurately predict postoperative hypothalamic-pituitary-adrenal axis function after transsphenoidal surgery for pituitary tumors. Pituitary 2010;13(3):249–55.

13. Klose M, Lange M, Kosteljanetz M, et al. Adrenocortical insufficiency after pituitary surgery: an audit of the reliability of the conventional short synacthen test. Clin Endocrinol (Oxf) 2005;63(5):499–505.

14. Hensen J, Henig A, Fahlbusch R, et al. Prevalence, predictors and patterns of postoperative polyuria and hyponatraemia in the immediate course after transsphenoidal surgery for pituitary adenomas. Clin Endocrinol (Oxf) 1999;50(4):431–9.

15. Adams JR, Blevins LS Jr, Allen GS, et al. Disorders of water metabolism following transsphenoidal pituitary surgery: a single institution's experience. Pituitary 2006;9(2):93–9.

16. Potts MB, DeGiacomo AF, Deragopian L, et al. Use of intravenous conivaptan in neurosurgical patients with hyponatremia from syndrome of inappropriate antidiuretic hormone secretion. Neurosurgery 2011; 69(2):268–73.

17. Wright WL, Asbury WH, Gilmore JL, et al. Conivaptan for hyponatremia in the neurocritical care unit. Neurocrit Care 2009;11(1):6–13.

18. Webb SM, Rigla M, Wagner A, et al. Recovery of hypopituitarism after neurosurgical treatment of pituitary adenomas. J Clin Endocrinol Metab 1999; 84(10):3696–700.

19. Nomikos P, Ladar C, Fahlbusch R, et al. Impact of primary surgery on pituitary function in patients with non-functioning pituitary adenomas – a study on 721 patients. Acta Neurochir (Wien) 2004; 146(1):27–35.

20. Neary N, Nieman L. Adrenal insufficiency: etiology, diagnosis and treatment. Curr Opin Endocrinol Diabetes Obes 2010;17(3):217–23.

21. Filipsson H, Monson JP, Koltowska-Haggstrom M, et al. The impact of glucocorticoid replacement regimens on metabolic outcome and comorbidity in hypopituitary patients. J Clin Endocrinol Metab 2006;91(10):3954–61.

22. Slawik M, Klawitter B, Meiser E, et al. Thyroid hormone replacement for central hypothyroidism: a randomized controlled trial comparing two doses of thyroxine (T4) with a combination of T4 and triiodothyronine. J Clin Endocrinol Metab 2007;92(11): 4115–22.

23. Mah PM, Webster J, Jonsson P, et al. Estrogen replacement in women of fertile years with hypopituitarism. J Clin Endocrinol Metab 2005;90(11):5964–9.

24. Arafah BM. Reversible hypopituitarism in patients with large nonfunctioning pituitary adenomas. J Clin Endocrinol Metab 1986;62(6):1173–9.

25. Molitch ME, Clemmons DR, Malozowski S, et al. Evaluation and treatment of adult growth hormone deficiency: an Endocrine Society clinical practice guideline. J Clin Endocrinol Metab 2006;91(5): 1621–34.

Index

Note: Page numbers of article titles are in **boldface** type.

Neurosurg Clin N Am 23 (2012) 691–696
http://dx.doi.org/10.1016/S1042-3680(12)00108-8

neurosurgery.theclinics.com

United States Postal Service

Statement of Ownership, Management, and Circulation
(All Periodicals Publications Except Requestor Publications)

1. Publication Title	2. Publication Number	3. Filing Date
Neurosurgery Clinics of North America	0 1 3 - 1 2 4	9/14/12

4. Issue Frequency	5. Number of Issues Published Annually	6. Annual Subscription Price
Jan, Apr, Jul, Oct	4	$346.00

7. Complete Mailing Address of Known Office of Publication (Not printer) (Street, city, county, state, and ZIP+4®)

Elsevier Inc.
360 Park Avenue South
New York, NY 10010-1710

Contact Person
Stephen R. Bushing
Telephone (Include area code)
215-239-3688

8. Complete Mailing Address of Headquarters or General Business Office of Publisher (Not printer)

Elsevier Inc., 360 Park Avenue South, New York, NY 10010-1710

9. Full Names and Complete Mailing Addresses of Publisher, Editor, and Managing Editor (Do not leave blank)

Publisher (Name and complete mailing address)

Kim Murphy, Elsevier, Inc., 1600 John F. Kennedy Blvd. Suite 1800, Philadelphia, PA 19103-2899

Editor (Name and complete mailing address)

Jessica McCool, Elsevier, Inc., 1600 John F. Kennedy Blvd. Suite 1800, Philadelphia, PA 19103-2899

Managing Editor (Name and complete mailing address)

Barbara Cohen-Kligerman, Elsevier, Inc., 1600 John F. Kennedy Blvd. Suite 1800, Philadelphia, PA 19103-2899

10. Owner (Do not leave blank. If the publication is owned by a corporation, give the name and address of the corporation immediately followed by the names and addresses of all stockholders owning or holding 1 percent or more of the total amount of stock. If not owned by a corporation, give the names and addresses of the individual owners. If owned by a partnership or other unincorporated firm, give its name and address as well as those of each individual owner. If the publication is published by a nonprofit organization, give its name and address.)

Full Name	Complete Mailing Address
Wholly owned subsidiary of	1600 John F. Kennedy Blvd., Ste. 1800
Reed/Elsevier, US holdings	Philadelphia, PA 19103-2899

11. Known Bondholders, Mortgagees, and Other Security Holders Owning or Holding 1 Percent or More of Total Amount of Bonds, Mortgages, or Other Securities. If none, check box ☐ None

Full Name	Complete Mailing Address
N/A	

12. Tax Status (For completion by nonprofit organizations authorized to mail at nonprofit rates) (Check one)
The purpose, function, and nonprofit status of this organization and the exempt status for federal income tax purposes:
☐ Has Not Changed During Preceding 12 Months
☐ Has Changed During Preceding 12 Months (Publisher must submit explanation of change with this statement)

PS Form 3526, September 2007 (Page 1 of 3 (Instructions Page 3)) PSN 7530-01-000-9931 **PRIVACY NOTICE:** See our Privacy policy in www.usps.com

---

13. Publication Title	14. Issue Date for Circulation Data Below
Neurosurgery Clinics of North America	July 2012

15. Extent and Nature of Circulation		Average No. Copies Each Issue During Preceding 12 Months	No. Copies of Single Issue Published Nearest to Filing Date
a. Total Number of Copies (Net press run)		735	585
b. Paid Circulation (By Mail and Outside the Mail)	(1) Mailed Outside-County Paid Subscriptions Stated on PS Form 3541. (Include paid distribution above nominal rate, advertiser's proof copies, and exchange copies)	274	249
	(2) Mailed In-County Paid Subscriptions Stated on PS Form 3541 (Include paid distribution above nominal rate, advertiser's proof copies, and exchange copies)		
	(3) Paid Distribution Outside the Mails Including Sales Through Dealers and Carriers, Street Vendors, Counter Sales, and Other Paid Distribution Outside USPS®	130	166
	(4) Paid Distribution by Other Classes Mailed Through the USPS (e.g. First-Class Mail®)		
c. Total Paid Distribution (Sum of 15b (1), (2), (3), and (4))	▶	404	415
d. Free or Nominal Rate Distribution (By Mail and Outside the Mail)	(1) Free or Nominal Rate Outside-County Copies Included on PS Form 3541	64	67
	(2) Free or Nominal Rate In-County Copies Included on PS Form 3541		
	(3) Free or Nominal Rate Copies Mailed at Other Classes Through the USPS (e.g. First-Class Mail)		
	(4) Free or Nominal Rate Distribution Outside the Mail (Carriers or other means)		
e. Total Free or Nominal Rate Distribution (Sum of 15d (1), (2), (3) and (4))	▶	64	67
f. Total Distribution (Sum of 15c and 15e)	▶	468	482
g. Copies not Distributed (See instructions to publishers #4 (page #3))	▶	267	103
h. Total (Sum of 15f and g)	▶	735	585
i. Percent Paid (15c divided by 15f times 100)		86.32%	86.10%

16. Publication of Statement of Ownership
If the publication is a general publication, publication of this statement is required. Will be printed ☐ Publication not required
in the **October 2012** issue of this publication.

17. Signature and Title of Editor, Publisher, Business Manager, or Owner	Date
[signature] Stephen R. Bushing – Inventory Distribution Coordinator	September 14, 2012

I certify that all information furnished on this form is true and complete. I understand that anyone who furnishes false or misleading information on this form or who omits material or information requested on the form may be subject to criminal sanctions (including fines and imprisonment) and/or civil sanctions (including civil penalties).

PS Form 3526, September 2007 (Page 2 of 3)

Moving?

Make sure your subscription moves with you!

To notify us of your new address, find your **Clinics Account Number** (located on your mailing label above your name), and contact customer service at:

Email: journalscustomerservice-usa@elsevier.com

800-654-2452 (subscribers in the U.S. & Canada)
314-447-8871 (subscribers outside of the U.S. & Canada)

Fax number: 314-447-8029

Elsevier Health Sciences Division
Subscription Customer Service
3251 Riverport Lane
Maryland Heights, MO 63043

*To ensure uninterrupted delivery of your subscription, please notify us at least 4 weeks in advance of move.

Printed and bound by CPI Group (UK) Ltd, Croydon, CR0 4YY

03/10/2024

01040355-0010